ON NEUROSES

Paul Schilder

ON NEUROSES

Edited by Lauretta Bender

INTERNATIONAL UNIVERSITIES PRESS, INC.
New York

Library of Congress Cataloging in Publication Data

Schilder, Paul, 1886-1940.
On neuroses.

Bibliography: p.
Includes index.
1. Neuroses—Collected works. I. Bender, Lauretta, 1897- II. Title. [DNLM: 1. Neuroses—Collected works. WM170.3 S3340]
RC530.S216 1979 616.8'5'08 78-61181
ISBN 0-8236-3810-3

Manufactured in the United States of America

CONTENTS

Preface

The papers selected for inclusion in this volume offer a comprehensive view of the neuroses. Written between 1929 and 1940, they are of both scientific and historical interest. Schilder's arguments for an organic and neurophysiological basis for the neuroses, for example, are perhaps even more cogent today than they were forty years ago. And some readers might be jolted to find that only forty years ago it was necessary to state that one did not have to feel guilty if one didn't love one's parents.

The earliest of these papers grew out of Schilder's work in Vienna in clinics and in private practice. Subsequent ones are based on his experiences in this country, at Phipps Clinic of Johns Hopkins, at Bloomingdale—now known as New York Hospital, Westchester Division—and later, at Bellevue Hospital and in private practice in New York City. As a collection, they offer a clear view of Schilder's concepts of the neuroses—how neurosis develops, what it means to the suffering person and to society, and what might be done about it.

Schilder was in Vienna at the time of the birth and development of Freud's and Breuer's psychoanalytic work on the neuroses; he explains how his own experiences led to some different views, although he agreed with Freud that the basic structure of a neurosis is determined by the family situation in early childhood. In his Foreword to *Mind*, he sums up his own way of thinking with his customary terseness: "Freud's work is an era in psychology. In order to utilize it fully, new, independent efforts are necessary." The reader will find a great many familiar names in these papers: Abraham, Adler, Alexander, Fenichel, Ferenczi, Hartmann, Horney, Jelliffe, Jones, Melanie Klein, Nunberg, Rank, Reik, and White, as well as unfamiliar ones—Schilder's reference list is an education in itself.

Schilder introduced group therapy to this country—and hence, internationally—with experiments described in this book. As Bernard Glueck wrote in his translator's Foreword to *Introduction to Psychoanalytic Psychiatry* (1925a), Schilder was also the first to apply psychoanalysis to clinical psychiatry. "Indeed," said David Rapaport, translator of Schilder's *Medical Psychology* (1924), "there is hardly any area of psychiatric and psychological problems which Schilder did not recognize, tackle, and illuminate; scarcely a syndrome which he did not study . . . few indeed are the problems with which he did not deal, whether they pertain to the form varieties of conscious experience, psychosomatic relationships, neuro-psychological interrelations, epistemological foundations of our relation to reality, or the nature of man's socialization; and exceptional the psychiatric phenomenon or symptom which he did not describe, whether depersonalization, *déjà-vu*, or body-image" (pp. 340-341).

Schilder has defined neurosis as "symptoms in relation to a past or present situation . . . a reaction of the individual as a personality [which causes suffering, but] retains a close relation to social reality. . . . Psychological processes are always psychophysiological . . . correlated with structures of the organism and especially in the brain. . . . However, neurotic attitudes and their psychogenic sequelae are not produced by structural changes, but from problems of the personality . . . that live[s] in a social milieu" (Ch. 10). Accordingly, some of the subjects discussed in this collection fall beyond the classification of neurosis. As

Schilder himself explains, alcoholism and homosexuality, for example, are considered from a similar point of view.

This is the final volume of Paul Schilder's collected papers. It has been preceded by *Brain and Personality* (1931a), *The Image and Appearance of the Human Body* (1935a), *Psychotherapy* (1938a), *Mind: Perception and Thought in Their Constructive Aspects* (1942b), and *Goals and Desires of Man* (1942a), all of which were edited by Schilder himself. In addition, the present editor has collected and edited *Psychoanalysis, Man and Society* (1951a), a revised expanded edition of *Psychotherapy* (1951b), *Contributions to Developmental Neuropsychiatry* (1964), and *On Psychoses* (1976).

Publishers of the original papers which are reprinted in this volume have been uniformly gracious in granting permission for such reprinting.

Thanks are due to Eleanor S. Lowman for typing and assistance with the manuscript. I am also grateful to Natalie Altman for helping to make the contents of this book, as well as of *On Psychoses*, as true as possible to the spirit and meaning in which they were originally written.

Lauretta Bender

July 1, 1977

CHAPTER ONE

Neuroses and Psychoses

It is to Freud's credit that today we can speak of the neuroses and the psychoses. Before Freud the neuroses were considered meaningless. There was either a spinal irritation or an anemia of the brain. It is true that Janet (1898) had already spoken of unconscious ideas in neuroses. According to him the hysteric patient forgot the most important events of his life because of an innate constitutional oral tendency to dissociation. This tendency was, according to him, a physiological state and not connected with what was going on in the psyche. It was a peculiarity of the brain and of the organism, without sense and without meaning.

Breuer and Freud (1893-1895) began their studies in hysteria in 1893 and found that hysterical symptoms occur when dammed-up emotions do not have an outlet because they are forgotten or locked out from consciousness by an amnesia. They did not think of the amnesia as a result of a psychological process, but postulated a state similar to hypnosis, a so-called hypnoid state brought on in a physiological manner. It was later that Freud (1915) found that the forgetting of the traumatic scene or, in a broader sense, of the disagreeable events and thoughts was due to a psychic defense. With that insight, psychoanalysis as such began. Freud (1894) gave one of his early publications the characteristic title, "The Neuro-psychoses of Defense" (*Abwehr-*

Appeared originally in *Psychoanalysis Today*, ed. Sandor Lorand. New York: Covici-Friede, 1933, pp. 293-306.

Neuro-Psychosen). In it he showed that neurotic symptoms are due to the self-defense of the individual against strivings, tendencies, desires, and experiences which are not in accordance with the conscious adaptation of the personality, i.e., the ego.

In "The Introductory Lectures of Psychoanalysis (1917)," Freud reported the case of a 30-year-old woman who suffered from a severe obsession. One of her compulsions, recurring several times a day, consisted of her running into the adjoining room, standing at one particular spot near a table, ringing for the maid, giving her an irrelevant order, and running back again. One day the insight into her action came to her, and she told the events which were at the basis of the obsession. More than ten years before, she had married an older man who proved to be impotent on their nuptial night. He had run innumerable times from his room into hers in order to try again, but without success. In the morning he said angrily, "One has to be ashamed before the servant girl who will make the bed." He took a bottle of red ink and poured some of it on the linen, but not quite in the right place. The cover on the table of the room into which the patient ran showed a similar stain. She also explained that the maid who was called in could not overlook the stain. This detail made it clear that there was a connection between the events of the nuptial night and her compulsion reaction. The patient played the part of her husband. She ran from one room to another as he did. The bed and bed linen are substituted for by the table and the table cover. The compulsion reaction appears as a repetition of this important scene, but there is a special importance in the fact that she wants to demonstrate to the maid that the stain is in the right place. The scene is not only repeated but also corrected, and she also corrects the impotency which occurred on the nuptial night. The compulsion reaction means, therefore, that it was not true that he was impotent and there was no reason to be ashamed before the maid.

Freud remarked that the effect of this compulsion neurosis was that the patient lived apart from her husband and made it possible for him to live a comfortable life, whereas she herself was compelled to remain faithful to him.

We see that the neurotic symptom had a meaning, but this meaning was not manifest. The patient did not know about it. In the course of the analysis the insight came more or less spontaneously. The meaning of the neurotic symptom was also unknown to the psychoanalyst. It was a hidden meaning or, in other words, a latent content in a neurotic symptom.

In the symptom mentioned here, table and tablecloth substituted for bed and linen. We may call this symbolization. If we summarize, we may say that the neurotic symptom did not have a meaning when we considered only the manifest content, but the manifest content hinted at something lying beneath it, or, in other words, it symbolized the inner meaning of the symptom. When we speak of the meaning of the symptom, we therefore mean only the latent content of the symptom.

But the example given is incomplete in some way. The meaning of the symptom seems here to be only connected with experiences very well remembered which belong to the adult life of the patient. Whenever we have the opportunity of delving deeper into a neurotic symptom, we always find that it is connected not only with experiences of adult life but with important childhood situations.

A neurasthenic patient I observed complained about itching sensations in his hands and genitals. He was very much disturbed about them. At the same time his hands and feet excited him sexually enormously. The analysis brought out that he had heard his mother moaning in giving birth to a sister four years younger than himself. He fantasied that the physician was tormenting his mother by brushing her feet with a stiff brush. He had seen his father occasionally cleaning his feet with his hands. The patient himself had suffered from an itching disease before the birth of his sister. His father also complained of itching on his back. The itching sensations on the hands, feet, and genitals therefore repeated early childhood experiences, and these early infantile experiences were of a sexual type. The boy, after having experienced these sensations following the birth of his sister, very often masturbated lying under the bed and fantasying himself or his mother being tormented. In his masturbation he used his hands. We now see more clearly that the symptom is a repetition of an infantile sexual experience, but it is a repetition which was changed. The most important parts of the early experience were omitted because they no longer fit with the strivings and tendencies of the adult ego of the individual. In other words, the repression caused the early sexual experience to return incompletely and altered. The incompleteness and the change had practically the same result and tendency as the symbolization. In brief, we may say that the symptom was a brief and incomplete and censored sex satisfaction of an infantile type. When one reads over the material given about this comparatively simple symptom, one immediately sees that there are many motives and many tendencies expressed in one symptom. In Freud's words, there is an overdetermination of a symptom.

But so far we have not spoken about the meaning of a neurosis, only about the meaning of the symptoms. Are the two identical? We know that there are many neuroses consisting of not only one symptom but many. Whenever we go more deeply into the structure of a neurosis with multiple symptoms we always find them centered around the same early infantile experiences and, very often, different expressions of the same basic tendencies.

In an anxiety-neurosis case which I observed many years ago the basic tendency was to see forbidden sexual things. In early childhood the patient was interested in his sister's genitals, in his mother's feet, which symbolized her genitals, and in the feet of their maid servants. He dated an early remembrance back to the time when he was one and a half years old. He was lying on the ground trying to look under the skirt of his wet nurse. The curiosity was in connection with the genitals of his mother and sister and with his enormous attachment to his mother which later prevented him from making sexual approaches to persons of the opposite sex who substituted for his mother. Since his curiosity was especially directed toward his mother's feet, he had particular difficulty in walking.

The description of one group of symptoms is practically the whole life history of a patient. When there are several symptoms, these are always connected with each other and lead back to the same basic situations in childhood. Freud has taught us that in the development of an individual, the Oedipus complex plays the dominant role. All of the pregenital activities reach their final formation in the Oedipus complex. We can judge a neurosis as well as a perversion only if we know in what way the pregenital activities have been resolved in connection with the dominant figures of father and mother and/or their substitutes. Therefore, we can also conclude that the symptom is a repetition of an infantile experience connected with the Oedipus complex. In some way the repetition satisfies the infantile desire, but the satisfaction is only incomplete and symbolic. This is the ultimate meaning of a neurosis, which thus becomes the expression of the basic tendencies of the personality.

It is not difficult to prove in criminal actions, in the actions of psychopathic individuals, and in perversions that the same infantile tendencies achieve their satisfactions. Psychoanalysis was first inclined to believe that the satisfaction obtained in a perversion is the satisfaction of an infantile perverse desire in a direct way. Newer investigations have taught us that the perversion, the criminal act, and the action of a psychopathic individual are all symbolic in the same way as is the neurotic symptom. We also find in such cases conflicts in the building up of the Oedipus complex. These conflicts finally lead to early repressions, which necessitate a symbolic expression of the primary wish. Overt homosexual activity, as well as any other perversion, therefore hides its real meaning in the same way as does a neurosis or a neurotic symptom.

All of these infantile desires belong to the system of the id. We know that the id has different strata, and in the different neuroses the different strata of the infantile desire find their symbolic expression. We know that in the obsessional neurosis, homosexual, anal, and sadistic tendencies are tied up in the Oedipus complex and find their veiled expression in the obsessive-neurotic symptom. The obsessional fear of one patient of being bitten in the genitals by horses was derived from an early scene where his father, in an outburst of anger, threatened to hit the child for putting a chair in his way. The same patient also had early anal-sadistic experiences in connection with a maid. Later on he felt under compulsion to think about streets entirely covered with feces.

Exaggerated cleanliness in an obsessive-neurotic case reveals itself as a defense reaction against the primary infantile pleasure in feces. It may be added that not only the neurotic symptom in the narrow sense, but also the symptom which the individual finally accepts and which we then call a character trend, have similar sources and similar meanings.

But whereas the meaning of the obsessional neurosis is to be found in the anal, homosexual, and sadistic sphere, the meaning of hysterical symptoms is based upon the heterosexual Oedipus complex. In hysteria there is already present a full genital sexuality. The hysterical symptoms constitute symbolic genital sexual satisfaction. The objects providing the sex satisfaction are the father and mother. In the hysterical attack we see a symbolic intercourse with the father. Hysterical anaesthesia shows the repression against the sexual satisfaction by the father. All this is very schematic. If one analyzes a case one sees that every neurotic symptom is, as we have called it, overdetermined. It combines within itself many experiences and many tendencies of the individual, like a lens converging the sun's rays to a focal point.

We may say that every neurotic symptom has a meaning from the point of view of the id, and that this meaning has not only theoretical significance but also dynamic value. Changes in the meaning are, at the same time and generally speaking, changes in the distribution of psychic energy or of the libido in each particular case. These changes in the libidinal situation find their immediate expression in physiological processes. We do not believe, as we once did, that a hysterical symptom is purely psychic. It also involves biological changes, a change in the somatic sphere. We know that the blood vessels and all of the organs affected by vegetative innervation undergo changes when the hysterical symptom occurs. We can even be sure that some of the so-called organic symptoms are due to dynamic changes similar to those which cause a hysterical symptom. One therefore has the right to consider some of the organic diseases an expression of a psychic meaning. It is not yet determined how far we may go in the understanding of so-called organic diseases. Jelliffe (1933), Groddeck (1923), and F. Deutsch (1922) have made important contributions in this direction. But at any rate we may form the hypothesis that the body in its structure and in its changes may have a meaning. We may understand this meaning better when we know something about the genesis of the neurotic symptom in general, and especially of the hysterical symptom.

When we study the psychology of persons who have an organic disease we immediately learn something new. The organic disease solves many problems for the individual. The sick person does not have to care for himself any longer. He also obtains a weapon in his fight for superiority in the family by achieving the right to be the center of the family's attention, to be taken care of. But still he suffers. He may feel, if he is pious, that he has been punished for a sin that he has not committed. Even if he is not pious, the disease may appear to him as a punishment, satisfying the feeling of guilt which is present in every person and which has its roots in the early development of the child (in the injunctions, punishments, and restrictions to which it has been exposed) and in the incorporation of the superego in its own ego.

The feeling of guilt is based on an ever-present tension between the ego and the superego. In it lies the basis for the Catholic belief in original sin and for Kant's concept that human beings are sinful and bad and that human nature is sinful and bad in itself. We try to escape this feeling of guilt by self-inflicted suffering. But there is also relief from this feeling of guilt when fate (the father) inflicts the suffering upon us. The organic symptom satisfies the desire to suffer.

Quite the same way is the neurotic symptom also the fulfillment of what Reik has called *"Straf Beduergniss"*—of the inner need for punishment. Reik (1925) and Alexander (1927) have shown that the neurotic symptom satisfies this need for punishment; it is a means of suffering which the individual inflicts upon himself. He partially assumes the suffering for the satisfaction he gets from the neurotic symptom, a condition which is particularly evident in obsessional neuroses where the sadistic impulse to kill the beloved person breaks almost openly into consciousness. The individual suffers enormously. We can therefore say, generally speaking, that the psychology of the organic disease has opened our eyes and has shown us that the neurotic symptom also has a meaning from the point of view of the superego or the ideal ego. It means the fulfillment for the need for punishment. Consequently, the neurotic symptom has a meaning for the id as well as for the superego.

But even these remarks do not exhaust the problem involved. I have mentioned already that a person who is organically sick becomes automatically the center of the family; he also gains many external advantages. Society usually takes better care of the sick than of the healthy. The neurotic symptom frees the individual from the struggle of life. In other words, the ego—the organization which maintains us as a unit and which maintains us in social life and in defense of our own existence—the ego, in the psychoanalytic sense, also uses the neurotic symptom. So the neurotic symptom has a meaning from the point of view of the ego. The meaning and purpose of the neurotic symptom are thus the same. We can not understand the neurotic symptom if we do not understand the meaning of the id, superego, and ego.

This point of view may be exemplified in the case of an anxiety neurosis. The patient mentioned above got his anxiety attack at first whenever he came near the districts where prostitutes lived. The analysis, we have heard, had brought out the strong attachment to his mother, and the fact that he wished to see the genitals of his mother and sister was one of the outstanding factors in the genesis of the neurosis.

Feet symbolized for him the female genitals. His fear of being castrated was extreme. Whenever he was obliged to walk he felt a heaviness in his legs. In "Inhibitions, Symptoms and Anxiety," Freud (1926) considered anxiety a danger signal that warns the ego of an inner or outward danger. The danger is, directly or indirectly, castration. The meaning of the anxiety in this case was: "Don't go into dangerous situations connected with sex; castration may be the result." From the point of view of the unconscious and from the point of view of the id, the patient gained the possibility of being closer again to his family, especially to his mother and sister. He satisfied some of the desires of the Oedipus complex. But at the same time the anxiety may be considered a substitute for sexual satisfaction. It is a product of the conversion of the libido. Freud himself was not sure whether his earlier statement that libido is converted into anxiety could be maintained.

I think that there is at least the probability that in anxiety we deal with something similar to a strong irritation of the vegetative system which is connected to sexual excitement. The patient pays dearly for the gratification he experiences by being more closely attached to the family, especially to the mother, just as he pays for the anxiety if it is a substitute for sexuality.

We may say that the meaning of the neurosis, in this respect, is that the superego obtains its satisfaction by self-punishment of the individual. We may look for this threefold meaning in every psychoneurotic symptom. In consciousness, the meaning of the symptom prevails. After all, the individual with his neurotic symptoms must maintain his position in society and in life, and the synthetic power of the ego makes it possible for the individual to keep in closer contact with reality.

Freud considered the neurosis the result of a conflict between the ego and the id. On the side of the ego is the superego. It is true that the defense apparatus—the expressive power—has to be exerted strongly against the id, and changes in this apparatus will be present in every neurosis. On the other hand, the neurotic individual obeys the law that asks for an adaptation to reality.

The fundamental difference between the neurosis and the psychosis lies in the fact that the neurotic person has maintained his adaptation to reality, that the ego of the neurotic has been able at least to achieve some synthetization of the three meanings of a neurosis. In a psychosis the situation is different.

In schizophrenia the individual goes back to the very early narcissistic stages of libidinal development. In a catatonic stupor the patient gives up the relation with the world; he enjoys his own body, and he may develop very primitive reactions by resisting every influence coming from the outside. The individual has sacrificed the ego organization. The whole state of mind has a meaning from the point of view of the id only. There is no superego of effective power; it has been pushed aside.

It is true, though not in all schizophrenic psychoses, that regression to the primitive stages and to the satisfaction of the id is very much in the foreground. Remainders of the ego functions and the superego functions are usually present to some degree. We generally believe that the ego in the schizophrenic is not destroyed, but is only deprived of its powers. Whenever the enormous stress to regression diminishes, the ego and the superego set up new defenses against the regressive tendencies, urging toward new relations with the world.

Hallucinations are often the expression of such a new interest in the world. The frequent schizophrenic hallucinations about snakes and worms signify a revival of sexual interests in love objects, a revival which is again partly regressed, partly projected by the ego. The superego has gained new strength.

One of my patients, dissatisfied with what he could achieve as a clerk, had started to study linguistic problems in his own way. All words which contained the syllable "po" (in German slang "popo" means "buttocks") interested him, especially the French word "pommes" (apples) which denoted to him the similarity between the roundness of the apples and of the buttocks. His linguistic studies signified symbolic satisfaction of his anal tendencies. He went back into a period in his childhood (around the fourth year) during which his interest in the buttocks was paramount. He even had experiences of eating feces. But the repression went further, and one day he went into a park and announced that the end of the world had come. This was the expression of the narcissistic repression when the world had lost its libidinal value for him.

Immediately afterward he announced that he belonged to the race of tigers, the leader of which had been crucified. The big tiger was his father, Christ. He, the patient, would now take his place. This psychotic symptom denoted that he wanted to take the place of his father. But his father, for whom he would substitute, was the Godlike father of his childhood. His own father, a butcher with enormous strength, had impressed him as a powerful animal. The name of the French statesman Clemenceau (tiger) always reminded him of his father whose name had been Clemens. In the psychosis, which lasted almost two years, the anal element came again and again to the foreground. He kept a piece of feces for himself because he thought he could rule the world with it. One of the attendants impressed him as being fair; he feared that this attendant would put a snake in his anus. The new interest he was gaining of the world was only anal to begin with, but gradually he gained higher levels of psychosexual integration, and recovered. It is easy to see here that the psychotic symptoms have a meaning. They satisfy deep-lying magical anal and homosexual tendencies.

When we deal with systematic delusions of a paranoid type, we have to reckon with the synthetic power of the ego and the superego, which try to unite the products of regression into some adaptation toward reality. We see immediately that only in the deepest catatonic stupors of schizophrenics, when they are motionless, stiff, cut off from every interest, would the meaning of the psychosis be completely understood. Probably such a case is only theoretically possible. In all other cases we meet again the threefold meaning such as we saw in the neuroses. In its whole structure, schizophrenia is much nearer to the neuroses than any other psychoses. We have in schizophrenia, too, the conflict between the ego and the id which provokes regression.

In manic-depressive psychoses, the interesting condition in which the individual is elated beyond all measure or equally depressed, there is also a meaning for the id. We know from Abraham (1924) that oral-sadistic features form the background of the depressed as well as the elated phases of the condition. The meaning of melancholia from the point of view of the id is the satisfaction of the oral-sadistic tendencies. The melancholic individual reproaches himself for it; the manic exults in giving free rein to oral and other impulses. From the point of view of the superego the meaning of melancholia is ruthless sadistic self-punishment. The manic has succeeded in getting rid of the infringements imposed upon him by the superego. Both phases have, therefore, clear-cut meaning for the superego.

In the life of a 26-year-old woman suffering from a depression which lasted about nine months, food and eating had played an important part from early childhood. She had always felt that food and eating were the most important part of life. The psychosis started when she had to leave the home of her mother and do the cooking for her husband. In the psychosis she saw herself being an enormous tube through which everything had to pass. All food for her meals was the flesh of persons she had killed. She accused herself of having bitten off and devoured the genitals of men. She said that she devoured a great number of human beings every night. But she thought also that she digested men through her vagina, swallowing them by way of her vagina. In connection with these fantasies and dreams she experienced an orgasm, which had never happened before. In her psychosis this patient therefore satisfied her oral-sadistic tendencies. It is understandable that she refused to eat and that she suffered an enormous feeling of guilt.

Finally, from the point of view of the ego, in melancholia we have the ego unable to stand the onslaught of the superego. It is lacking in the power of synthesis. In the manic, the ego is liberated from the superego and is unable to resist the onslaught of the libidinal tendencies. In both cases we have serious disturbances between the relations of the ego and the superego and in the ability of the ego to adapt itself satisfactorily to reality. One sees immediately that the ego is seemingly the mechanism that makes adaptation possible. Psychoses are characterized by deeper disturbances in that organization. But one sees that even if the ego does not fulfill its function—giving up partially or completely—there is still a meaning in every psychotic symptom. There are unconscious tendencies that want to be fulfilled—tendencies of the superego—so that it may generally be said that the psychotic symptom also has meaning, although this meaning is sometimes very difficult to determine. There is not only regression in the psychosis, but there is also serious trouble in the adaptation to reality.

Whereas in schizophrenia and in the manic-depressive psychoses the disturbance of the ego generally results from conflicts, regressions, and the overflow of libidinal and sadistic tendencies, there is a group of psychoses in which it seems that the function of the ego is disturbed in a more or less direct way.

In so-called organic mental confusion, the individual is unable to orient himself in the world; he cannot differentiate among or integrate the impressions he receives; he does not see the *Gestalten*. Freud believed that in mental confusion a conflict existed between the ego and reality. I would prefer to say that the ego is no longer able to maintain its organizational function in perception.

When there is severe destruction of the brain, as in general paralysis due to syphilis, arteriosclerosis of the brain, or senility, the ego loses its capacity for organization, especially in relation to cognition, but maintains its relation to perception. In some of these cases we find that perception is subject to troubles of an agnostic type. Certainly, patients with agnosia are unable to organize their perception. But this trouble is different from the perceptive difficulties in the case of confusion, where only the higher synthesis is disturbed. We cannot say that dementia as such has meaning. We can only say that the individual has lost the possibility of achieving closer contact with reality. Whenever such an impairment of the ego occurs, libidinal tendencies which have hitherto been repressed come to the surface and have a meaning which we can only understand by using analysis. But we cannot say why the ego in mental confusion or in general paralysis either gives up its functions or ceases to exert them in a proper way. We do not know why the ego resigns, but we do know that when the ego can no longer maintain its functions the id and the superego will have a freer range and will express themselves more unrestrainedly than before. In other words, the organic lesions of the brain bring the unconscious tendencies and their meaning nearer the surface so that they become more understandable.

Neuroses and psychoses thus become manifestations of life which appear in every normal individual; they become as meaningful as life itself. Life reveals its meaning only in the concrete life of concrete personalities. We must try to understand the personality of the neurotic and psychotic so that we may learn to understand the meaning of their symptoms.

In general paralysis there are ideas of grandeur in which all wishes and daydreams reach their fulfillment. The patient is king, emperor, general; he has enormous sexual potency and has relations with the most beautiful women in the world. But more or less infantile wishes are also fulfilled: he is taller than anyone else; he has more stools than any other person; he can urinate streams. Such ideas of grandeur fulfill all the infantile and puberty wishes life has denied.

One knows that perverse tendencies which were not active through an entire life may appear in senility. So even the organic destruction of the brain brings out the early problems of the individual. The infantile wishes and the early experiences are still present. In other words, the life of an individual is an entirety even when an organic brain disease interferes. The id will still strive for satisfaction, and will succeed even more when the repressive forces are impaired by brain disease.

Every personality possesses deep-reaching tendencies and desires rooted in the psychosexual and ego constitution and formed by the experiences of life, especially by the experiences of infancy and childhood. Our character and our actions, the whole aspects of our lives are all the expression of these composite inner desires. Actions, feelings, character have, therefore, a profound meaning from the point of view of the personality as a whole. They are also symbolic in the normal person in that here, also, they point to deeper and more hidden dynamisms and experiences.

CHAPTER TWO

The Somatic Basis of the Neuroses

If one asks whether a neurosis has an organic background or not, one must answer that of course every neurosis must have an organic basis because normal life, normal psychic life, also has an organic background, and one cannot make a distinction between the organic and the psychic. It is a necessary conclusion that changes in the psychic life of an individual are accompanied by changes in the organism.

This is the point of view of psychoanalysis, and when in psychoanalysis we speak of a change in the libido, we must be aware that this means that something is taking place in the body. When Freud (1905b) speaks about libido he includes in this some products of the metabolism of the sex organs. He is of the opinion that when we speak about sex constitution, about sex development, we include somatic changes in the metabolism of the sex organs and that we deal with processes which sooner or later will also be understood from the point of view of physiology. He himself was of the opinion that the neuroses are connected with changes in the organism.

We therefore have to ask ourselves, what do we know at the present time about the bodily changes in the neuroses and how

Appeared originally in *The Journal of Nervous and Mental Disease,* 70:502-519, 1929.

can we make use of this knowledge for the interpretation of the neuroses. The first attempt to approach this problem was that of Eppinger and Hess (1911), who developed the concept of *vagotonia*. They had the idea of a special type of human being in whom the autonomic nervous system is in a condition of special tone, special excitability, and they believed this vagotonia to be the cause of neurotic troubles. But we find difficulty with this concept because observation shows that vagotonics usually have rather large pupils, and this is the opposite of what we should expect in people who have a true hypertonus of the autonomic vagus system. The symptoms of vagotonia are mostly combined with symptoms of *sympathicotonia*. For this reason Bergmann (1930) developed the concept of stigma in the vegetative nervous system as a substitute for the notions of vagotonia and sympathicotonia (*vegetative stigmatization*). In connection with these changes in the vegetative nervous system, we may observe vasomotor troubles. These individuals blush very easily, they have an increased perspiration, the pulse rate is increased. In some cases we find extrasystoles, and respiratory arrhythmias are common. Among the cases I have observed, there were two rather clear instances of extrasystoles. One case was a person who had difficulties in living with his older sister. He also had rather marked vasomotor trouble, especially in the nose. When he became excited he frequently had noticeable extrasystoles. The other patient suffered from an anxiety neurosis and frequently got extrasystoles in connection with the situation at home. He developed this symptom and palpitation of the heart whenever he felt neglected by his mother. Hansen (1927) reported similar cases.

These symptoms of the vasomotor system are, however, not the only ones we find in neurotics. We can observe very similar symptoms of disturbed motility, of stomach secretions, of bowel movements, and of urination. We could say that there is no vegetative organ which is not affected in one neurosis or another. The changes are sometimes more or less marked, but I would like to stress that one does not find these changes in every neurotic case. If one studies cases of obsessional neuroses particularly, one observes that many of these cases do not show changes in the vasomotor system or in other parts of the vegetative nervous system. We know, on the other hand, that there are many persons who show a rather high degree of lability of the blood vessels and of the vegetative nervous system who are nevertheless not neurotic. It is not possible to interpret the whole problem of the neuroses in terms of the vegetative nervous system. The greater frequency of vegetative troubles in neurotics is still an important problem, but the vegetative system is only one part of the system which regulates the metabolism of the body.

In this respect I would like to call your attention to the ideas of F. Kraus (1927) who formulated the hypothesis that irritation of the vagus is in many ways similar in its effects to the administration of potassium. The effect of calcium is considered identical with the influence of adrenalin, which irritates the sympathetic system. He was of the opinion that the ratio of calcium to potassium in the tissues is the real basis of the personality. He also speaks of the "deep personality" (*Tiefen Person*), and develops the point of view that all toxins which influence the vegetative nervous system are in some respects similar to potassium or to calcium (adrenalin). One of his experiments, which will perhaps best portray the trend of his conceptions, is the following. When mesothorium (a radioactive substance) is placed upon frogs, the spinal cords of which have been removed, these animals act, as Kraus puts it, as if they were under the influence of calcium. If potassium is first injected into the lymph sac of such a frog and then mesothorium is put on the back of the animal, the animal does not act as if under the influence of calcium.

These are the types of experiments that Kraus quotes toward the solution of the problem of the neuroses. For him the problem is whether or not there is an equilibrium between calcium and potassium in the tissues. These might be interesting facts, but it is not true that they have anything to do with the problem of the neuroses, and all this speculation on the "deep personality" in Kraus's sense does not lead us further into the problem at hand.

It is true, of course, that the vasomotor vegetative functions are very closely related to another group of bodily activities which are very important from our point of view, i.e., the glands of internal secretion. You know, for instance, that in tetany the change in the calcium component of the blood plays a very important part. It is very likely that in many of the disturbances of internal secretion the relation of potassium to calcium in the blood is of great importance (cf. Zondek, 1923). But even in organic disturbances of the endocrine organs we never find a complete analogy to the neuroses.

It is interesting from this point of view to study cases of hyperthyroidism and to compare them with cases of neurosis. To begin with, the whole structure of a case of hyperthyroidism is very different from that of a true neurosis. I refer especially to those cases of hyperthyroidism which we so frequently meet in countries where goiter is prevalent. It is indeed true that a neurotic patient can also develop symptoms of hyperthyroidism, but in such a neurotic case we can easily distinguish a rather close relationship between the special complexes of the individual and the symptoms of hyperthyroidism, whereas the hyperthyroidism will have quite a different relation to the whole personality and the life problems of the patient in a case of hyperthyroid disease or exophthalmic goiter of organic origin. I believe that some of the cases of true exophthalmic goiter have at least a psychogenic component in their etiology. In many cases the cause is organic in the usual sense. Some cases of so-called polyglandular insufficiency may offer some similarities with cases of neurosis. A girl whom I had observed was always fatigued, could never work, felt a marked degree of slowness in all her movements. Examination disclosed rather clear signs of polyglandular insufficiency. In this case organic treatment changed the situation rather quickly, but all her difficulties and symptoms had quite another role in her psychic life from what one observes in neuroses. These cases of polyglandular insufficiency are in no wise identical with cases of true neuroses. Succinctly, there is no doubt of the existence of some relationship between the glands of internal secretion and the neurotic picture, but there is no complete identity, and we cannot understand the neuroses if we approach them only as a disease of the glandular system.

Great attention has been paid to thyroid changes in neuroses. Some investigators (Dattner, 1929) have stated that there are changes in temperature in every neurosis, or that there is some variability in the regulation of the temperature. It is quite true that in some neuroses (and I shall refer later to an instance of this kind) we find a great variability in temperature regulation. This is doubtless due to the vasomotor lability of the patient. It is certainly not true, however, that such findings are at all the rule among neurotic patients. The percentage of such patients in whom such changes of temperature regulation are found is rather small, and not infrequently we find such deviations among patients who have no neurotic signs at all. It has also been said that it is possible to cure neuroses by the administration of small doses of iodine, but I do not think that this observation is true. I think that the use of iodine in such cases has a purely suggestive influence. In short, I think that also from this point of view we cannot reach an understanding of what takes place in the course of a neurosis.

There have been other attempts to find out what takes place in the course of a neurosis. It has been emphasized that there are changes in the electric excitability of the nerves. Hopmann (1926), especially, has stated that a high percentage of the cases of neurotic patients show such changes in electric excitability. But we must say in this respect that our methods of electric investigation are very unreliable. In several of his papers, F. Hartmann (1902), has attempted to connect some of the neuroses with an organic change of the skin, but no one other than Hartmann has ever observed such changes in the skin. In respect to the electric excitability, we know that it varies in different countries. In countries where tetany is more or less common we often find a decreased electric threshold of the nerves. Nevertheless, the average number of neuroses is not greater in such places than in other countries. I am therefore of the opinion that the neuroses cannot be more deeply understood from the point of view of electric excitability or the endocrine function of the parathyroid gland. An examination of every glandular function from a similar point of view will lead us to the same conclusion, and we must say that neurosis can be understood neither as a change in the vegetative system nor simply as a change in endocrine function.

I wish to mention, however, in this connection, the interesting studies of E. Jaensch (1930) and his brother, W. Jaensch (1930), in the attempt to distinguish different constitutional types among normal persons and neurotics. These two different types comprise persons who are inclined to have *eidetic* pictures. Eidetic pictures are such as stand between an optic image and an optic perception. One can produce them if one asks a person to look at a picture and then to close his eye. Such pictures have in part the characteristics of a perception, and it is sometimes possible to mix colors in the same way that colors are mixed in perception. Also, one finds these eidetic pictures marked by characteristics peculiar to perception in space and not to pure imagination. Jaensch and his brother now state that there are two different types of such eidetic pictures. The one is called the B or basedoid type (exophthalmic goiter type) and the other the T or tetanoid type (connected with tetany). These authors claim that the type of eidetic pictures is quite different in these two types of cases. The eidetic pictures of the exophthalmic goiter type are very fluid and vivid in color. All persons who perceive pictures of this nature are, according to the authors, of the basedoid type, that is, they have a more mobile facial expression and brighter, more lustrous eyes. The other type has more rigid eidetic pictures, they are not so well colored, nor are they subject to such fluid changes. The individuals who produce this latter type of picture are also more rigid in the motor sphere, and they also have a more rigid facial expression. These two types react in a different way to the same drugs. According to the authors, iodine has a special effect on the eidetic pictures of the exophthalmic goiter type, whereas the eidetic pictures of the tetanoid type may disappear under the influence of calcium.

The psychological findings of these authors are doubtless of importance and certainly contain much truth, but their statements concerning the constitutional relations of their psychological types have provoked justifiable criticism. S. Fischer (1925) has shown that the statement of W. Jaensch that the T type has an altered nervous irritability is not correct. Karger (1925) disproves the existence of a relation between constitutional type and a special type of eidetic picture. We might therefore say that there is no complete justification for this attempt to connect a special type of psychic life with a special part of the glandular system. We are thus not able to make use of these descriptions in a real classification of the neuroses from a physical point of view. A further difficulty of the Jaensch conceptions lies in the fact that these eidetic pictures are usually not present during the entire life of an individual, but that they generally occur just before or during adolescence, and it is not definite whether they can be found similarly in children. It is possible that there are special phases in childhood in which these pictures could not be found, and that they may not be present during the whole of childhood. We frequently see persons with vivid optic pictures of the eidetic type who do not suffer from a neurosis. And, on the other hand, persons suffer from a neurosis who do not have eidetic pictures in one or the other sense. It is thus also impossible to solve our problem from this point of view. Succinctly, this conception is akin to the point of view of Kraus (1927), that the content of calcium or potassium ions in the tissues determines the problems of the personality and thus closely connects the neurosis with endocrinological disturbances.

We cannot interpret what takes place psychologically in a neurosis by changes in the vasovegetative system. But perhaps we can interpret the changes in the vasovegetative nervous system by studying the neurosis and the psychic problems which take place therein.

What takes place when we are under the influence of an emotion? Every emotion has characteristic reactions in the whole vegetative system. We cannot expect to learn anything very characteristic of an emotion if we study only the blood pressure, only the volume of the arms, or only the skin resistance. We know that in many of these reactions there is nothing very characteristic of any special emotion. The psychogalvanic phenomenon, for instance, changes in the same way if the individual experiences great joy or depression. Many other emotional changes in the body are also not specific. If we were to study all the reactions at the same time, the reactions in the vasovegetative system and in the glands, in the secretions, in the stomach, and in breathing, then we would find a picture which contains a living situation either perceived or imagined, real or represented, fully conscious or unconscious, and also our attitude toward this situation. The attitude is accompanied by feelings and is, together with them, an immediate inner experience. We can suggest an emotion to a person by evoking the life situation which calls forth the attitude.

In this respect I would like to call your attention to some experimental facts which will illustrate these ideas. Gigon et al. (1926) succeeded in suggesting a change in the blood sugar of diabetic patients. Such an influence cannot be demonstrated in normals, but the experiences of Knauer (1915) and others show clearly that the emotions have a strong influence on sugar metabolism. Anxiety is often accompanied by glycosuria. I have only to point to the experiments of Cannon (1932). The calcium metabolism can also be influenced by suggestion, as Glaser (1924) has shown. These experiments were repeated with similar results by Kretschmer and Krueger (1927), who show that such changes do not occur in every subject. The vasovegetative system is different in different persons, and suggestion to different persons does not act in the same way on the vasovegetative system. The influence of the emotions on the vegetative system is a fact. Those functions not directly under the influence of the will, such as the calcium and blood-sugar metabolism in the blood, can be changed by suggestion. We know, also, that the blood pressure is dependent upon psychic factors to a very great extent, and that such changes take place not only when physical work is suggested to the individual but also when emotions, such as anxiety, are present. In suggestion as well as in emotion, the special life situation is the important influence. The bodily answers vary according to the life situations which are either perceived or imagined. Hansen (1927) was able to achieve the same temperature regulations not only by cooling off the body but also by the mere suggestion that the body found itself in cooler surroundings. I might also mention that the basal metabolism can be altered to the extent of 30 percent by psychic influences. In such a case, also, one has to suggest a life situation in order to get the desired result. Felix Deutsch (1933) has shown that the unconscious life situation has the same, or even greater, influence than has the conscious one. It is possible, according to Astruck (1923) to provoke rapid and irregular action of the heart in hypnosis, so-called palpitation. No one else has as yet been able to observe the same results. It is, of course, well known that in hypnosis one can change the secretion and motility of the stomach and duodenum, and these changes are closely connected with the special situation you suggest to the individual. Suggestion and the neurosis have in this respect one thing in common. They refer to an important situation, and the psychological result to be derived from this connection is that the emotion can be understood only in relation to life situations and must have a specific content.

When we come to consider asthma, we find that psychic influences here also interfere with bodily changes. In one respect asthma is partly an allergic reaction, but at least in a certain number of cases the allergic disposition provokes symptoms only when a change in the psychic attitude of the individual is also present, and it is this psychic influence in combination with the allergic processes which provokes the bronchial asthma. If the psychic component of such a condition is treated by psychotherapy, then the bronchial asthma may, in some cases, be seen to disappear, although the organic allergic processes have not been changed. Nevertheless, it is also likely that the allergic processes themselves can be psychically influenced.

If in neurotic cases we find changes in the vasomotor

system, the glands of internal secretion, in the innervation of all the organs which are under the influence of the vasovegetative system, we will then have to consider whether all these changes may not be secondary to changes in the psychic make-up of the individual. We will, of course, not deny that there may be some general change in the vasovegetative or glandular system, but the special character of the vegetative disturbance in any neurosis will very largely be influenced by the specific problems in the lives of such patients.

At this point I wish to go somewhat deeper into the analysis of what might happen to the emotions and the vasovegetative system of such neurotic patients. An emotion does not only cause a general reaction. That would not be a sufficient description of its effects. If we study the secretion of the stomach, for instance, we find that it varies in character and quantity according to the specific content in the suggestion. If it is suggested to a patient that he is going to eat meat, the secretion of the stomach will be different from the secretion produced by the suggestion that he is going to eat fat. The great question is, how can we suggest to an organ. We may suggest to the patient, "You will now experience a change in your stomach," but he would not react to that. We have to suggest to the patient some food which he wants to eat. We have to deal with a special life situation, and it is only by the suggestion of such a life situation that we are able to bring the individual to all these responses in the area of the vegetative system. We cannot, for example, influence the secretion in the kidneys by suggesting a certain quantity of urine, nor will the urine content of phosphates be thus changed. The individual would not know what to do with such a suggestion. But we can suggest to the individual, as Heilig and Hoff (1925), as well as others have done, that he has drunk a great quantity of water. The living situation thus provoked will then bring about a special adaptation in the secretory apparatus, and there will not only be a change in the quantity of the urine, but the phosphate and chloride content of the urine will also be increased. In short, the suggestion as such can have an influence only if we deal with a suggestion which fits a special biological situation and not if the suggestion concerns or is directed at a special organ. Our task is to find the special life situations which are connected with a change in the vegetative nervous system and in the system of endocrine glands.

The question arises whether the life situations in neurotic patients have a greater influence on this system than in so-called normally adjusted persons. We certainly cannot deny that such a possibility exists. It is possible that neurotic persons are those in whom the physical changes in the vegetative system occur more easily than in the average person, but we must also reckon with the possibility that the neurotic person is an individual who already in childhood was under the influence of marked emotions. The organ in question might have been trained in the pathological direction. We have to reckon with the fact that every neurosis consists of a special psychic training to a specific psychic situation, and the special emotional training in this regard will necessarily have an influence on specific vasovegetative organs (cf. F. Deutsch, 1933). Some of the symptoms of the isolation in the vegetative nervous system that we meet in neurotics are doubtless connected with events of early childhood which, in the course of time, have created an entirely different state in the vasovegetative nervous system.

We thus come to the conclusions which are very similar to those we would have achieved if we had considered the neurosis strictly from the point of view of psychology. Looking at the neurosis from the psychoanalytical point of view, we state that there may be some constitutional change in the sex make-up in the whole vasovegetative and glandular system of the individual, but this whole system can also be influenced by the events of the individual's development and life. Psychoanalysis states that the events of childhood have a special importance in this respect. Every emotion which arises in our adult life has, as I have already pointed out, a special expression in the vasovegetative system, depending entirely upon the personality. The vasovegetative and the glandular systems are connected with every part of the body. We know that there is some relationship between the sympathetic and the parasympathetic system and the motor system of the striped muscles, and we know that there is no organ in the body that is not under the influence of this vasovegetative system. This influence, as you all know, is very complex. For example, I might mention the interesting experiment of Loewi (1921) which shows that when the vagus nerve is irritated the heart produces a substance that influences the vagus nerve itself. Probably every function of any organ produces substances that change the function of that selfsame organ.

Now we must also reckon with the emotion itself and with the changes resulting in the vasovegetative system. We know from a psychoanalytical and a psychological point of view that every emotion simultaneously reactivates the appropriate infantile emotions, and that every emotion of childhood is in turn related to some process in the vasovegetative system. The other experiences of life, with their emotions, of course, tune in. Succinctly, any present emotion sums up all the emotional influences which the vasovegetative system has undergone since childhood. The affective value of every event in life is not only determined by the actual event itself, but is also dependent on what has actually taken place in the previous life of the individual. Every experience of life leaves its traces in the vasovegetative and the glandular systems of the individual, as it were. I emphasize again the fact that the problems of life are closely interrelated with all the problems of the sympathetic and parasympathetic systems. Any special reaction to a specific situation is built up on the more general attitudes of the individual and the organism.

I might mention in this connection the interesting ideas of W. R. Hess (1925). He has developed the theory that the sympathetic system has to do with the catabolic processes, the processes of life which spend energy, and that the parasympathetic system regulates those processes of life by which we spare and build up energies to be used later. He has pointed out that cocaine, which excites the sympathetic nervous system, provokes in us a great expenditure of nervous energy, an excitement which may become almost manic. Ergotoxin, on the other hand, which paralyzes the sympathetic nervous system and also probably excites the parasympathetic nervous system, provokes the phenomenon of sleep, especially when, according to Hess, it is injected into the third ventricle in small quantities. The parasympathetic action of the organism builds up energy; it is anabolic. According to Hess, sleep is the expression of the forces in us that try to build up and save energy. The sympathetic and the parasympathetic nervous systems, all our vegetative activity, are closely connected with the rest of the activities of life, which are intimately related to the actual situations in life. Certainly the problem of the neurosis has something to do with all these systems, but we will doubtless come much nearer to these problems if we dispense with the mechanistic idea of some change in the nervous system as a cause for the neurosis and consider the neurosis as a change in the individual's whole attitude toward life. This, of course, is a difference which we can at the present time understand much better from the psychological point of view. The difference in the individual's attitude brings with it all these important changes in the functions of life which are connected with the vasovegetative nervous system. Each emotion provokes some change in these anabolic and catabolic processes. We do agree, however, that such an attitude might be partly due to a specific situation in the vegetative system.

Here we must consider some interesting psychological data by Weinberg (1923, 1924). He has found that with every increase of attention, i.e., of the level of consciousness, there occurs a reaction of the sympathetic nervous system which is followed by a reaction of the parasympathetic system. The parasympathetic reaction is then again followed by an increased activity of the sympathetic system. We see here that every action of life is accompanied by general changes in the body and that the vasovegetative system reflects our psychic activity. In addition to such a general change, however, there is a specific vasovegetative change commensurate with the specific life task.

Perhaps we should not have begun our examination of the

organic basis of the neurosis with the vegetative system but from the point of view of the so-called conditioned reflex. Let me first describe again what a conditioned reflex is. Pavlov (1927) found that when he fed a dog and simultaneously produced some other sensory stimulus such as ringing a bell, playing a tune, or flashing a light, this combination, when repeated frequently, soon provoked the secretion of saliva in the dog when the secondary stimulus alone was produced. Such a reflex is called conditioned because it varies from the innate reflex which, in this case, would consist of the secretion of saliva upon the sight, taste, or smell of food. The light flash or the sound might be called the signal stimulus and the food the unconditioned stimulus. Some time later, Pavlov connected the signal with the production of an artificial reflex of a similar type by injecting hydrochloric acid into the animal's mouth. Such conditioned reflexes follow special rules which are of considerable interest. In the beginning of training or conditioning the reflex is rather generalized. Taking a sound of 200 wavelengths per second, for example, it will not only at first provoke salivary secretion in the animal but will also affect other movements. It will also be possible for a sound of 300 wavelengths, for example, to produce the same results, but in the course of time the conditioning becomes very specialized, and the animal will react to a sound of only 200 wavelengths per second and no more or less. I repeat that the conditioned reflex is at first a very generalized one, and that only later does it become more specialized. In this respect, I might mention that Beritoff (1926) found that if the successful signal is combined with some other unknown stimulus, the result is a weakening of the conditioned reflex, although in the course of time the added stimulus loses its disturbing effect and the combination between the new stimulus and the former signal is as efficient as the old stimulus alone. Still another factor is quite important. If, for example, I offer the animal the combination of sound and acid rather often, the conditioned reflex will be formed, but if I then offer the animal only the sound, continue it rather frequently, and in some way also frustrate the animal, the conditioned reflex will disappear entirely in the course of time. If we want to have a conditioned reflex which lasts, it will be necessary for us to repeat that combination of the sound and the unconditioned stimulus again. If, however, the conditioned reflex is provoked too frequently, the sound or the signal as such will not bring about any further reaction. In other words, the signal irritation has to be proved as a real signal.

The effort has frequently been made to prove the neuroses of children as due to such conditioned reflexes. If, for example, the child has been frightened by something having to do with the father, perhaps the very sight of the father will again cause fright. This response may also spread to all adults who at all resemble the father. This would be a conditioned reflex brought on by experience, and the conditioning might become even more efficient if the father had beaten the child very often. There can be no doubt that such a mechanism exists, but we easily recognize such mechanisms as those we study every day in psychoanalysis, and we can understand them in psychoanalysis much better than in animal reactions. The animal is not able to tell us what is taking place.

I have made a study of conditioned reflexes in man from a similar point of view (1929a). I offered my subjects the optic stimulus of a light, and five seconds later I sent a strong electric current through the right hand so that they were compelled to withdraw the hand. After ten or more days of such experimentation, I then offered them only the light, and it very frequently occurred that the subjects would suddenly withdraw their hands five seconds after the light had appeared. I had built up a conditioned reflex. Now, if I asked the subjects what they had experienced during the period in which the conditioned reflex had been built up, they stated that they were under the influence of fear. In the beginning of the trials their fear occurred simultaneously with the signal, but when the trials were continued it appeared immediately before the electric shock was expected. They felt queer sensations running through their hands, the sensations being the representation and the anticipation of the shock itself.

Finally, they would withdraw their hands, feeling that the current might come through their hands again. Conditioned reflexes take place only when there is an urgent biological need, and the withdrawal of the hand was conditioned in these cases because it was in the interest of the individual not to keep it in position as soon as they felt the shock coming. It was rather interesting to note that in my human subjects it became very difficult to get the conditioned reflex again when such a reaction had taken place. If, immediately after such a reaction, I showed them the light again without turning on the electric current, they did not withdraw their hands. It became rather manifest that psychic processes were very closely connected with this reaction because the subjects always said that they were angry at having withdrawn their hands without actually having felt the shock. They would reproach themselves and resolve not to do such a thing again. In some way there was a struggle between their ideal ego and the tendency to withdraw. In other words, in the simple experiments of conditioned reflexes the individual reacts as a whole, the personality and all of its problems are contained in the conditioned reflex.

Every conditioned reflex already contains the elements of the psychological problem as its basis. We therefore cannot expect to be able to interpret the neuroses by means of the conditioned reflexes. On the contrary, we must interpret the conditioned reflexes on the basis of the mechanisms we have studied in the neuroses. Conditioning is a process which is at least psychic and can only be understood by studying the psychic motivation behind it. It is only natural that we can find all the phenomena of the neuroses in experiments with the method of conditioned reflexes. When Pavlov, for instance, had built up a conditioned reflex of a positive type to a sound of 100 wavelengths and a conditioned reflex of a negative type to a sound of 104 wavelengths, and then produced these sounds together, the animal subject would be filled with considerable struggle. The dogs became very restless, and some of them even developed eczemas in connection with these conditioned reflexes. Now, these are precisely the mechanisms we know from the neuroses, and we can understand them as the indication of a struggle, a conflict between different tendencies in the individual. It is this conflict between the different strivings of the individual which leads to physical manifestations, as I have already mentioned. We therefore have to consider all these reactions neurotic reactions, but such neurotic manifestations in the conditioned reflexes would be much better understood if studied carefully by the psychoanalytic method in the neuroses. We must certainly not be astonished to notice all the mechanisms of the neurosis appearing in the conditioned reflexes. I might mention here that when a great flood took place in Leningrad, all of Pavlov's dogs lost their conditioned reflexes. Emotions very frequently destroy the system of our attitudes and customs. Some time after the flood, the conditioned reflexes returned again, but when someone spilled some water in the laboratories the dogs again lost their conditioned reflexes. The spilling of the water was manifestly symbolic of the flood.

These important experiments of Pavlov and his school can be understood only if we look upon them in the light of our experiences in the neuroses. We cannot interpret the neuroses by means of the conditioned reflex. But, by means of the psychic mechanisms we have studied in the neuroses, we can certainly very well interpret what takes place in a conditioned reflex. There is therefore not much hope of interpreting the neuroses on the basis of the conditioned reflexes. The latter are psychic attitudes which we can understand only if we study human beings from the psychic point of view. There is also no hope of our finding a bodily interpretation of the neuroses from this point of view. Many important relationships between body and mind may be studied and clarified by the method of Pavlov, Bechterew (1911), and Beritoff (1926), but not the central problem of the neurosis.

In every neurotic action there must be, of course, a change in the action of the brain function, too. It will, however, be very difficult for us to say that there is any change in this or that part of the brain structure. We can only say that the total action of the individual has been transformed and that, along with this change in the action of the individual, the transpositions or connections in the brain have also been changed. This does not mean that a complete change in one or another function has taken place, but simply that the union of function is not what it formerly was. I am of the opinion that in a normal person all the functions of the brain are in action whenever any attitude is taken or any experience is made. The whole body is, as it were, in tune with the brain. In the neurotic person, on the other hand, one or another brain apparatus may be functioning differently, but this difference in the functioning of that particular brain apparatus need not be at all connected with any organic lesion, but rather with the individual's previous experiences. Just as the brain functions of the normal person and the neurotic individual are not fundamentally different, so there is also no psychic content which is essentially different in the neurosis or in the normal personality. It is only that some psychic constellations are somehow more active in the neurotic than in the normal person. The neurotic individual does not differ from the normal person in the sense that he is suffering from an Oedipus complex, for instance, whereas the normal person is not, but only in the sense that the neurotic person suffers from some specific expression of the Oedipus complex.

We might also hope that a careful study of the functions of the brain would disclose that organ as the somatic basis of the neurosis. C. and O. Vogt (1920) have supposed that some hysterical phenomena might be based upon a diminished function of the striopallidal system, and indeed, the study of lethargic encephalitis has revealed to us many symptoms resembling functional ones. We find, for instance, that a hyperkinesis checked in one limb will appear in another. There is a possibility of shifting energy from one place to another provoked by some psychic influence. Such experiences only show that we have hitherto looked upon an organic lesion as a simple loss of function. But the more closely we study these problems, the more we shall find that the laws we have seen in studying the functional neuroses by the psychoanalytical method are also the laws which we find in organic lesions of the brain. According to Magnus (1924), we find a shifting over even in the spinal cord, a condition very similar to the displacement of libido or anxiety in the neuroses. The result of an irritation to the foot of a spinal frog will be different depending upon whether the leg is flexed or whether it is extended. Goldstein and Riese (1923) and Hoff and I (1927) have shown that the reaction to a change in the position of one extremity differs according to different positions in parts of the rest of the body. In a cerebellar case I observed with Hoff, supination of the right or left hand gave an impulse to the right or left side, and the patient moved either forward or backward. We can state generally that if the special shifting closes off one pathway, the energy will run into other paths. In other words, the laws of the physical and psychic flow of energy correspond to a high degree. If energy is spent in one place, it appears again in a corresponding pathway. Even special motor attitudes are connected with special psychic contents. Hyperkinesis and organic tics of the labial muscles very frequently provoke coprolalia. We also find this to be true even in the psychogenic tics. In cortical lesions, too, we find interesting analogies to what takes place in the neuroses. When there is a lesion of the visual centers of the cortex, we find that the perceptions of such a patient reveal condensations and symbolizations quite similar to the phenomena of dreams. In a case of cortical blindness, the patient will take the whole of a perception for a part, or a part for the whole. If we show him a picture of a mouse, he will call it only by the general name "animal" or he will call it a cat. The same changes occur in the expressions of aphasic patients. In short, changes due to cortical lesions, the expressions of the dream, and the neuroses follow the same laws, and it is valuable to study these laws even in organic cases. The difference is that in the neuroses we can go deeper and find out the motives, why these condensations and symbolizations take place, and why the whole cannot be differentiated into its parts or the parts integrated into a whole.

There exists in the posterior wall of the third ventricle a sleeping center. This sleeping center is very likely only one of many centers which spread from the medulla oblongata to the diencephalon. These centers regulate the consciousness of psychic activity, and any physical change in them causes some psychic transformation which is identical with changes in the neuroses. We nevertheless never get a complete picture of a neurosis in such a brain lesion, nor can we say that the psychic changes involved depend solely upon the changes in the function of one brain apparatus. We may understand the functions of the brain apparatus better by studying the neurosis and its laws, but there are certainly important and complicated relations between the cortex and the subcortex in every psychic process. The brain acts as a whole. The diencephalon and mesencephalon influence the cortex, but are also influenced by it. Changes in the extracortical brain mechanisms change the efficiency or the effective value of the emotions. On the other hand, the emotions and the psychic content of the individual can also change the subcortical functions. We very likely have here a dynamic pendular process, and it is very probable that the neurosis provokes changes in this creative organic rhythm. It is to be expected that the changed attitudes of life must influence the complicated interrelationship between cortex—diencephalon—mid-brain—medulla oblongata. (I might mention in this connection the changes in vestibular function which occur in the neurosis and, on the other hand, the provocation of neurotic attitudes by organic disturbances of the vestibular nerve.) Such a change in rhythm will certainly vary according to the organic state of the brain apparatus connected with the function of consciousness. We thus see how the study of the brain apparatus as well as of the neurosis both point to the unity of the organism and its integrative power. At the present time, however, the study of the neuroses from the psychic point of view provides us with a more effective approach to the principles of organic life.

One more example will show us that what psychoanalysis has found to be true of psychic energy also holds good for physical processes. If we inject an animal with ergotoxin we block the paths of the sympathetic system. If we then inject adrenalin, the latter drug will not be able to travel along its ordinary pathways, i.e., it will not be able to provoke an increase in the pulse rate or the blood pressure. It will provoke just the opposite. In other words, if the sympathetic system is blocked, adrenalin will irritate the parasympathetic system. E. Pick (1919) prepared animals by giving them drugs which irritated the parasympathetic system. As soon as the parasympathetic block was released, the adrenalin was able to take effect.

We must not consider psychic problems from a static but rather from a dynamic point of view. Changing attitudes toward different situations is characteristic of psychic life. The events of childhood always interfere with and determine one's actual experiences. One or another infantile experience is always revived by any immediate situation. The dynamic relations are influenced by the brain, by the sympathetic nervous system, by the whole body. All psychic experience takes place within the organism and is therefore dependent upon it, in one respect, while influencing it in another. The various apparatuses of the brain are similarly interrelated. They are also closely connected with the body as a whole and with the vasovegetative nervous system. We have gained insight into some of these laws by studying the neuroses from the psychological and the psychoanalytical point of view. We have also found the same laws throughout all the functions of the organism. We have found organic changes in the organism of the neurotic individual, but we found them partly dependent upon the special psychic attitude. We have seen changes in the brain mechanisms of neurotics as well as in their vasovegetative system, the glands of internal secretion, and in the entire metabolism. But the study of the psychic life and the experiences of the neurotic individual lead us to an even deeper understanding of the neurotic make-up than does the study of organic symptoms in the neuroses. Even these symptoms themselves can be better understood from a psychological point of view. Psychology and psychoanalysis afford us not only an insight into the psychic life of an individual, they also give us an approach to the understanding of the organism.

CHAPTER THREE

The Unity of Body, Sadism, and Dizziness

Helen Hoffman, 45 years old, had been under my observation in Vienna for several years. Her family history was of some importance in that a daughter of her sister had a chronic psychosis. The patient complained that she had terrible states of anxiety, especially when walking on the streets. "When I get this anxiety state I cannot walk further. I run into myself. It breaks me into pieces. I am like a spray. I lose my center of gravity. I have no weight. I am quite mechanical. I am broken in pieces. I am like a marionette. There is a lack of something that could keep me together. I am not on the earth. I am someplace else. I am in between. I am rigid. I cannot cry. Once I had an uncanny dream. I floated without any feeling of belonging anywhere. In the morning when I awakened, all was flown away. I have no time before me. I don't know how it will go on. I am turned upside down and wrong side up. I am only half a human being. I have been pushed back in school. Even as a child I felt I was not a whole being. I never was as happy as the others even when I was eight or nine years old. I have been happier."

She knew when nine years old—she had a premonition—that two sisters were going to die. "Indeed they died afterward.

Appeared originally in *The Psychoanalytic Review*, 17:114-122, 1930. Reprinted through the courtesy of the Editors and the Publisher, National Psychological Association for Psychoanalysis, New York, N.Y.

That is a terrible feeling. They suddenly looked blue and yellow." She couldn't stand hearing talk about natural death. "If I hear about it, I melt away and remain so for several weeks. I am completely in pieces. There is no ground under the feet when you are not on the earth. I feel the ground very rarely." She also knew about the death of her mother and her sister beforehand. "When I am melting, I have no hands. I go into doorways in order not to be trampled on. Everything is flying away from me. In the doorway I can gather together the pieces of my body." When she passes wooden fences, the boards tear her head. "It is as if something is thrown in me, bursts me asunder. Why do I divide myself in different pieces? I feel that I am without poise, that my personality is melting, and that my ego disappears and that I do not exist anymore. Everything pulls me apart, therefore, I do not like the saying 'to jump out of one's skin.' The skin is the only possibility for keeping the different pieces together. There is no connection of the different parts of the body. Sometimes the roof of my skull flies away. When it does not come back, then I stand on my head immediately, and it tears me to pieces. When the anxiety on the street catches me, I do not feel anything. So I hurt myself with my nails in order to feel myself. Then I do not see human beings, but only unlikely beasts such as kangaroos, rhinoceri and prehistoric animals." In the public school the teacher told about the kangaroo carrying her babies in her pouch. She had been very much impressed by that fact. Once her skull fell from her body, she related, and lay before her feet. She felt she was in danger of stepping on it. She felt some pulling in her body, then the upper and lower parts of her body separated from each other. Then the roof of her skull would go away. Once, there was an icy coolness. Another time the roof of her skull remained on a tree. "I felt it there on that tree."

She feels light, then her body flies up and down. "Is it possible that the head is growing and then becomes smaller again?" she asked. "When I am lying in bed, the bed flies with me." She could not fly over bridges and open places. She had the feeling that she had to float with the water. She had dreams of a similar type, e.g., she saw many big lions in her dreams. One of the lions opened its jaws, and she put her head in it; then it closed its mouth. The whole yard was full of lions. "I would take the risk." Once, she dreamed that her head was battered against a wooden chest. For months she saw five big heads before her. They came nearer like bells. "They went through me. They became bigger and bigger until they were one and a half meters in diameter. They had a vivid blue color. Then I have no self. I am not of the world. I am beside myself." She was, as always, afraid that somebody would step on her limbs.

She heard voices behind her right ear. There was a bad voice which ordered her to pull down the clothes of others. She felt the wish to strangle people on the street. Then she said to herself, "My God, give me strength to stand what the voice is saying. No, that's the devil in me. I have to fight against my own self, and I have no self."

In the evenings she saw in her fantasy wonderful things: landscapes, foreign cities, boats, garlands. In her dreams she did not walk; she flew.

When the roof of her skull got higher, she felt a devil in it. He spoke to her very clearly. He was her second self. "You cannot before you have pulled this hook three to five times." She could not resist this voice.

This report describes the patient as she was in 1929. Her comments did not vary much from time to time. She had a kind and amiable personality. She often came alone to the University of Vienna Clinic, although she felt anxiety. She was very easily hypnotized, sinking quickly into a deep hypnosis with marked suggestibility, and got considerable relief from hypnosis. She wore gloves from fear of dirt. She was a virgin, and was extremely shocked when sexual matters were discussed. "Those feelings do not have to exist." She would have liked to eliminate sexuality. In spite of being over 45, she behaved like a shy coquettish girl.

She gave the following history of her life. She had spasms at two years of age. At three or four years she became frightened for fear she could not find her way home. At this same time she was afraid of ghosts, and cried for weeks. At four years a pea got in her nose. In the second year of public school, the teacher told her that parents usually die before children do, which also frightened her. At fifteen she had her first menstruation and thought she would die. Her father died when she was about eighteen. She began then to feel anxiety when alone. She would go on the street only in the company of two persons. She could not do anything with knives and scissors because she was afraid she would do something wrong. After three years she felt better, but she did not feel strong enough for marriage. She went often to cemeteries. "When I go there the corpses come out; it is a noise as if of silk, and something is floating around me. It is transparent. The dead talk to me." When she was 30 years old an uncle of hers died. She said that the dead man lay beside her during the night and grasped her with his arms until she felt as if driven into them. She felt it also on the genitals. She saw skulls of the dead. But after that she felt well for some years.

She had only a few obsessions. She did not like to be left alone by her sister. When she was 42 years old, a mother of a friend died. When this woman was sick, she felt a compulsion to drill a hole in her skull and to suck her brains out. She felt also a compulsion to bite the forehead of the dead—"that's also the voice." She had wanted to get into the woman to get her brain. She had always been very fond of this person. When she died, her head always came back and drilled itself between the upper and lower part of the patient's body. At that time she could not eat any meat. She felt disgust, yet at the same time had an impulse to put all things into her mouth.

She could not listen to anything about operations. She felt that the souls put the operated part (whether the genitals, leg, etc.) into her mouth. "Are you afraid of me?" she often asked. Once she told her mother that she should have been ashamed of having given birth to her. At that time she again felt as if she were falling to pieces. She was very fond of her sister, but sometimes she swore at her and felt the impulse to throw her against the wall, to stretch out her arms and finally to tear out her arms. After the death of this sister, she started to pick up useless things. She felt not only that the dead woman was between the two parts of her body, but that her dead uncle also was with her.

She picked up all kinds of dirty objects from the street. She dug holes in order to find something. She picked up dirty papers and stones, brought them into the entrance hall, wanted to put them in her mouth. In the meantime, the dead began to stick on her. This obsession grew. She could not go into the first street car, but had to wait until five had passed. She had to clean the sewer gates. She had to count the number of buttons on men's suits. She was interested in whether others had the eyes of murderers. In the church she tore off the altar covers and wanted to see what was in the statues of the saints.

She was obsessed with the question of how one gets children (she was told in her childhood that children were fished out of the Danube). She had to touch everything. She forced her friend to allow her to touch her tongue. She felt the compulsion to tear it out in order to have something of the friend. She was completely perverted. She was compelled to touch everything in the shop of her friend. She touched the statues of the saints and also of Christ. She felt compelled to touch his genitals. All things had relation to the mouth. She was compelled to stare at shops, to look at ties, dolls and linen.

There is no doubt that in the history of this case sadistic features prevailed. It was a neurosis. She sometimes touched the borderline of psychosis, but never transgressed it. Her voices were not like real voices, but were like the voice of conscience. All her delusions about her body never produced a full conviction in her mind. Believing one moment, she disbelieved the next. Her superstitions did not win a real influence on her life. She always remained sociable, even amiable. One could be in doubt whether it was an anxiety neurosis or an obsessional neurosis. But the anxiety, at least in the years I saw the patient, was incidental to the queer delusions concerning her body. Still, I would never classify the patient as pure obsessional neurosis. Her hatred did not reach the heights it reaches in classical obsessional-neurosis cases. Her amount of love was greater than in such cases. There was also the fact that she was so easy to hypnotize. Her strong repression in all genital matters fit into this scheme. She had certainly a fixation in the area of the Oedipus complex in addition to her fixation in oral and sadistic spheres, which was even more important.

We understand now that the anxiety was a part of an hysteria. Her fixation on her father must have been a strong one. It is remarkable that the first attack of neurosis followed the death of her father. Since every relapse of her neurosis followed the death of a loved person, we have a right to suppose that she had a special attitude towards death. If she believed she was able to know beforehand who would die, and when, she must have had wishes concerning the death of other persons, especially loved ones. Her superstitions dealt with the death of other persons too. Her interest in cemeteries belonged to this group of phenomena.

In this case it is necessary to make use of interpretations. The sadistic tendencies are the overt content of her compulsions. We can see in an especially clear way that the compulsion to touch had the same basis. The primary impulse was that of tearing and breaking to pieces, but her strong ego ideal prevented her from doing it and even from wishing it too openly. It is remarkable that these cruel impulses were not impulses of tearing, but also of biting and sucking. It was an oral sadism. One remark of the patient deserves special attention. She said, "Whatever happens, I feel it in my mouth." She felt compelled to put into her mouth parts of the body cut up by operations.

We see that, always, whenever a partial libido prevailed, it applied to all events of her life. Every interest, every emotion got connected with the partial desire and with the special organ of it. One of my patients with impotence told me, "Whatever emotion may go on, I feel it in my genitals; they shrink in." It is as if there were one deep canal attracting all the water. Her sadism had a special direction against the genitals; she wanted to tear out Christ's genitals. The tongue of her friend was a substitute for genitals. Behind that lay the childish belief that girls have a penis.

Her childish curiosity was destructive too. She wanted to tear the statues of saints apart in order to see what was in them. Of course in such a picture the anal features must be present. She did have them. The dirty objects she picked up and brought in the doorway represented the anal penis, and the doorway the vagina as well as the anus. Poking the holes in sewer grates with scissors again added the cruel note to the anal tendencies. But I would not have reported this case solely for this reason. Such things are well known in psychoanalysis, although maybe this case shows them in a clearer way than usual.

What is remarkable is that this sadism directed against others affects her own body too. She does not feel a tendency to hurt herself, but she feels her body falling to pieces. In other words, there is a mechanism of conversion instead of a mechanism of compulsion. Still, we see again that sadism, as I put it, is a borderline phenomenon. When there is a sadistic tendency, it is likely to be directed against the object as well as against the subject (masochism). Psychoanalytic opinion as to what is primary—sadism or masochism—has changed during the course of the years. Freud stated (1920a) that there is in every individual a primary death wish, a primary masochism or a tendency to self-destruction. He believed that sadism is secondary to these self-destructive tendencies. Self-love (narcissism) turns the destructive tendencies from the self against others. I personally do not believe that masochism or sadism are either primary or secondary. They are both. They are just as well primary as secondary. They are both borderline phenomena. The same is true about reproaches. There are self-reproaches as well as reproaches against others.

Another borderline phenomenon to be mentioned is dizziness. This lies in between subject and object and wanders from one to the other. We shall soon discuss the importance of this fact that both sadism and dizziness are borderline phenomena.

As I have often emphasized, there are some points in the

world where subject and object are closer to each other. In pain, for instance, the hurting object is not so important as the feeling on the body. Patients with agnosia concerning their own body are also disoriented about the bodies of other persons. Right and left are concepts concerning the outer world, but in a specific relation to one's own body. Many psychic phenomena lie in between subject and object, and according to the situation and the psychic need, they are either *appersonated* or *projected*. It is of importance that one's own body is often treated like an outer object. The patient's feeling as if she would fall to pieces is also a sadistic attitude against her own body. There is another important point. When she has these feelings that her limbs are separated from her and that there is danger that somebody may step on them, one could call that a projection of her own body. Maybe she did not want to have her limbs.

It seems that from a psychological point of view we overrate the cohesion of the body. In spite of the patient's tactile and kinesthetic perceptions, she did not only imagine, but she also felt her body to be outside. Another patient of mine, who was in the course of a gonorrheal infection, felt pains in his glans, felt that while eating at a table that his burning penis was in a glass. The same patient also had the feeling that his bladder was on the street, and that a street car was crushing it. Sometimes he felt that dogs on the street would carry away his penis like a sausage. Afterward the picture changed, and he had a similar feeling about his feces. These were not hallucinations. They were vivid optic imaginations, but accompanied by a queer exteriorization of feelings that made him feel that out there on the street were parts of his body. It was an obsession. Obsessions very often have this queer vividness which makes the content of the obsession almost an hallucination.

The important conclusion we may draw is that feeling our body intact is not a matter of course. It is the effect of self-love. When destructive tendencies go on, the body is spread over the world. One could doubt the strictness of such a conclusion. One would like to say that we lose the unity of our body only under special pathological conditions. But we have to remember also how much the feeling of our body varies under normal conditions. When touching an object with a stick, we feel with the end of the stick. We feel that our clothes become a part of ourselves. We rebuild the picture of our body over and over again. I have shown this with E. Klein (Klein and Schilder, 1929), studying the mistakes one makes in localizing one's fingers when the hands are doubly crossed. There are forces of hatred scattering the picture of our own body, and forces of love putting it together. H. Hartmann and I have shown (1927) that we perceive our body as we would perceive any other heavy substance. If we perceive that heavy substance as our body we have to build up the knowledge of our body over again. Neither the optic nor the kinesthetic nor the tactile impression gives us a ready-made impression of our body. We have to build it up continually and give shape to vague material. The shaping takes place according to biological needs.

The fantasy of cutting one's own body to pieces is accompanied by some interesting sensations in our patient. She felt her body was lighter, as if she were flying. The patient also had some flying dreams. We know that when we are dizzy we cannot maintain the unity of our body. The parts of the body seem dislocated. When in an airplane that is descending, one feels suddenly lighter, as if the substance of gravity would leave the body eddying upward.

The destructive tendencies concerning one's own body are aroused by excitation of the vestibular nerve. In this respect the multiple hallucinations of the patient are very remarkable. There are five large heads. Hoff and I (1928) have shown that polyopia is not uncommon in vestibular lesions. With Eisenger I have shown (1929) that in dreams of patients with vestibular problems, multiplication of sensations is the rule. We have the right to suppose that conversion in this case affects the vestibular apparatus too. The connection with anxiety would point in this direction. But we do not have definite proof for this idea.

I have pointed out on different occasions, initially in my

book *Selbstbewusstsein und Personlichkeitsbewusstsein* (1914), that there are very close relations between the vestibular apparatus and depersonalization (cf. E. Stern, 1919 and Stengel, 1935a, 1935b). It is remarkable that our patient complained about herself in the same way as do cases of depersonalization. On the other hand, many patients with depersonalization complain that the poise of their body is altered. I may mention that our particular patient, as all patients with depersonalization, complained that she did not know how time would go on. The relation of vestibular sensations to time should be studied more carefully than has been done. We know that every negation of one's self is connected with troubles in the perception of time (cf. E. Straus, 1928 and Minkowsky, 1923). But the important thing is that, in this patient, depersonalization was a sadomasochistic negation of her own body in connection with vestibular mechanisms.

Now we come to the last point of importance. Goldstein (1927) and especially Hoff and I (1927) have shown that the perception of one's own body is dependent upon muscle tone. The tone also changes the perception of the heavy mass of our body and its limbs. Vestibular irritation which changes muscle tone has, in many ways, a similar effect.

Certainly, there are many primitive tonus tendencies which drive the limbs away from the body. Goldstein spoke about an outward tendency of the body. The cerebellum prevents this outward tendency. With cerebellar lesions this outward tendency recurs. Goldstein ascribes to the cerebellum the function of keeping the body together. There must be some truth in the statement. These centripetal and centrifugal tendencies which Goldstein discusses in motility and tonus are present in the postural model of the body too. The centrifugal and destructive tendencies are in connection with sadistic tendencies, the centripetal with narcissistic ones. We find it important that these centrifugal destructive tendencies concerning the postural model of the body exert a conversion influence on the vestibular apparatus which, from the organic point of view, has to do with a tonus in the medulla oblongata which is at least partly centrifugal.

There is still another detail in this case history which should be discussed. The patient saw the faces of those girls who were doomed to die as though they were changed in some way. Their faces had a yellow and blue hue. Of course her prophesy concerning the death of these persons meant that she had sadistic death wishes against them. But the patient also had optic visions of faces colored blue. The multiplicity of these hallucinations was a hint to us that the vestibular apparatus was involved.

In the course of a relatively short time I observed two cases in which the colors blue and yellow played a special part. One case was a typical picture of a 50-year-old man with a mild depression. He had been in the state hospital several times before, and came for treatment at the onset of another such depression. At that time he had the following dream: He was in the asylum. Attendants caught him. He felt inferior. He recited a poem about Neptune. He suddenly saw a corner of a pillow colored bright yellow. This was a sign for him that immediate dissolution and death were imminent. He would suffer terrible torments.

The yellow color here had a seemingly symbolic value. Of greater importance was the next observation concerning a woman of 53 whom I observed in another hospital. Her illness started several months before admission. The world was unreal as though everything was upside down. It was completely different. It was the same way with objects. Faces of men looked like murderers. Faces were distorted, even those of her children. She felt sucked down into a pit and felt that she was drowning in a terrible whirlpool. Terrible things were whirling around. She was alone in a corner. All things looked eerie, yellow, and in a cold blue. She was afraid to sleep. She did not sleep at all because she feared she would lose her personality in sleep or even die. A frightful burning came all over her body. It burned under her skin like fire. When she closed her eyes there was red fire before them. Ideas passed like pictures in a kaleidoscope, awful ideas, burning thoughts. She could not stop. Something gripped her. She thought she had syphilis and gonorrhea. She thought she would infect everyone else. She thought she was a murderer. She murdered the city and would be electrocuted. Afterward she felt pregnant. The shape of her body changed. She did gymnastic exercises. She felt a rupture. She thought that she had killed her child. She murdered the city. She did not look at her body. It was as if mind and body were separated. "I do not feel at home in my body, as if I might be an alien object. I am really almost convinced that it is not only the feeling, but that it also looks queer."

This patient had had a depression when she was about fourteen. She was married and had two grown-up children. She had been divorced long before, and had had an intimate friend since.

In this case, too, the colors blue and yellow were in close relation to the patient. This case also teaches us something about the mechanism of the psychosis which started with the picture of depersonalization. It is noticeable that she did not want to sleep, fearing that she might lose her personality completely, thus showing that the mechanism of sleep and depersonalization are in very close relation to each other.

A lesion near the sleeping center can provoke a picture similar to depersonalization. In a case of oculogyric crisis, a similar change in the personality occurred. All cases of depersonalization see the world changed in a "different light." The distorted faces of her children are the expression of her dissociated emotions. When the faces of men on the street look like those of murderers, she projects her own sadistic tendencies into other persons. One sees that the world, as far as optically perceived, is changed according to the emotions of the patient. That is typical for depersonalization. Others see the objects flat, like pictures without a third dimension. Or the objects are remote. They appear smaller. Colors lose their brightness. Sometimes they are even without any color.

Lemos (1906) described cases of melancholy with complaints

that all objects were colorless. Here we come to the problem we are interested in. The way we perceive colors is dependent upon our whole emotional life. Colors have an emotional value. According to Froebe (1923), yellow is serene and clear. When one rides by a landscape, it becomes a warmer hue. Blue seems to recede; it is the color of remoteness and profundity. It makes one long for softness. But in patients it is the color of horror, fright, and despair. Maybe there are different hues.

In the first case I mentioned, these colors are the color of death, the colors of the corpses. If the case here described sees the world in such colors, she sees a dying world. There is an associative basis for why she sees the world in these particular colors. Very likely in the hues of the colors, as such, there is something inducing fear and fright. The associative mechanism is induced over the physiological mechanism. Emotions change the perception of the colors.

A. Pick (1908) and I (1914) have emphasized the similarity between the pictures of depersonalization and optic agnosia. But the optic agnosia concerning colors is quite different from the change in color described here. In the one type, the perception of yellow and red is impaired; in the other one the perception of blue and green. The emotional changes in the perception of color are different from the "agnostic" changes.

Let us stick to the observation that, in some cases, the colors of yellow and blue are related to sadism and death.

CHAPTER FOUR

Neurasthenic Hypochondriac Character

The neurasthenic patient has always been a riddle from the psychological point of view. Beard (1869) believed in a spinal irritation. The psychoanalyst Landauer (1927) considered neurasthenia an organic toxic state that could not be understood from a psychological point of view.

Freud (1916) included neurasthenia and hypochondria under the group of *actual neuroses*. He held that there was an actual neurosis when there was a difficulty in living out one's sexual tendencies. These difficulties might consist either of abstinence, coitus interruptus, condomatus, or frustrated sexual excitement. Freud even had the idea that special forms of *actual neurosis* followed the various types of somatic sex dissatisfaction, that dissatisfaction had an immediate toxic influence which provoked anxiety, neurasthenia, or hypochondria.

Stekel (1923), Jones (1929), and Schilder (1924) have stated that anxiety was not provoked by an immediate toxic influence, but followed a repression and was a conversion symptom. Freud, meanwhile (1926), no longer believed that anxiety developed from somatic toxic effects; instead, he saw in anxiety a psychic reaction to a dangerous situation. The danger might be from outside or from within. He was not concerned whether or not there was a conversion of libido into anxiety. His concept of

---

Appeared originally in *Medical Review of Reviews*, 36:164-176, 1930.

anxiety had undergone important changes. Nevertheless, he maintained his opinion that neurasthenia and hypochondria were caused directly by toxic influences of sexual energies and sex products not properly used.

Reich (1927) showed that neurasthenic troubles occur following a sex conflict. By means of this conflict the unemployed sexual energies were converted into something else. To him, the neurasthenic symptom was not the immediate effect of sex products, but the result of the conversion of this sex energy.

The chief symptoms of neurasthenia are: fatigue, inability to concentrate, pressure on the head, dizziness of a mild degree, trouble in sexuality (impotence), spermatorrhea, and sleep troubles. Hypochondriacal fears and hypochondria sensations often occur.

When one reviews the superficial clinical facts, two things become obvious. Neurasthenia, in the first place, occurs in a much higher percentage among men. Secondly, there are especially two ages at which men seem to be predisposed to the acquisition of neurasthenia: puberty and the age of 40 to 45. These are two ages in which special psychosexual developments take place. Puberty is the age of adaptation to a new sex task. It would be too narrow to suppose that there is a single sex task to be solved in puberty. The whole life has to be repatterned and rebuilt. The way has to be found from exuberant daydreams to the narrower paths of reality. The ego ideal undergoes changes. The whole process is not a continuous development, but proceeds in phases. Genital sexuality pushes forward, breaks through, and is immediately pushed back again by an ego ideal which is extreme in its repressing power. Irregular waves of unlived-out libido are then converted into neurasthenic symptoms. The unsatisfactory release brought by masturbation sets free sadistic tendencies, which, incorporated in the superego, increase the feelings of guilt which come from many sources.

The increased pressure of the ego ideal converts the unlived-out libido into the manifold neurasthenic symptoms of youth. The common fears in connection with masturbation are that one will lose one's mind, that one will become weak and unable to work. All this is very closely connected with the castration complex. There is even the fear of losing every possibility concerning sex, what Jones (1929) called aphanasis (disappearance of sexual potency). Hypochondria traits are common. All activities in connection with sex are watched with suspicion by the patient. These neurasthenic and hypochondriacal symptoms are primarily an expression of a desire to enjoy one's own body without caring much for the outside world. It is a regression to the narcissistic stage. At the same time, the ego ideal forbids its enjoyment in an open way. There is even a desire to get rid of a body which, by its high libidinal pressure, endangers the adaptation to outer reality demanded by the ego ideal. This is the theory of the genesis of hypochondria which Freud has given. He compares the organ that is in the center of the hypochondriacal attention with the genitals, which also always furnished sensations that try to take possession of the whole personality. What I want to emphasize is that, in puberty, there are many factors that prevent the realization of the libido, which is therefore stored in the body and provokes the neurasthenic symptoms. There remains only the question of why neurasthenia and hypochondria result in these particular symptoms. But we will postpone this question until we discuss the psychic situation of men during the ages 40 to 45.

Forty to 45 is the age when in men a strong ego ideal has been built up. A definite position in society has been reached. A facade has been built up which shields one from the uncontrolled tendencies of childhood and adolescence. In order to climb the social ladder, in order to built up this façade, many renunciations have been necessary. Perhaps too many. The chase after social honors and wealth is partly due to the compensation of libidinal tendencies. The ego ideal at 40 enjoys control over the ego. There is a great amount of self-love in the successful business man at this age. His activities in the practical life, it is true, partly satisfy his sadism in a sublimated way. His ceaseless insistence on work is partly a satisfaction of sadistic tendencies against objects and co-workers and partly a sadistic self-punishment directed against the ego. But these self-punishments make it possible for him to achieve great self-esteem. After self-punishment, he can enjoy himself in a narcissistic way. Of course there is some danger that if this facade is impaired, there will no longer be any possibility for object cathexis. Neurasthenia never occurs from overwork alone. Only if there is failure in business or such success that further progress is no longer attainable will the man get a "nervous breakdown" and finally declare that it is not worth while to continue putting his whole libido into work.

Certainly, it is a problem to understand why people work too much. It is a question of the greatest importance why, in modern civilization, labor has become of value in itself. The same processes repressing the genital libido, increasing sadism, sublimating sadistic tendencies in work and self-punishment by means of work, which take place in single individuals, also occur, as far as I can see, in the mass, and give to our era the stamp of restlessness, simple-mindedness, hurry, and ceaseless labor. Insofar as this is true, present civilization is responsible for the increase of this particular type of neurosis. When the individual feels that it is not worth while to submerge the better part of his personality in work and to renounce love, neurasthenia sets in.

This psychic development can be understood only if we get an inside view of the love life of the average successful man of 40. He generally has not the courage requisite for a real deep love. He prefers eroticism of the superficial type. He frequently attains his love objects directly or indirectly much more by his social position and wealth than by his personality. He debases his love life.

The very fact that so many sadistic tendencies are satisfied in social activities takes energy from the genital libido. We know that connected with the sadistic tendencies of "grasping" and "overwhelming" are tendencies of "keeping" and "retaining." Here, the interest in money comes in. The connection with the anal tendencies of retaining is obvious. No wonder that, sooner or later, difficulties with potency occur. It is from this point that neurasthenia often starts. We now understand better why neurasthenia at this age is especially a disease of men. These are the actual situations which determine the outbreak of neurasthenia.

As has been mentioned, hypochondriacal tendencies are also common. The borderline between hypochondria and neurasthenia is not at all sharp. The hypochondriac is in fear of a serious somatic disease. He has sensations which justify this suspicion. Mostly, he does not actually believe this, but he is very near to this belief and is afraid lest he be convinced of the fact. At the same time, it is not possible to persuade him that his fears are without basis. His actual complaints are not so far different in their nucleus from the neurasthenic complaint. When there is not only belief but conviction, hypochondriac psychosis begins.

When there is true hypochondria, the relation to reality is not as close; the ego ideal is not as strong as in neurasthenia. Hypochondria is at any rate nearer to psychosis. The actual cause of hypochondria is not always as clear as in neurasthenia. Its relation to the "successful age" is often absent. Constitutional factors may prevail. What this means from a psychological point of view will be discussed later.

The hypochondriac, as well as the neurasthenic, will not agree when he is told that he has problems of psychic adaptation. He believes, rather, that there is something going on in his body; in other words, neurasthenic and hypochondriac symptoms are projections from the psychic sphere of central interests to another sphere, which is at least felt as somatic and does not belong to the nucleus of the personality. It is felt to be on the periphery of the self.

We should not deny that a real somatic change takes place when hypochondria and neurasthenia symptoms occur. Freud (1914) and Ferenczi (1926) believed that in hypochondria there was indeed too much libido in the organs; libido was dammed up there. And libido was also a somatic agent. We have at least the right to speak about a tendency to conversion of symptoms, although the final proof that there is some change in the body cannot always be given. Vasomotor changes are often obvious. Constipation and spastic states of the bowels exist, as well as impotency, spermatorrhea, and prostatic oversecretion. Conversion does not take place only in hysterias, but also in neurasthenia and hypochondria. It is worth while to compare these two types of conversion.

TABLE 1
A COMPARISON OF
SIGNS OF CONVERSION IN HYSTERIA AND NEURASTHENIA

Hysteria	*Neurasthenia*
Amnesia Hallucination	Lack of Concentration
Spasms, Paresis, Fits	Pressure on the Head
Disorders in Sensibility and Sensation	Dizziness Fatigue
Hysteric Points and Phenomena of Spontaneous Pain	Hypochondriac Sensation Hypochondriac Pain
Vaginal Anesthesia	Troubles in Potency, Spermatorrhea
Vasomotor Troubles	Vasomotor Troubles
Organic Diseases	Constipation and Spastic States of the Intestines Palpitation

This table shows that hysteria and neurasthenia have in common the tendency to conversion. But it becomes immediately clear that the hysteric gets rid of his psychic problems by a mechanism which is more careless of reality. Amnesia and hallucinations neglect reality more readily than, for instance, lack of concentration or pressure of the head. The queer feelings of the nuerasthenic are not as far removed from reality as the hysteric anesthesia. This difference probably has something to do with the tendency of the male, especially at the age of 40, to stick to reality. But hysteria as well as neurasthenia reach into the organic depths of the body, into the world of real symptom conversion. Doubtlessly, the conversion is very closely related to projection. In comparison with our innermost feelings and strivings the body is outside. When conversion takes place, what had been a psychic problem now becomes a disease of the body which belongs partly to the outer world, although not so far out as are other objects. Hypochondriacal and neurasthenic disorders are therefore described as if there was an object in the organs. Patients speak about sensations of a ring constricting the head, of lead in their limbs, of something solid in their liver or abdomen, of bubbles under their skin, etc.

Neurasthenia and hypochondria are like other neuroses—ways of getting rid of tormenting conflicts. Their mechanism is one of conversion, which tries to keep in closer touch with reality than does the hysteric mechanism.

Hypochondriac and neurasthenic symptoms must, therefore, have an unconscious meaning.

Let us reiterate from this point of view the different symptoms of neurasthenia. The various troubles of potency such as premature ejaculation, incomplete or absent erection, inability to enjoy orgasm (*"orgastische impotenz"*—Reich, 1927) are the expressions of renouncement of genital libido for social activity, which is, as we stated, partly sublimated sadism of a more primitive origin. In adolescence it is often very clear that the progress from partial desires to genital sexuality has been checked. Sadistic urinary and anal fantasies can be easily demonstrated.

In one of my patients with premature ejaculation and occasional spermatorrhea, eneuresis had persisted a long time. In one of his fantasies, a man refused a girl who was in extreme sexual excitement after he had torn off her clothes, and had an ejaculation turning away from her. Another of my patients, a student of nineteen, complained that he was unable to study as others did. Once, with a prostitute, he felt disgust at her greasy body and was impotent. He always felt tired. He would have liked to sleep the whole day. He always wished he could rest. His head would get heavy and droop. Fantastic ideas about sexual inferiority and the inferiority of his body existed. He was discontented about not having enough hair on his body and therefore of not being sufficiently masculine. He believed that he looked like an hermaphrodite, that he was too ugly. The patient was a very tall, stooped fellow with an infantile face. His genitals were normally developed. He had had epileptic fits at the age of two that he did not know about. Behind this neurasthenic and hypochondriacal façade were very strong sadistic tendencies. He got erections when he heard children crying. He had played sadistic games with a cousin between twelve and fourteen years of age. There were many ceremonies concerning urination and defecation. In early childhood he refused to go to the toilet. Before he went to a party he had to urinate again and again. He also wanted to have everything, including feces, pressed out. Sometimes he felt as though he should pull something out of his head. Sometimes he had to blow his nose. He got an urge to urinate and defecate. Of course this was an extreme case, but it shows clearly the mechanisms behind neurasthenia and hypochondria of adolescence, and especially the motives of impotence. There is a denial of genitality, but it must not be forgotten that the neurasthenic and hypochondriac of later life still has his developed genitality. It is not so completely abandoned as in schizophrenia, and the regression to anal and sadistic tendencies is not so tenacious as in obsession neurosis.

Whereas the impotence of the neurasthenic indicates his denial of genitality, the fatigue is the renouncement of sublimated sadistic activities. It is in some ways a phenomenon with a background similar to that of melancholic inhibition and the apathy of the compulsive neurosis. Finally, the type of sadism which is turned into a symptom is different, and also the structure of the ego ideal and the adaptation to reality is different in fatigue, apathy, and inhibition.

Difficulties in concentration in neurasthenia are a constant complaint of those who believe that they have ruined themselves by masturbation. It reveals itself as a feature of the castration complex transferred from below upward. In my experience, the frequent complaint of schizophrenics that somebody is taking their thoughts away has a similar basis in the castration complex of being cut to pieces, and of mental and physical mutilation. But, of course, the withdrawing of thoughts in schizophrenics and the lack of concentration in neurasthenics take place on different levels.

Dizziness does not need an elaborate discussion, since it is well known that dizziness occurs when there are antagonistic tendencies in the psychic system.

Constipation and spastic states of the intestine may be an expression of the same tendencies of keeping and hoarding which led to accumulation of money and social prestige—another illustration that interest in money and anal tendencies are closely connected. The youth about whom I have reported was extremely close-fisted and thrifty. But it seems that this interpretation is based on what we know from other experiences rather than what we actually know from neurasthenia.

Hypochondria symptoms will be found in organs especially important to the individual. In one of my patients, hypochondria occurred after a slight injury to a thumb; she had always cared especially for her hands and had manicured them oftener than others of her social standing. Singers develop hypochondria about their beloved voices and throats. In another case of mine, an actor got hypochondriacal sensations in his mouth after one of his teeth had been removed and had been replaced with an artificial tooth in order to give him a better appearance on the stage. Hypochondriacal sensations symbolize the genitals. The sex pleasure no longer experienced in the genitals is now experienced in the symbolic genitals by way of the hypochondriac's beloved organs. In my experience, the hypochondriacal sensation symbolizes the male genitals much more often than it does the female.

One may ask whether or not this helps us understand the common hysterical symbolization of the penis. The answer is that in hysteria the *clavus* and *globus hystericus* and other sensations of this kind symbolize the genitals of special persons. The penis is not normally regarded as an isolated organ but as a part of a personality that is loved and appreciated. The hypochondria symptom is the symbolization of sex tendencies concentrated only on the genitals as such and not in relation to a special person. It is even probable that the genitals symbolized are the genitals of the hypochondriac himself. Of course there are also female organs symbolized in the hypochondriacal sensations. There are caves in the body, wasting of organs, empty spaces. But we hear much more often about stiffening in the body, tight muscles, a piece of something sticking somewhere. Hypochondriacal sensations are felt mostly a centimeter or two under the skin. There is no organ which cannot become the seat of hypochondriacal sensations and fears. In two hypochondriacs I have observed, there were special hypochondriacal fears about blisters on the mouth. Both patients reproached themselves for either cunnilingus or penilingus.

There remains the question along what line does the conversion take place? We shall never understand either the hysterical or the neurasthenic and hypochondriacal conversion symptoms if we do not know how one's own body is experienced. We have a picture of our body, the so-called postural model (*Koerperschema*) or body image (Schilder, 1923, 1935a). It is illustrated in the phantom of an amputated hand. This picture of the body is the basis for our narcissism. Our self-love is attached to this body image, and only self-love keeps the body image intact. Self-love replaces the amputated limb in the phantom, which contains not only the experience of the immediate past, but also the experience of childhood. If the phantom persists for a while, the hand becomes smaller and becomes like the hand of a child.

The body image is built up in several "time layers." It follows our everyday knowledge of the body. The differentiation of left from right is acquired rather late in the individual experience and therefore can be rather easily lost. We do not have a fair knowledge of our own skin. If we close our eyes, we feel our skin, paradoxically, "under the surface." The tonus of our muscle influences our body image, our postural model of the body.

Whenever there is, for instance, increased tonus of the postural and righting reflexes, the postural model gets distorted in the direction in which the increased tonus tries to pull the limb. Every sensory experience we may have is brought in relation to this body image. We experience our body, not in accordance with our present sensations alone, but according to a scheme which we build up from childhood. In the building and rebuilding of this scheme, narcissistic libido plays an important part.

In one of my cases, sadistic fantasies of cutting and tearing others to pieces were very strong. The patient felt that she, too, fell to pieces. She felt the inner part of her body only as a heavy mass. Inner sensations normally are felt only a centimeter or two under the skin's surface. That is why the hypoesthesia of internal organs is projected toward the surface of the body. My preliminary experiences suggest that the pain in neuritis and also in other internal diseases is mostly projected against the surface of the body but does not reach it.

We must not believe that the visual impression of our body is accurate and conforms completely with reality. If we keep our limbs in unaccustomed positions, we lose power over them. Finally, we never know how we really look. The more we look into the mirror, the stranger we seem to look to ourselves. We never can perceive what is going on in our skin. We do not even know how the skin of others looks. One is always astonished about the colors and lines of naked bodies. Therefore, as might be expected, the condition of the skin is an inexhaustible source of hypochondriacal complaints. There are complaints that the skin does not look right, and also that there are queer sensations in the skin. We understand these complaints because even the normal individual does not feel a distinct smooth surface of his skin, but, instead, is aware of a rather blurred borderline. The relative vagueness of our body image makes possible the conversion of symbolic representations of parts of the body, i.e., such as the genitals, into somatic symptoms. Special attention should thus be given to the representation of the genitals in the body image.

We know that in the body image all of the erogenic zones

are especially marked, the nipples, for instance. Every organ has a special representation in the body image. This representation is changed by personal experience. The actual body image of an individual in some way represents the balance of the current stage of the distribution of his libido. Conversion symptoms take place mostly along the lines of the individual body image, which contains the history of our libido development.

If we compare, from this point of view, the hysterical conversion symptoms of neurasthenics and hypochondriacs, one noteworthy feature appears. The hysterical conversion occurs in much closer connection with the individual's experiences. Hysteria takes place in the part of the body image which has been built up personally, whereas the conversion of the neurasthenic and hypochondriac has less to do with the personally built-up part of the body image but rather with the part that is common to all of us. It is interesting to compare the variety of hysterical symptoms with the uniformity of neurasthenic symptoms. Single cases of neurasthenia are much more similar to each other than are the individual cases of hysteria.

I have frequently emphasized that uniformity of the mental pictures in mental disease points to a situation which is either organic or near the organic sphere, or at least which develops very early in infancy or is prenatal or phylogenetic. Neurasthenia and hypochondria are also, in this sense, narcissistic. The narcissistic stage occurs when self-love is given to the whole body and the body is loved like one's own genitals. But we have to assume that those persons who get hypochondria or neurasthenia associated with real difficulties in puberty, or later, have a body image which is labile and weak either due to early experiences we do not know about and which are perhaps beyond our descriptive faculties, or due to a constitutional weakness. We can better imagine this constitutional weakness of the body image if we know that the functions of the parieto-occipital lobe are the basis for the building up of the integrated perceptual experiences of the body image. Perhaps this weakness of the body image, however, is less a weakness of the integrated perceptual experiences than of an inability to put enough libido into it. We speak of the point of fixation in psychoanalytical terminology as meaning the level of the psychosexual development which, due to either constitutional or individual experiences, has arrogated to itself too much importance. The point of fixation for neurasthenia or hypochondria lies in the early stage of development of the body image. By constitutional or acquired weakness in neurasthenia or hypochondria, single parts of the body image are chosen out of the whole bodily picture and attract more libido than they should. Neurasthenia and hypochondria are thus diseases where the floating of the libido to the different parts of the body image has been directed to selected parts. We have to imagine that the libido is always floating to and from the genitals to other parts of the body and back. The flow of the libido is changed with actual events of life which accord with early infantile weakness of the body image. Of course individual experiences will give particular coloring to individual cases of neurasthenia and hypochondria. Besides the principal fixation mentioned above, there will be fixations in more recent layers according to experiences in stages of life which can be more easily understood from the purely psychological point of view.

The body image transfers its activities to the life centers in the diencephalon and the midbrain. The stream of the vasovegetative innervation is shaped and directed by the body image. Thus, we understand better now why we believe from the psychoanalytic point of view that neurasthenic and hypochondriacal symptoms are also organic.

There remains only the question about why the point of fixation lying in such a primitive layer in neurasthenia as well as in hypochondria allows such persons to behave normally and not as a psychotic would. Generally, we can assume that when a repression goes to a very primitive layer, there will not be a neurosis but a psychosis. This point of view is thoroughly justified, but we have to ask not only how deeply the repression goes, but also whether the total personality is involved in the repression. The answer is rather simple. The repression in neurasthenia and hypochondria goes to a very primitive level, but only in the special field of the body image. I may add that, in the end, every conversion, including the hysteric, affects the body and runs into the early infantile period. But in hysteria, the major part of the personality remains directed toward the heterosexual love object, whereas in neurasthenia and hypochondria the individual continues to pursue his social aims. In brief, we could characterize neurasthenia and hypochondria as diseases of the body image, or, in order to make use of a term which would be in accordance with Wernicke's (1906) terminology, they are somatopsychoneuroses.

Since, according to this psychogenetic scheme of neurasthenia and hypochondria, we can grasp the actual psychic causes of neurasthenia and hypochondria better than the point of fixation in the body image, it will be generally sufficient to explore the actual psychical situation of the individual. Where secondary points of fixation in the infantile period are of importance, complete psychoanalysis will be necessary.

Since the body-image model of the individual is affected so much in neurasthenia and hypochondria, and with it the love for one's own body, we know that caressing the body surface by means of baths, showers, and massage are often successful. At the same time the rest forced on the patient makes it impossible for him to use his libido for work (sublimated sadism) and for making money (anal tendencies).

From the psychoanalytic point of view, we should consider that the somatic treatment—massages, showers, douches—generally alters the distribution of the libido. This change goes on both in the conscious and the unconscious, but also very likely goes on in the somatic sphere akin to this conscious and unconscious activity. Here lies the connecting link between somatic medicine and psychoanalysis. Perhaps we shall understand the vasomotor effects of hydrotherapy better if we know that, in the psychic sphere, hydrotherapy increases the individual's love for his own body.

CHAPTER FIVE

The Organic Background of Obsessions and Compulsions

Obsessions and compulsions have been repeatedly observed in epidemic encephalitis (Schilder, 1929b). They may occur in acute cases as in the observation of Mayer-Gross and Steiner (1921). The majority of cases are either subacute or chronic (cf. for instance Herrmann, 1922; Bürger, 1928; Bromberg, 1930; Jelliffe, 1932; Bender, 1937). Of particular interest are the obsessions and compulsions observed in cases with oculogyric crisis (F. Stern, 1928; Stengel, 1928; and Jelliffe). Jelliffe has not only collected the whole literature on the subject, but has also added valuable observations of his own, and has especially pointed to the personality factors which determine, in connection with the encephalitic process, the oculogyric crisis and the contents of the obsessions and compulsions in these cases. The subject has lately been reviewed by Wexberg (1937). It is obvious that organic disease of the central nervous system is an indispensable factor in the genesis of the psychic symptoms. If one reviews the cases in the literature carefully, and compares them with one's own experiences, one sees that although infantile experiences and situations have created a pattern, it finds its expression in compulsions on the basis of the organic processes involved. Such a statement cannot be fully substantiated since no reliable

---

Appeared originally in the *American Journal of Psychiatry*, 94:1397-1416, 1938.

methods are available at the moment by which we are able to predict the consequences of infantile patterns. Comparative studies of analyzed cases of obsession neuroses and obsessions and compulsions on an encephalitic basis have led me to the conclusion I have formulated.

The encephalitic process liberates motor impulses and motor innervations. Release phenomena of this kind are, for instance, the oculomotor spasms, the palilalia, the ticlike movements, the choreic and choreiform phenomena, and finally, all the impulse phenomena comprised under the heading of hyperkinesis. Forced movements of any type, even when they occur on a purely somatic basis, represent increased innervation and increased activity, and have their reflection in the psychic sphere as an increase of impulses which reinforces sadistic attitudes. This is true concerning epileptic attacks (which do not concern us here) as well as for oculogyric crises. Akinetic states and rigidities which restrict impulses and movements dam up impulses which may originate in other levels. These dammed-up impulses will finally break through with great violence. Impulsive actions of more or less sadistic character are common in these cases. When they are checked, compulsive phenomena may result. Hyperkinetic phenomena of all levels may lead to compulsions and obsessions. Akinetic phenomena, however, may lead indirectly to the same result. Compulsions thus may originate from motor sources in the widest sense. It is necessary to keep in mind that a direct connection exists between compulsions (the urge to actions against which the individual resists) and obsessions (thoughts and representations which maintain themselves in the consciousness of the individual contrary to his intention). A Polish Jew felt the urge when crossing a street to call out that he was an illegitimate child. He suppressed this impulse, and was afterward tortured by the obsession that he had done so. The obsessive thought substituted for the repressed impulse.

I have observed postencephalitic cases in which obsessions had a different genesis. In these cases the patients experienced a change in the state of consciousness in which thoughts and representations were going through their minds and persisted against their wishes. The change in consciousness during oculogyric crisis is a factor which has to be considered for the genesis of compulsions and obsessions. Stengel (1930) has proved that the vestibular function is changed during the oculogyric crisis. The vestibular function influences the tone and the motor impulses. Studies of Hoff (1928) and myself have shown that the change in the function of the vestibular apparatus changes the state of consciousness. There exists, therefore, a close interrelation between the impulses, the tone, the vestibular apparatus, oculomotor mechanism, and consciousness. Such considerations may lead to the better understanding of a postencephalitic case in which the patient complained that she saw dirt everywhere. She said that everywhere there were dark spots. She had to clean her house continually although she was rather convinced that there was no dirt. She felt particularly uneasy when she saw regular patterns on the pavement or somewhere else, and dizziness followed. There was a similar uneasiness when confronted with any complicated optic situation. When she was turned around on a swivel chair she saw more and more dirt. Irrigation of the ear had no specific effect. The patient showed a mild akinesis and rigidity and a particular difficulty in her eye movements. She improved with fever therapy, but came back later complaining that everything was glittering before her eyes so that she felt dazzled.

The following case may illustrate the relation between impulses originating from encephalitis and compulsion phenomena.

Yvette R., 30 years old, complained that she was compelled to think the whole day thus: "It is not true that I am lazy—it is not true that nothing interests me! It keeps repeating in my mind. I keep on telling myself the cockeyed world can go to hell! I have to count the pinholes in everything I see. When I look at something I say, 'How many pinholes are there?'" The patient complained that she asked herself, concerning every object, how many pinholes it consisted of. However, she did not try to count them.

The patient had a typical encephalitis when she was fifteen years old. She was sick for six weeks. A slight rigidity and akinesis remained. She married five years later. She worried all her life, even before the encephalitis. After being married two years she gave birth to a boy. During her pregnancy she worried that she wouldn't be able to take care of the baby. When she came home from the hospital she was so upset that she tried to kill herself with roach poison. She was then sent to a sanitarium. There she developed the fear that she might go crazy. She blamed herself that she was the most selfish person in the world. At this time, one of her sisters told her that she had been lazy all her life. Another older sister admonished her that she should have more interest in the world. Immediately after that, the compulsions to say "It is not true that I was lazy all my life," and "It is not true that nothing interests me" developed. When she complained to her husband, he said that she should send the whole cockeyed world to hell. This led to the other compulsion. Several months later she accidentally stuck a pin through the bed sheet in her child's crib. She developed the compulsion to count the pinholes immediately after that. It turned out that she was afraid she might stick a pin into her child's body.

When the obsessions started, she also began to repeat words and short orders again and again. Her appetite disappeared, and she didn't sleep well.

During the discussions she talked in terms of exaggerated affection for her husband and for her child, whom she called "honey" and "darling." She showed a very outspoken palilalia. This became particularly manifest when she told about her obsessions. Sometimes she repeated the beginning of the text, but more often the end. She also repeated orders she gave to her baby, especially when they were short. She reported that she gave up religion when she married since her husband was her God. She declared that she loved her child and her husband dearly, and that she loved everybody. "I love the whole world." She complained that she was slow in her movements, and that sometimes she remained for a long time in frozen attitudes.

The somatic examination showed that the patient had a typical Parkinsonism of medium degree. The rigidity of face was outstanding. The palilalia was severe. There were no other somatic findings.

The psychoanalytic approach was difficult, but a strong attachment to the father, dating from early childhood, came to the foreground. She was his favorite child and worried very much about his diabetes, to which he had succumbed when she was thirteen. She was occasionally spanked by her mother whom she often disobeyed. She had little contact with two brothers and a sister much older than herself. She had many fights with a sister who was four years older and a sister who was four years younger. She slept with the younger sister in one bed and often hit her sister when the younger girl didn't obey.

One of her earliest remembrances is that her older sister wanted to cut off the finger of her younger sister and was spanked by her mother. She remembers being hit often by her older sister. In one of her dreams, one of her nieces wanted to marry another girl. One of the patient's friends appeared continually in her dreams, which were filled with much activity. There were also dreams of being held against her will. In one of them, she said to her older sister, "The whole cockeyed world can go to hell, and you too." This sister kicked her out of the house and told her not to come back again. Her early history was filled with accidents. At three, the stick of a lollypop pierced her lips. Then she burned herself with hot tea and ripped her behind when she slid down a staircase. She hurt her head when she was five. The patient thinks that she was wonderful before the baby arrived. There were frequent worries about money at the beginning of her marriage.

The patient was a lively and aggressive child. We have reason to believe that there were homosexual trends present in her relations to her sisters. She had a great amount of hostility before she acquired encephalitis and before she gave birth to her child. The hostility against her child was obvious in the pregnancy, to which the patient responded by self-accusation and depression. After the birth it finally led to a suicidal attempt. It is probable that the akinesis was present before her pregnancy. Her fear of laziness and inactivity came into appearance with childbirth. There was an increase of impulses in the speech function, which led immediately into the compulsions expressed directly and indirectly as hostility against her sisters and her child. She overcompensated her hostilities against others by praising them beyond measure. She put all the blame on herself. Psychotherapy and benzedrine did not cure the patient, but she learned to send the cockeyed world to hell with greater ease.

It is easy to see in this case the relation of the change in motility to the expression of hostile impulses and compulsion. The connection between compulsion and obsession and the motor impulses is not always so clear, but more careful examination of these cases often shows an intimate relation between impulses and compulsion.

In spite of the fact that such an obvious connection exists between the impulse disturbance on an organic basis and compulsions, the question rarely has been raised whether it is possible to find an organic background for obsessional neurosis cases in general. Naturally, in the majority of instances there is no history of epidemic encephalitis. If one examines a large number of obsessional neuroses, one not so rarely finds organic symptoms identical with those found in chronic encephalitis. In the comparatively short time of about two years, I have seen seven cases in which slight organic signs could be found in careful examination, and in two other cases there was at least some clinical evidence that impulse disturbances on an organic basis were present. The symptoms which are of particular importance in this connection are the following: (1) Rigidity of the face and masklike facies. It is true that an objective appreciation of the mobility of the face is not always easy. When two independent observers agree on this point, one might use this symptom. (2) Evidence of flexor rigidity in the arms. We shall generally not expect that cases of this type will show a very outspoken Parkinsonism. Even the cogwheel phenomenon may not be present. Hoff and I (1927) have described the convergence phenomenon of the arms. The phenomenon has to be tested as follows: The arms are outstretched parallel to each other, and the patient is ordered to keep his eyes closed. The sign is positive if the hands come nearer to each other. This sign is due to a flexion in the elbow. When merely one arm is tested, the flexion is present too. If both arms are tested, one has to take into consideration that the arms diverge in the normal subject. The normal divergence and the convergence on the basis of flexor rigidity may compensate each other. The sign is a reliable help in detecting slight Parkinsonian features, and points to an organic lesion of those parts of the brain which are affected in Parkinsonism. The sign is present in alcoholics when in the state of an acute intoxication and may disappear with the recovery. Although it is very often combined with tremor it may be present without tremor, and tremor may be present without convergence. (3) Tremor of an organic type is an important symptom, even if the tremor is slight. (4) If the convergence of the eyes is impaired (when exophoria is not present) further evidence for an organic process is hardly necessary. However, in the majority of the cases studied here, a decided evidence of impaired convergence could not be given. (5) Great urge to talk and propulsive features in speech are of paramount importance. (6) Hyperactivity and motor urges of higher degree should be considered confirmatory evidence. Also, the history of hyperactivity in childhood should not be neglected. (7) Outspoken rigidities, propulsion and retropulsion, higher degrees of akinesis and catalepsy can hardly be expected in cases of this type. Persistence of tone described by Hoff and myself has not been observed in any one of these cases.

I have observed seven cases of obsession neurosis in which organic signs of the type described here were present. Only a few of these cases will be discussed in detail.

Emanuel P., 26 years old, came with the complaint that he was afraid of dogs and cats. They instilled awe and disgust in him. Since the age of five he has been afraid that dogs might come near him and bite him. He was particularly afraid that his penis might be hurt. By mere contact with dogs his skin might become like the skin of a dog. His fear of cats was less intense. For many years he could not eat food if his mother tasted it before serving it. He feared the food might be infected by her saliva. Furthermore, he was continually plagued with the idea that he might not be clean enough, and he spent hours in the bathroom washing his hands again and again. Fears of this type went back to age fourteen.

The patient was small, almost dwarfed. His movements were quick and jerky. He talked incessantly in a loud voice and in a propulsive manner. He often repeated what he said, but this was not a palilalia. He salivated and spat a little while talking. His face was somewhat rigid. There was a slight tremor of the head and of the fingers. There was no convergence of arms. The eye convergence was good. The pupils reacted, but during an examination three years before the pupils were found slightly irregular and almost stiff. When the patient was twelve years old he suffered from a period of sleepiness; at school he was called "sleepy head" and "dopey." A tentative diagnosis of encephalitis was made but not definitely substantiated. As the later discussion will show, he was at that time under a particular psychic stress. He complained often about a pain in his left side, about headache and dizziness. A careful checkup showed that there was no somatic basis for these complaints.

The patient lived with his family who were of rather low social status. He had two younger sisters who worked. The father was often unemployed. The patient himself worked for only a short time during his life as a messenger boy. He lived in constant conflict with his family. For years he was treated in different outpatient departments, and was for several months in a state mental hospital.

As mentioned, he stayed in the bathroom for a long time and could not stand any interruption. He could not defecate thoroughly when someone was near the bathroom. He washed very carefully and was in fear of being contaminated by germs. When the process of washing was interrupted, he began all over again. He was very sensitive. He felt continually attacked by everyone. If people on the street said to him, "Hey, Red," he was afraid they might beat him up. He was also afraid that the analyst might make fun of him and that the other patients might laugh at him. He usually came to his appointments late and reacted with great anger if the physician was not able to see him when he came three or four hours late. He left the treatment in great anger. During the treatment, which lasted several months, his ambivalence was very outspoken. Love for the analyst was combined with fear and violent outbursts of hate when he felt rejected. It was always difficult to finish a session because he clung to the analyst, asking question after question, and demanding that the answers be repeated again and again. The patient repeated everything he said several times, insisting that he had to repeat in order not to be misunderstood. He liked to write, and wrote a long autobiography and long reports in which frequent repetitions occurred.

I quote a few sentences in a report he wrote about an encounter with a cat. "I opened the door and the cat ran out and when I saw the cat run out I ran also because I was very much afraid that the cat is after me and will attack me if I do not run. Then I saw the cat run away from me. I ran after the cat so that the cat will not be at the building where I live, so as not to come into the building where I live. Then I felt my legs shaking and I felt my legs weak." The patient also repeatedly dreamed the same dream twice in one night. I do not hesitate to consider the motility and the impulses of this patient as organically determined. However, the ambivalence and his doubts and his tendencies to questioning reinforce many of his motor trends.

His whole sex interest centered around the anal region. He was particularly interested in the anus as such and in the region between the buttocks. This attitude can be traced back to his fourth year when he had scarlet fever and was given an enema by his mother. He could not urinate at that time and an onion was put on his penis. When he came to the hospital at age eleven because of functional heart trouble he was greatly interested when he saw the nurses give enemas to other children. He liked to fancy himself in the same situation and got sexual pleasure out of such fantasies. Ever since his fourteenth year he has masturbated thinking of a teacher's rectum, "associating her rectum with a female nurse who gave a child an enema which I had observed." He also had a fantasy of a female giving him an enema. He felt that the rectum of females was broader, and by getting an enema his rectum would become broader too and be more like the rectum of a female. He would thus be transformed into a female. He was extremely interested in seeing these parts of women. He was also interested in smelling the places where women had been sitting. This interest went back to his fifth year. He often wished and fantasied that his father would insert his penis into his rectum. Many dreams and fantasies make it clear that the muzzle of the dog, the dog itself, the penis, the feces were equivalent to him. He therefore tended to be passive toward his father and his sex organ and toward women who were endowed with a symbolic penis—the nozzle of the enema.

He reported that he loved his father very much when he was small, and that his father was very good to him. He occasionally had sexual dreams about his father, spilling semen on his father's chest. Around his fifth year his father became a menace to him. He was afraid of his father's looks, and when his father was angry, he was afraid that his father might bite off his penis. The patient reported this with decided gusto, and even reported that he had voluptuous sensations in his sex organ when threatened by his father or anybody else. Even the repetition of the story gave him sexual pleasure. He often had the wish to attack his father with an axe from behind and kill him. Sometimes he wanted to choke his father, and was afraid his father might choke him. He also had hostile impulses against his mother and sisters. His fear of dogs went back to his fourth year. He said that dogs have a grim expression on their faces, and in a description of dogs he used the same words he used in describing his father. He was also afraid of being infected by dogs and of becoming like a dog if he touched one.

The patient was conscious of being short, weak, and helpless. His autobiography began "When I was born I was told by my mother and father that I was a short baby. . . . I used to throw my feet up and down nervously and to make nervous motions with a rattle."

The parents obviously were very conscious of the size and weakness of the child, and later on became annoyed by his hyperkinetic aggressiveness. Around his fifth year the counteraggression of the parents was in full swing. At this critical age a scarlatina occurred, which led to his mother's handling of his penis and anus. The passive attitude of the patient mingled immediately with anal and especially sexual motives to establish a definite pattern. The persistent hyperkinesis sharpened the conflicts with the parents. The sexual problems awakened in connection with the scarlatina experiences before puberty reinforced the anal pattern and sexual excitement. Masturbation led to preoccupations and sleepiness. His attitude toward dogs ran parallel to his attitude toward his parents. An early love for a white dog was substituted for a fear of brown dogs. He was in a world which continually threatened him. The threats coming from father and mother were that he might be cut to pieces and dismembered, and especially that he might be deprived of his sex organs. He was furthermore threatened by the saliva of his mother which was poisonous and contained germs. Uncleanliness became the general expression of threats coming from excretions of any other person's body. Semen and feces also became formidable. Animals were a combination of the danger coming from direct attack and secretion. They bit and were unclean.

It was obvious that in this psychological development the increase in motor impulses was of paramount importance. However, the body configuration of the patient in its effect upon the parents and the attitudes of the parents in general was of decisive influence on the further development of this severe neurosis. This is the only case of this group in which the therapeutic effort was without any result.

The obsessional neurotic patient who complained of being

too small, mentioned in my paper on ideologies (1936a), had compulsions to curse God and at the same time make movements with his feet, showed a rigid face, a propulsive speech, a slight tremor of the hands and especially of the eyelids. His cursing was obviously in connection with strong motor impulses, not only concerning his speech but also his feet. In his early history, consciousness of his small size, homosexual attachment to his father, as well as fear of the father played an outstanding part. He made movements with his toes three times. He had the urge to touch everything, especially the female breast. There were compulsions to use obscene words. The verbal attack was obviously the precursor of a physical attack which ended in anal intercourse with the defeated love object.

Thirty-three-year-old Fram M. suffered from severe anxiety states. He had been analyzed for about two and a half years by other physicians. He had compulsive fantasies about cutting women into pieces, tearing out their sex parts and devouring them either in part or as a whole. He had similar impulses toward the analyst. He had a compulsion to count. "I count and think in my mind. Also Napoleon had counted windows. I count the corners and borders of every piece of paper. Then I count the planes and break everything in my thoughts. I would like to smash everybody to pieces and urinate on them." For this patient counting meant to tear and break into small pieces. This meant also a destruction of the human body. The patient had a rigid face and an enormous urge to talk. In his childhood he was exposed to the attacks of older brothers. He was weak and continually threatened. In addition, he was a hyperactive child and continually came in conflict with his mother.

Thirty-four-year old Archibald B. had the urge to assault women and to kill his wife. Sometimes he wanted to assault women sexually. The idea of killing appeared initially four years previously in a dream. The patient had a slight quick tremor in his left hand, which also had a tendency to convergence. There was also a tremor of the eyelids.

Frank B., 30 years old, complained about slight depersonalization symptoms. He said he had to count his footsteps. He could not decide in what direction to walk. He had the urge to explain his symptoms continually to the doctor. Physical examination showed a tremor of the hands and a decrease in the associated movements of the right arm. There was some stiffness in the posture and in the face. The convergence of the left eye was decreased. His speech was slurred and propulsive, and his face had a staring look. There was no history of encephalitis. This case had not been fully investigated from a phylogenic point of view. There were slight compulsion symptoms (counting steps) obviously in connection with an impairment of the motor function. The patient complained bitterly that he had to give constant attention to his staring and to his stiffness. This case reacted obviously to the impairment of the motor function with a compulsive attention to this function.

Alfred R., 30 years old, had the compulsive thought that he was an illegitimate child, that his mother had had sex relations with another man whom he identified. He had the compulsion to kill his mother. The borderline from compulsion to delusion was not sharp. There was a slight tic movement of the head which disappeared. Later, he felt the urge to move his head in this direction without giving in. The patient had a rigid face. The right side of the face was particularly akinetic.

Edward T., 21 years old, had an outspoken compulsion to wash. He had a rigid face, a tremor of the outstretched hands, a marked degree of akinesis, paralysis agitans posture without rigidities but with a slight convergence of the arms. In the early history, anal and sadistic trends were outspoken. It was not possible in the comparatively short observation to establish a psychological connection between organic impulse disturbances and the washing compulsion.

In all the seven cases cited, organic signs were present, pointing to organic lesions of the brain, partially identical in localization with the symptoms of encephalitis. Four of the cases showed evidence of an increase in impulses which were in obvious connection with the psychological determinants of the compulsion. In two of the other cases, the self-observation of disturbances in motor impulses formed the basis for obsessive self-observation. However, the connection with impulse disturbances and obsessional symptoms was not as obvious as in the other cases. In the seventh case, no definite psychological connection could be made between the motor disturbance and the obsessive picture.

If one studies the characteristics of these cases in which organic signs are obvious, one sees in many other cases clinical and psychological characteristics which make it at least probable that a similar impulse disturbance on an organic basis is at work.

Ruth S., 32 years of age, had been in analysis for more than five years before she came to my observation. She suffered from a fear that she might have killed others with poison. She thought she might have gone without realizing it into a drugstore or into the bathroom and mixed some drugs. When she passed a drugstore she was not sure whether she had not gone in. She was also haunted by the obsessional fear that she might have kicked automobiles and automobile drivers, causing terrible accidents. Furthermore, she believed that she had kicked persons in manholes and had destroyed gas pipes and electric wires by her action. The obsessions went back to her eighteenth year. She often had death wishes against her husband, the relatives of her husband, and her mother. She was otherwise a good hater. In connection with her obsessions she suffered from time to time an indescribable pain which was localized in the abdomen but was different from somatic pain. It was more akin to a feeling of terrible emptiness. She experienced this pain for the first time when she was six years old and looked into a garden. The world appeared to her so beautiful that she wanted to take it in as a whole. She would like to die but was afraid to kill herself because she might kill others in the act of killing herself. In early recollections, blood poisoning of her brother, who was two years younger, played an important part. She felt that she had caused it by scratching her brother's arm. She felt that her mother had mistreated her in early childhood. There was a strong affection for the father, who died of general paresis when she was twelve years old. She was an extremely lively, active, and outgoing child. At the age of twelve, one of her teachers, obviously seduced by her, tried to make love to her; however, there was merely petting. Her strong sex wishes were incompletely satisfied by her husband. Her extramarital experiences were few and disturbed by repressions. She was extremely gifted as a writer and was full of energy if not too much hemmed in by her obsessions.

A physical examination was negative. However, her motility was exaggerated. She was continually in movement, did not sit still for a minute, and was afraid that with every movement she might have kicked something or might have spilled poisons.

The result of therapy which showed the connection of her impulses and drives with her motility was very satisfactory, and the obsessions went more and more into the background without disappearing completely.

Her brother, who was two years younger, showed an excessive sex drive and potency. He acted out his sex urge without any inhibition. He was an extremely severe alcoholic and was analyzed for more than three years in Germany with no therapeutic results. He had a slight diabetes. He was under observation in Bellevue Hospital, but was only seen for a short time.

The history makes it at least probable that we deal with an impulse disturbance in the sense of hyperactivity based on organic factors. The possibility cannot be denied that the brother's and sister's sex urges may have been increased. Ruth's repression of these urges may have been a contributing factor in the structure of her obsessional neurosis. It is interesting that the symptomatology of the case is specifically based on motor impulses which find their psychic fulfillment by contracting space and bringing objects which are merely in sight within the reach of her immediate action.

Marvin B., twelve years old, suffered from obsessions for more than two years. A letter had arrived from his mother's sister inviting them to Europe. He pictured Europe vividly, thought how nice it would be to play with other children there, and could not get rid of this thought. He was so bothered by this continuous desire that he hit himself four times on the left arm, telling himself that he would die if he continued to think of Europe. An obsessional fear of death set in. He had to hit himself four times on the shin bone with his leg before crossing the street because he thought he might otherwise get killed. When walking on the street he felt an extreme pain when he was by chance touched by passers-by. He was afraid that they might wish his death and infect him with their touch. The patient had a severe infection of his arm one year after his obsession had started. When he asked questions, he had to repeat them four times. Four is an even number, which has something restful about it. Three had something unfinished about it, in his opinion.

There were no organic signs.

Psychoanalysis, which was conducted partially in a group, showed that he had always been an aggressive and violent child who was often hit by his father and mother. At six or seven he stole repeatedly and was severely punished. At the age of five he played with other boys on the street and tortured cats, tying them, pressing their muzzles together, pinching them, and pulling their tails. However, he protested when another boy was treated in a similar way by his friends. During the night he often had nightmares that an enormous cat was sitting on his chest. When this happened he went into his mother's bed. He liked to fight with his older sister. When she made him angry, he felt like killing her and wished she were dead. He acted similarly to his friends with whom he still liked to wrestle. When he wrestled with them he was not afraid to be touched, had no pain and no fears of infection and death. He started to masturbate before age ten, and just before the outbreak of the obsessional neurosis he felt that he might harm himself and tried to stop masturbation, without success. He was particularly afraid that the loss of semen which occurred during masturbation might do him irreparable harm. There was a strong sexual curiosity and sex urge.

After three months of treatment when he was twelve, the

patient was completely free of symptoms. However, treatment was continued for six months.

The parents were obviously of an aggressive type. The mother had been so during several interviews. A brother, five years older, was in Bellevue hospital with the diagnosis of schizophrenia and was under treatment at the same time as Marvin was. He had started around his twelfth year with a complicated obsessional picture in which obsessional thoughts about vampires were paramount. He complained about a vibrating sensation near his heart which reacted especially to noises. The observation was far from being finished. I was more inclined to believe that we dealt with a complicated obsessional neurosis. The face of the patient was decidedly rigid. There were no other neurological signs.[1]

In Marvin's case, violent aggression was in the foreground. There was a tendency to actions and to repetitions in which the number four and counting played an important part. Aggression and fear of infection were present. The child was lively and very active. In this case, I was also inclined to believe that we were dealing with an organic motor factor. It was remarkable that obsessional features were also present in the brother, although the brother's aggressiveness expressed itself in fantastic fears and preoccupations.

When Marvin was fourteen, he broke his arm while jumping from a trolley car on which he was hitching a ride. He was aware of the danger of hitching rides on trolley cars, but he could not resist the impulse. The healing of the fracture was uneventful, but he became preoccupied with hypochondriacal ideas; for instance, that his arm was weak, that there was a red mark, and that the veins "stuck out." He felt like a cripple; he wished that everybody else had a broken arm. His apprehensions expressed themselves in dreams. He also worried that his breasts were too large and that his hand might fall off at the red line. However, these symptoms disappeared

[1] [This older brother was able to maintain himself in the community while he received group therapy with Schilder. After Schilder's death, he became progressively more disturbed and was institutionalized. A diagnosis of schizophrenia was made, he was given shock therapy, and later, a lobotomy, after which he deteriorated.—Ed.]

after he realized that his fears were punishment for his aggression. He wanted to kill people who pushed him in a crowded subway. He bought a gun to compensate for his weakened left arm, and then felt that nobody would touch him. At the age of fourteen, he had his first sex relations with a prostitute. He felt he would like to go to a prostitute every day. He showed his penis to a woman looking out of a window. Both he and his family decided that he should be sent to a boys' institution for a while. When this was decided, he demanded of the physician that it should be done immediately. Meanwhile, he and some friends broke open a parcel-post package in the hope of finding candy and money. He had continuous fights at home. He said he would like to kill his teacher, who had a grudge against him, or run over him with a car. He finally was placed in an institution, but he soon felt that he had to go home again, and he repeatedly ran away. He was then discharged. He complained only of his strong sex urge; however, he was fairly well adapted. His dreams were of the following type: "There was war in this country, and they gave everybody a revolver in school. They gave me a .38 revolver. I felt very happy. Maybe I want a girl more than a gun."

When he was sixteen, he came to the clinic again, complaining that his brother was "butting in" on his girl friends, and that he also made him nervous by talking about spooks all the time. Marvin said that he was losing interest in school, and wanted to quit and join the army.[2]

In a short paper dealing with the psychoanalysis of geometry, arithmetic, and physics, I (1936b) reported two cases of obsessional

[2] [This follow-up report was obtained after Schilder's death. Marvin did join the marines, just before Pearl Harbor, thinking he could get away from home, travel, and have a gun. When the real war started, he became frightened and anxious, and got a neuropsychiatric medical discharge. He returned home, married, and had a son. He remained dependent on his family and his wife, and was anxious and hypochondriacal. In July, 1953, Marvin, then a young adult, again came to us for psychiatric help because his obsessional thinking was threatening to overwhelm him and ruin his life. He had become so increasingly absorbed with gambling on horse racing that he was neglecting all his responsibilities. Abandoning his schooling (under G.I. benefits), he became desperate for money, sold his home, and exhausted his wife's funds. She had consequently left him and taken their only child. Regretful over these results, he nevertheless was helpless to control his obsessional drives.—Ed.]

neurosis which did not show any organic signs, but showed a particular relation to numbers and reacted to symmetry and asymmetry and to specific numbers with actions which were repeated five times. I came to the conclusion that obsessional counting and counting in general is an action of an aggressive type. Counting and dividing into parts have a very close relation. To divide into parts means tearing and destruction. Activity and aggression very often combine with oral and anal tendencies. The relation to genital tendencies is not as close. The aggression is obviously not merely derived from oral and anal tendencies. It serves orientation and self-assertion in the world. The intake of food (and its excretion) and the eroticism connected with it is merely a part of self-preservation and of adaptation to the world. Whereas numbers serve as preliminary points of orientation in an almost amorphous world, geometry comes to life in other compulsions. Symmetry and asymmetry in the surroundings provoke, as is well known, changes in posture and attitude. Asymmetry is a definite threat to the body, acting on the inner organs and sensations and on the sexual functions. Symmetry and balance are motor phenomena which ask for definite moral attitudes that express themselves in the muscular system but also influence the intestinal system. There is no doubt that counting and the reaction to symmetry, asymmetry, and gravity belong to the fundamental functions of the ego. The functions of the ego are connected with activity and aggressiveness. They serve not only to maintain equilibrium, but also as a defense against hostile attacks and possessiveness, and oral and genital tendencies.

I am inclined to believe that in many cases of obsessional neurosis, organic factors are at work which influence these fundamental functions of the ego. In a great number of cases, a direct proof can be produced that the impulse disturbances are in connection with organic changes in the brain. In other cases, probabilities can be offered. It can be shown that the organic impulse disturbances lead to a specific compulsive symptomatology. The inference may be drawn that cases which show an identical structure of compulsions are based on motor impulses of the same type. We have reason to believe that there are cases in which psychogenic factors, as commonly defined, are at the basis of the impulse disturbance.

I come, therefore, to the conclusion that there exists a group of obsessional-neurosis cases in which the motor impulses are disturbed. Compulsions are in the foreground of these cases. There is repetition, counting, and a special relation to symmetry and asymmetry. There is distortion of space. Only E. Straus (1930) has so far drawn attention to the space disturbances in the symptomatology of obsessional neurosis. I want to be more specific insofar as I endeavor to elucidate the relation of space (Schilder, 1935b), geometry, arithmetic, and physics (Schilder, 1936b) to a specific organic apparatus. I want to emphasize that these remarks point to a specific group of compulsions. Obsessional neuroses exist in which such mechanisms are not present. From a psychoanalytic point of view, it has to be emphasized that we deal primarily with changes in the ego functions. These ego-function disturbances are in intricate relation to libidinal structures. The details of this problem cannot be discussed in this clinical paper. Wexberg (1929), starting from the experiences of encephalitis cases, has also come to the conclusion that there is an organic nucleus in obsessional neurosis. I point to a more specific mechanism of a specific group. There may be other organic mechanisms in obsessional-neurosis cases. Goldstein (1924) remarked that there is a symptomatic similarity between the basic tendencies of the obsessional neurosis and a striopallidar case which he has observed. He sees the common factor in a tendency to persistence. My observations do not substantiate this mechanism.

The organic factor, found in this group of obsessional neurosis cases, is not the only factor. In many such cases, the state of consciousness changes when the obsession occurs. The imagery which represents the obsession becomes plastic and exceptionally clear. Kauders (1931) very aptly characterized this state in obsessional neurotic cases as a visionary state. Such a case was observed by Curran (1938) in a paper on bromide intoxications. The patient, an elderly Italian lady, found herself thinking continually of the sex parts of her daughters, on whom she wanted to perform cunnilingus. The patient finally took, on her own counsel, a great amount of bromides and developed a bromide psychosis in which there was deep clouding of the consciousness. She heard voices and saw her daughters killed. With the disappearance of the bromide psychosis, the obsessions disappeared completely, and the patient remained well for several months. We need observations on more patients before it can be determined if we are dealing in such cases with organic factors regulating the state of consciousness.

It is difficult to appreciate the number of obsessional-neurosis cases in which organic factors are of importance. Preliminary impressions let me believe that organic signs can be found in about one third of the cases. In another third the symptomatology arouses the suspicion of an organic background, and in the last third merely psychogenic factors as commonly defined are of importance. This statement does not pertain to the general question of the constitution of the obsessional neurotic case but merely to definite neurological mechanisms. In the majority of our positive cases, we do not deal with sequelae of epidemic encephalitis but with organic changes similar to those observed in encephalitis but of different origin. They may be constitutional or they may be due to lesions in the fetal life, to birth traumas, or to early toxic and infectious processes of unknown origin.

It is worthwhile mentioning that, with the exception of the first case, satisfactory therapeutic results were obtained when the patient was either taught in individual analysis or in group psychotherapy what the connections were between his motor drives, his compulsions, and his libidinal structure.

CHAPTER SIX

The Structure of Obsessions and Compulsions

Freud stated (1916-1917) that the system of conscious experience has perception and motility as its basis. According to him, access to motility is through consciousness. Consciousness and motility are the nucleus of the ego in the psychoanalytic sense. Psychoanalysis has given attention to the more complicated functions of the ego and has neglected the study of primitive motor function in connection with problems of the ego. The works of Jelliffe (1932) and Stengel (1935a, 1935b) are exceptions to this general neglect of organic motor functions. The general psychoanalytic literature does not sufficiently emphasize motor problems in relation to obsessions and compulsions. Compare, for instance, the papers of Federn (1933), Bergler (1936), and Goldman (1938). The more general discussions of Nunberg (1932) and Fenichel (1934) mention Freud's fundamental discussion of the defense reactions in obsession neurosis—isolation and undoing — but do not stress the motor elements in the psychology of obsessional neurotics.

On the other hand, neurological literature on epidemic encephalitis offers extensive and interesting data on obsessive and compulsive phenomena in acute and chronic encephalitis. In these cases there is direct evidence of a change in motor drives. Compare, for instance, Jelliffe. My own studies have shown me

Appeared originally in *Psychiatry*, 3:549-560, 1940.

that about one third of the obsessive and the compulsive cases show organic signs pointing to pathology with the same localization as that found in encephalitis [see Ch. 5]. However, there is no indication that these cases have a process in any way comparable with the process in epidemic encephalitis. These changes may be constitutional or they may be due to lesions in fetal life, to birth traumas, or to toxic and infectious processes in infancy. Kehrer (1938) has recently pointed to the coincidence of true obsessions and compulsions with chorea and ticlike hyperkinesis. I have found great psychological interest in the motor factors in obsessional neurosis because they not only show the relations of drives to perceptions, but also prove an excellent approach to the fundamental therapeutic problem in obsessions and compulsions.

The material on which this discussion is based comes from approximately twenty cases which have been treated either in group psychoanalysis or in individual analysis for a minimum of several months. Many cases have been treated for two years and more. Some of the cases have been seen after they had previously had long individual analysis with other analysts.

The Motor Drives

Among the more primitive drives to be found is the impulse to throw things. For illustration, E. S., a girl of eighteen, was afraid that she might throw knives at people, or an icepick-like instrument with which she worked. She felt she already had thrown it at somebody. The same patient also had the feeling that she stuck a knife into the back of any person whom she faced. Furthermore, she had fantasies of breaking a string of pearls offered to her by her lover and throwing them in his face. She feels she may even have stamped on the pearls.

Another patient had a compulsion to kick others in the shins or genitals, or at least to touch the latter.

H. H. had impulses to tear, to break objects into pieces, to bite and to suck. Furthermore, she wanted to touch and tear out the genitals of Christ [See Ch. 3].

Other patients counted, thus isolating one part of a whole from another. It was, as one of my patients formulated it, a tearing to pieces.

S. H., a young man of 28, first came for treatment for a tic of turning the head, opening the mouth, and swallowing. Later on, he felt that he had to curse people against his will.

The motor impulse may lead to a more indirect form of destruction. E. S., as an example, thought that she might have taken a kerosene lamp into a street car, knocked it over, and set the street car on fire. Sometimes she thinks she has done this with matches. She and another one of my patients felt that they had set God on fire. Her fantasy of using knives implies the use of weapons to indirectly increase her power of action.

A. L., a man of 30, is afraid that he may put wrong objects into printing machines and so cause disaster.

The wish for action arouses in patients a fear that they may have gone longer or shorter distances and committed aggressive acts. E. S., for instance, thought she may have gone to a policeman, taken his gun out of his pocket, and shot him down. She was also afraid she might have put cockroach powder into the hems of her clothes, might have taken it out later and put it into people's drinking glasses. R. S. believes she has gone into drug stores and mixed medicines together or interchanged them.

All these are more complicated actions in which the patients overcome space by the force of a motor impulse. Their impulses transgress distance and time.

Very similar tendencies to movement are used as defenses against obsessive and compulsive ideas. A. L. is sometimes struck with a destructive idea while he has a paper in his hand. He has to tear this paper into pieces and throw it into the toilet. A pencil in his hand has to be thrown away when an uncanny thought occurs at the time he is holding the pencil. For similar reasons, he and another patient discard wearing apparel of all kinds.

He says: "God be damned. This has no sense, but I think it and act it out with my toes. I make three taps with my toes when I say 'God be damned' and that contaminates things I wear. If these things are indispensable I continue wearing them. If they are not, like socks or handkerchiefs, I discard them and throw them away. Sometimes I actually do say the words 'God be damned.' I say it after contemplation." When asked: "Why do you tap your toes?" he replied: "I do it three times because it is for each word. I throw away these objects because I feel that I'm removing the possible cause for punishment. When I move my toes I don't feel like kicking anybody." "At present I feel like throwing my belt away, having just experienced such a sensation. By discarding it I will have purified myself. In some cases I wash myself over this same area covered by the belt."

A 33-year-old woman, T. H., suffering from a severe obsessional neurosis for many years, has to make pushing movements with her hands. She thus pushes buildings away or otherwise she would have to confess her sexual transgressions. Since the second finger means masturbation, the third finger homosexuality, and the fourth finger marriage, she can only take things with her first and fifth fingers. She defends herself against the pushing notion by a formula which she says to herself, moving her lips: "Overhead, underhead, underground." This patient also used a great deal of obscene language. She not only pushed with her hands, but also with her eyes and with her teeth. She pushed away curtains which meant condoms, ivy and orange color which meant prostitution, and candies which meant masturbation.

E. P. could never end a session. He had to ask the analyst one more question. The patient repeated everything he said several times, insisting that he had to repeat in order not to be misunderstood. He also repeated himself continually in writing and rationalized this action by saying that he did not want to be misunderstood. He even repeated one dream twice in the same night. Another patient, C. B., also repeated over and over again, but his repetitions were due to dissatisfaction with his formulation. A. L. had to put his hand in his pocket several times in order to see whether it was still there.

In all compulsions and obsessions, one finds endless repetitions which never completely satisfy the patient; the same urge always remains.

BALANCE AND THE OUTWARD WORLD

S. C. complained that he had to put every package exactly in the middle of the table. If he did not do so, he would get sick and die. If he touched an object on one side and not on the other side, he felt empty inside. At five years of age he had to touch his head on the other side after he had touched one side. If he did not he felt that he had made a hole in his skull. Asymmetry in the outside world made his body asymmetrical; it pulled him to one side, which seemed overweight. E. M. had anxiety when he was in the middle of a room. If he touched something with his right hand, he became anxious unless he made movements with his left hand or left foot (Schilder, 1936b).

The geometrical or physical qualities of the world may become signs of threat which emanate from the world. Patients may defend themselves by new geometrical arrangements, or they may defend themselves by counting and by numbers. A. L. had to sit in a specific way. He could not stand disorder of any kind. Things should not be out of balance. Only a regular world gave security. Sharp angles were felt as a particular threat. Neatness, orderliness, and regularity in the world thus become conditions for security. One might interpret this tendency as a projection of excess potential activity out into the world. The world thus appears in continual danger of getting out of equilibrium. A. L., accordingly, wanted everything in the outside world compact and neat; he was also interested in technocracy. E. S. also wanted order and was interested in mechanics. However, E. S. took pleasure in seeing blocks toppling down.

These tendencies come out very clearly in the drawings of obsessives. We find endless repetition of the same motif; great regularity and order. A. L. particularly enjoyed drawing cherries with very sharp and clear outlines. Things which were not clear in outline, such as spots on the street or in wood, reminded him of syphilis and cancer. E. S. liked to draw almost abstract pictures in more or less symmetrical wavy lines. Furthermore, she liked to represent sharp contrasts, as day and night, in pictures. The urge to symmetrv was very outstanding in her drawings. The wavy lines represented the energy of an orchestra conductor or the energy of waving arms. A. L., in an abstract drawing, came to the conclusion that a border is like a fortress, especially when the border had sharp angles outside. Curved lines suggested a swinging waltz. He was also interested in walls made of brick where everything was standardized. Obsessive and compulsive patients have a particular sensitivity to angles, sharpness, lack of symmetry, lack of equilibrium, and disturbance of balance. The world thus becomes a continuous source of danger.

Thoughts

A. L. thought that all his movements were unnatural. Without his knowing, they served as a signal which might be appreciated and perceived by his enemies who might, in turn, punish him cruelly—especially by cutting off his hands and arms. He felt that his unnatural motility was a result of his attempt to avoid spots which meant syphilis and cancer. He sometimes had frightening thoughts concerning the results of actions he had forgotten about. Such thoughts were particularly terrifying to him. He tried hard and in vain to remember them. It seemed that they had something to do with fire and with hurting somebody. His tiniest movement while writing made the writing and letters unnatural, and they became signs by being unnatural. It is conceivable that the particular strength of these archaic thought flashes was due to their being imbued with motor power and drive. I have mentioned the episodes in which R. S. and E. S. felt that they had performed complicated actions which catapulted them through space to the object they were to destroy. The motor impulse, when checked, was transformed into an obsession. Motor power can be transposed from motion to thought and thus change the importance and persistence of the thought. A thought endowed with motor power may become omnipotent or may become obsessive.

A. L. thought many things at once. The thought had a dreamlike character which made the occurrences seem like signs which could be read by others and answered with counteraggression. He developed the concept of a secret language and a special code. The thought became a substance which, once connected with an object, became a part of the object which then had to be destroyed. The destruction was, however, a real action, as had been mentioned. The pencils were thrown into the toilet, the paper was torn and also thrown into the toilet.

It has not generally been appreciated that omnipotent magical thoughts act irrespective of distance in space on the basis of motor power or dreamlike powerful imagination.

E. S. was very nearsighted. She did not like to look at people carefully. It was all right as long as she did not get a clear picture of the faces of other persons. If she saw the face clearly, she had to imagine it distorted and in agony, and then thought that she had poisoned the person or murdered him in some way. A superior optic memory was here the condition for the obsession. However, the mere fact she saw a person once and not again was sufficient for her to imagine that she had killed this person. The optic impression had to reassure her of the other person. A. L., in contrast, was afraid to write since this would leave a permanent record. This permanent record might be a sign of his permanent aggression. He found it admirable, however, when something was kept forever in books and dictionaries. The problem of duration and change was therefore an important problem for these patients. The patients had the tendency to destroy, and felt that if they destroyed, the proof of their guilt would be lasting.

Some Ideas of Obsessional Neurotics

Some patients were not convinced of their actions and had to repeat them. One patient was afraid that she might not have closed the gas jet. She had to go back to it, open it, and close it again. The motor impulse had not been exhausted and went in the opposite direction. The repetition of the thought and action was comparable to the purely organic repetitions to be found in the palilalias and palipraxias of encephalitis cases. I have mentioned before that some of these patients repeated because they felt that they had not been understood. In all their turmoil, the patients want orderliness. In thoughts, also, they do not want imbalance to exist. A. L. said that he should stand in the right proportion to space. Some like to think in opposites. E. S. drew day and night, light and dark, rain and shine, which spoke of love and hate. A. L. liked machines, compactness, technocracy and was for a very strict division of right and wrong. He, of course, was always right, and he became very violent in discussions. He could not understand that others could not see that he was right.

Things in the thought world of the obsessive neurotic are very well separated from each other. However, this wish for orderliness, separation, isolation, and absoluteness is partially a reaction against the fact that one's actions, which are of magical character, bring everything into connection with each other. T. H. said that white chicken meat reminded her of a white breast, and a white breast meant homosexuality. Since she did not want to be reminded of homosexuality, she could not eat white chicken meat. If she were reminded of homosexuality she might have to confess to her mother. Her brother-in-law's penis reminded her of the color of peaches; therefore she could not eat peaches.

Her world had too many connections, and things were not isolated enough. I said to the patient: "You take away independence from the world; things are for themselves and not merely in order to remind you of something. There is too much meaning in your world." For the patient, a connection in thought was a connection of real things. She actually connected things by touching them, and separated them afterward by pushing them away. It was not easy to ascertain in this case whether the obsession started from the motor impulse. This patient at nineteen had obsessional homosexual feelings and later on had a delusion that she was licked by and had intercourse with a dog. During the stay in the sanitarium she succeeded in having sex relations with the head nurse.

When there was a tendency to isolation in these cases it was an attempt to counteract the connection of thoughts, which in turn was a connection of things by action. This can be expressed paradoxically in the following way. Everything is connected with everything else by touching, pushing, and throwing. This means destruction. Therefore, everything should be kept separate; or, still better, the whole world should be separated into its parts.

It is furthermore characteristic that so many obsessive patients take every possibility as a reality. They say, for instance: "But it is possible that I went into the drug store and mixed all the poisons together so that a catastrophe will follow." E. S. also said that it was possible that she kicked a passing car which may have done something to the gas tubes and which may have killed hundreds of persons. Possibility meant for these patients a connection of ideas which was powerfully cemented by motor or libidinal ideas. The interchange between possibility and reality was another form of the magical power of thoughts.

For almost every obsessional neurotic, numbers and counting have a special importance. M. O., a 28-year-old married woman, had to repeat things ten times. A. L. repeated actions three or six times, since two or four times would mean that his arms and legs would be cut off. For S. C. one meant the father, two the mother, three the family, five death, and six somebody else. E. M. makes five movements with his left hand after he has touched something with his right hand. Bergson (1910) is right when he states that the number is in the closest relation to action. M. L. very often had to think over every detail of an argument or of a scene. She had to say to herself "things forward and backward." Sometimes during intercourse she had to remember a scene in all details before she could have an orgasm. When she argued with her husband she had to think what he would do in her place and what she would do in his. However, this patient had no manifest motor symptomatology. A great deal of her difficulty was related to her having observed intercourse between her parents, and her tendency to put herself in the role of her father as well as of her mother. Furthermore, her mother was extremely jealous and continually had scenes with her father.

To sum up, the motor-obsessive-neurotic cases, in their thinking, connect everything with everything else since they have the urge to reach everything by action. They try to isolate the objects by restraining their actions or by making counter movements of pushing away. Their thoughts, loaded with motility, transgress spatial distances. They have, furthermore, a magical power. Their thinking, which consists of action and counteraction, is reflected in thinking in opposites. There are, furthermore, preferences for machines, for neatness and oppositions of right and wrong. The ideas of justice and punishment gain importance.

One may wonder why I have not used the term "ambivalence." To be sure, the patients vacillated between love and hate. However, this was in no way a primary, mysterious quality of ambivalence of feelings, but was an expression of impulses coming from the different layers of the personality and could only be understood as the expression of drives in connection with situations of the past and of the present. Ambivalence is a mixture of actions and drives belonging to different historical layers or to different layers of the personality. I think the term has outlived its usefulness.

The Symbolism of Motor Drives

When E. S., at twelve years, thought of intercourse, she defended herself against this thought by spitting. This corresponded to an ejaculation on her part. Her most aggressive thoughts were of pushing a knife into somebody, of shooting or throwing an ice pick. These were all symbols of attacks with the penis. Motor drives blended with aggressiveness of the sex organs. According to her obsessions, she carried blue powder in her clothes. This probably meant, partially, the destructive fluids of her body. A. L.'s fear that his aggression might be punished by having his arms cut off was obviously a castration fear. E. K. had the wish that something should be pushed into his anus. In other words, the motor drives were psychologically blended with erotic drives connected with protrusions and with openings.

The motor drives also lend themselves to severe aggressiveness. As mentioned above, C. B., a patient with hypochondriacal trends and outspoken obsessional thinking, was ordered to draw a human figure again and again. In the first picture he drew a human figure standing, but in the following pictures the figure became increasingly motile. Finally, there were two figures swinging in the air fighting each other; a man hangs himself, and wild motion results.

Drives and counterdrives were present not only in the field of motility but also in the field of thinking. C. B. clung to his parents, on the one hand, and, on the other, he hated them. He once attempted to strangle his mother. He wanted to be dependent upon the analyst and wanted to be reassured concerning his hypochondriacal symptoms; but he also wanted to show that the analyst was wrong, and he wanted to find contradictions in his statements. Furthermore, he could never finish. Whatever he did had the character of incompleteness to him. The overwhelming motor impulse was stopped by counteraction, but it had not lost its motor power. There was a tendency to repeat over and over again. Doubt and clinging are thus in close relation to motility.

The so-called "elliptic technic" consisted in omitting a part of the obsessive thought. A. Z., a 23-year-old housewife, had the obsessive fear that she might be a homosexual. She continually had to say to herself "I am," which meant, "I am a homosexual." To be sure, this was a patient without manifest motor signs. However, this was an interrupted spoken sentence. When she was a burlesque dancer at sixteen, she particularly enjoyed kicking with her legs.

The Evidence for the Increase of Motor Drives

I have shown previously [Ch. 5] that in many obsessive-neurotic cases, neurological signs were present which pointed to parts of the brain that have to do with the distribution of impulses. To mention a few of them: tremor of the eyelids and arms; propulsive speech; rigidity of the face; lack of convergence of the eyes; convergence of the arms and elbows; minor changes in the postural reflexes. In another group of cases, the symptomatology pointed to an increase in the motor impulses.

Furthermore, there have been a great number of cases of encephalitis which showed obsessional phenomena, partially in connection with palilalia and palipraxia. One must point to the coprolalia observed in tic cases. My own material contains a case in which a tic was converted into a compulsion to curse and to use obscene words.

Activity, Aggression, and Sadism

Most of the theories of instincts do not take into consideration that motility is an outlet of the needs of the total personality. Every instinct therefore has access to motility. Sexuality in the narrower sense carries with it its own activity just as well as the ego instincts, however one may define them. Also, the conscious organization of the ego in the analytic sense is an organization with motor implications. Besides these more organized forms of activity and motility, we often have to deal with changes in the part-function of motility, as, for instance, in the changed drives of postencephalitics. Increased activity and motility are directed toward other persons and will sooner or later lead to problems of superiority, inferiority, and to problems of aggression and submission. Sexuality has motor outlets as well as the ego instincts and the ego, and aggression may be connected with either of them. In the previous discussions we were chiefly interested in an increase in the motor drives which were seen as part functions. It has been shown that such an increase in motor drives leads to aggression. Aggression may come from sexual, genital, and pregenital drives; internal drives or motor drives proper; and external drives. The drives in connection with the organization of the total personality—the ego—stand in between.

Aggression is a quantitative increase in activity beyond the usual which leads to a fight for superiority as well as to a destructive attitude toward persons and objects. If one uses this formulation, one would say that normal sex activity does not include aggression. Aggressiveness in connection with internal drives is called sadistic.

One may have the opinion that in sadism an admixture of external aggression to internal aggression can always be found. One may have the opinion that internal aggression is sufficient. One may say that the phenomenon of sadism occurs when sexuality is added to external drives. I am, indeed, of the opinion that sadism may start either in the internal or external sphere. At the height of the aggression coming from either sphere, an admixture of the other sphere probably does occur. Furthermore, strong external drives blend with internal drives partially by way of symbolism.

Obsessions and Compulsions by Internal Drives

It seems that several types of internal obsessive and compulsive neuroses can be differentiated. A. B., a 21-year-old student, had the fear of impending orgasm in the presence of men. He had to think about it continually in the presence of men. At the age of five he became aware of his erections and began masturbating by squeezing his penis between his thighs. He fantasied intercourse between his parents, which he had witnessed. The squeezing of the penis between the legs signified his fear of, and wish for, passivity. From an early age he had felt his body to be inferior: his penis too small (examination showed it to be of average size), his hands too small, his body flabby, his skin too white. He felt he had insufficient hair on his chest and that his buttocks were too prominent. He felt that all these were feminine characteristics. The only compensatory feature he could point to was his deep voice. In early childhood, because of a faulty circumcision, other children referred to his penis as "chopped liver." He was also poor in games and clumsy in manual training.

Although the patient's analysis showed many anal trends, the genital components were prevalent in this picture. He felt more feminine than anal.

M. O., a 29-year-old woman of inferior intelligence suffered from the fear that she might have a bottle of benzine in her vagina which might explode. Only rarely was she afraid that this bottle might be in her anus. She was furthermore afraid that she might be raped on the street, so did not dare go out. At the age of seven she had a vaginal discharge, the treatment of which was very painful. In her marriage, intercourse was very painful until her child was born.

A woman of 32 had impulses to drown her boy in the bathtub or to stab him. Her chief problem in life was that she did not get enough of anything. She wanted more luxury and more pleasures. She felt that her parents never gave her what was her due. Since puberty she had had fantasies of keeping a brothel in which she treated the girls very severely and forced them to submit to the rape of men. In her earliest childhood she had many fantasies of nursing, was interested in the udders of cows, and in her dreams the motive of nursing repeatedly occurred. Her unsatisfied oral libido led to hate of her parents and to the supposition that the parents hated her since they withheld their love and approval. She had the obsession that she did not want to give anything to her children: neither clothes nor food. Especially, she did not want them to grow up. When she drank water she was reminded of the wish to drown her child. Her satisfaction would be the death of her child. The patient always felt inferior by being too fat and especially by having breasts that were too large. One might consider this case chiefly oral in character.

E. P. complained chiefly of fears of dogs and cats. In this case, motor components were prevalent. However, on the side of internal drives, anality was paramount.

M. C. had developed his motor drives, which were very strong, as a particular defense against anal aggression.

A. K., a 25-year-old man, had to think continually about the analyst catching gonorrhea and syphilis. Unconsciously he feared anal passivity against which he defended himself by vigorous counteraggression.

E. B., a 21-year-old girl, at first had an obsessive fear of being pregnant—she hadn't had any kind of sex contact. Later she developed the obsessive fear that she might get hydrophobia. For a long time this had been a firm conviction. Her earliest memory was that her uncle raised her skirt and "spit" on her buttocks.

Although in the majority of cases the anal drive prevailed, I do not doubt that there are cases in which the neurosis was chiefly based upon oral and genital drives and their transformations. Although my own material did not contain instances of this type, Hitschmann (1920) stressed the importance of urethral tendencies. The question of why these drives become the basis for an obsession remains. We have comparatively little indication for a particular constitutional strength of these internal drives. It seems that these internal drives are closely connected with aggressive drives.

A. Z., at the age of five, observed her father trying to push her mother out of the window. She had arranged with her husband to tell him before intercourse that she had had sex relations with other men. The husband then started to upbraid her and to call her all kinds of names. The intercourse was then very satisfactory. The husband, however, was inclined to treat her badly outside of the intercourse situation; this she did not particularly enjoy. This patient was afraid that she might be a homosexual. She thought female homosexuals have a growth which they use for intercourse. She did not consider the passive female homosexual a homosexual at all. The patient had homosexual play with her sister in her later childhood. The problems of sexuality were in the closest relation to submission and revolt. She used her obsessions as a method of fighting against her husband and her mother-in-law. It had been mentioned that in her sex fantasies she was dominant over the girls in her brothel; and, furthermore, that the girls were forced into submission by the men.

R. U., a 32-year-old man who was very proud of his athletic ability, developed a hernia and had to be operated on. He felt that he had lost his potency and developed an obsessional fear of being infected in the wound. He had fears of bacteria, and believed that he was the only one who adequately appreciated the danger of bacteria and infection. His pride in his athletic ability was extended to his pride in his intellectual capacity. This feeling not only gave him intellectual superiority but also the possibility of dominating the whole family.

K. L. was always afraid that her husband might get the upper hand, and continually asked herself what she would do in his place or what he would do in her place.

In the obsessive and compulsive neurosis, the individual often wants to gain the upper hand by his internal drives. The internal drives come in close relation to the problems of inferiority and superiority. These, in turn, are dependent on general human relations between the child and his parents. These human relations are also of a libidinal—pregenital and genital—type.

The internal drives are never isolated. They are in close relation to factors of interpersonal relations and defenses—the ego in the psychoanalytic sense. The ego, as well as the internal drives, has its own motility. Out of the interaction of the human relations and the internal drives arise problems of superiority and inferiority, activity and passivity, aggression and submission. Conflicts between the ego and internal drives will finally lead to an expression in the motor sphere. These expressions in the motor sphere are more the result of general human problems than of the increase in motor drives described above.

The Symbolism of Internal Drives in Relation to Motility

When an individual, like M. C., felt overpowered by his mother, he feared that her protrusions might be pushed into his openings. For various reasons, the anal opening offered itself particularly to such usage at a time when the child had not yet discovered the vagina or felt uncertain of the distinction between the two openings. Aggression may, and does, emanate from parents of both sexes. The aggression-submission problem transgresses sex differentiation. Aggression and protrusion are then very often used as signs of masculinity. The openings and interest in openings become signs of femininity. Whenever the aggression and submission problem becomes paramount, insecurities concerning one's own sex and the choice of one's sexual partner are liable to occur. One may speak about problems of defense against an overpowering and intruding parent. The interpersonal ego problem seems to be sufficient to explain the psychological complications concerning anality and bisexuality occurring in obsessive and compulsive neuroses. However, the particular course of the psychological problem may be connected with constitutional factors concerning internal drives. We know, on the other hand, that superiority and inferiority problems are in close relation to the external drives. One can prove that these external drives are, at least in some cases, organically and constitutionally changed. The internal drives, in turn, have their own motor power, and the conflict between these motor powers and the motor power emanating from the ego and the external drives are of fundamental importance. The external drives serve as reinforcement of internal drives as well as of interpersonal drives.

The obsessive-compulsive neurosis in which motor phenomena are of proven importance, and the obsessive-compulsive neurosis in which the internal drives are paramount lead to a very similar picture. One cannot even say that compulsions have a closer relation to external drives. In the long run, motility belongs to every part of the personality.

The Genesis of Aggression

E. P. felt constantly attacked by his parents, especially his father. He was afraid that he might be cut to pieces and dismembered, and that his father might bite off his sex organ. This fear was transferred from his father and mother to cats and dogs. It was a fear in connection with motor aggression. He did not only fear motor aggression, he also feared aggression which might come from the excreta of his parents, from saliva, from feces, and from urine. This corresponds to the findings of Melanie Klein (1932).

He was in danger of being pushed into a definite inferior position by such an attack. Something might be pushed into his openings; his penis might be bitten off, and he might be contaminated by what was put into his mouth. There was, of course, the greater danger of the dismembering and destruction of his body. Although the patient experienced the attack by motor forces and poison directed against the outside and inside of his body as fear and anxiety, he nevertheless got satisfactions out of the inferior position, and was partially inclined to submit. He wished particularly that something should be pushed into his anus. He was inclined to face neither the danger nor his drives, and had to experience them in a symbolic way. Animals were substituted for the parents, and hygienic motives were given as the reason for his fear of his mother's saliva.

The counterreactions were manifold. The patient ran away from cats and dogs in a phobic way. He considered some of his thoughts as not belonging to him, and experienced them as obsessions and compulsions. He was very much inclined to counteraggression, and felt justified in being aggressive. He accepted many of his internal drives and enjoyed them again and again. He discharged some of his aggression in motor urges and in repetitions. Furthermore, he showed strong tendencies to identify himself with another person who was given an enema or had anal characteristics which interested him. This identification gave him a greater anal satisfaction. However, his fear that by touching an animal his skin might receive animal-like properties showed that he experienced identification as a danger even though it also gave him satisfaction.

This patient, as well as other patients, derived a part of his aggression from preceding attacks of others. Aggressiveness is therefore experienced by the patients as reactive aggressiveness.

It was also the case with M. C. These patients even experienced an aggressiveness based upon increased external drive as counter-aggression. Obsessions and compulsions come from a double source: from the fear of being attacked and from the continued preoccupation with such fear; from the countermeasures against dismembering, castration, poisoning, and contaminations. Attack and counterattack are not tolerated by the total organization of the personality. To be sure, this is only a very superficial and incomplete discussion.

Guilt Feelings

Aggression and submission are closely related to each other. By projection and identification one regularly plays both parts at once. It seems more than plausible that aggressiveness and increased destructive tendencies are a child's answer to the fear of destruction and to the fear of being pushed into the inferior role. Since the threatening forces which demand submission are still present and are incorporated into the personality by the projection, a strong but dissociated superego will force the individual to develop strong feelings of guilt in connection with aggression. The feelings of guilt will be increased when the individual becomes aware of his normal or reactively increased internal drive. Alexander (1927) and Bergler (1936) have particularly pointed to the fact that a very severe superego puts unjust demands on the individual. Finally, the individual succeeds in evading exaggerated demands. These authors, as well as Federn (1933), have described in detail the complicated reactions and counterreactions between internal drives, interpersonal drives, and the superego. It seems that the individual demands from himself absolute exactness, isolation of the obsessions from other parts of the psychic life, and absence of doubt. I have shown above, in discussing the motility of obsessive neurotics, how the increase in motor drives makes it impossible to act as a unified individual. Drives fight continually against the forces which counteract the drives. The drives—internal and external—are also a part of the personality and try to devaluate the severity of the demands of the superego.

The State of Consciousness

The general picture of obsessive neurosis seems to show a patient who is clear and reasons with particular perspicacity. Furthermore, it has been stated that the obsessive and compulsive neurotic patients are always aware that the contents of the obsessions and compulsions are not part of their own strivings or of reality. Even superficial observation shows that, at the height of the obsession, the patients lose their judgment. They become delusional. For instance, R. O. believed, even in quiet times, that he would be a victim of bacterial infection. B. O., a 21-year-old girl, was convinced that she would die from hydrophobia. Torn between impulses and counterimpulses, the patients answered with confusion. Obsessions very often have a dreamlike quality, and representations have particular intensity and clearness. The patients saw themselves perform the act which they dreaded.

T. H. was convinced that a dog had performed cunnilingus on her. A patient, mentioned in my previous communication, experienced the contents of obsessions as hallucinatory reality with the help of drugs. Even patients without primary motility disturbance spoke forbidden sentences to themselves. A. K. had the analyst continually with him, and conversed with the analyst as if he were present. One can generally say that obsessions and compulsions lead to an intensification of representations which receive eidetic and sometimes hallucinatory characteristics. The motor impulses express themselves in actions or speech of low intensity. The dreamlike state, as such, facilitates the breaking through of forbidden impulses.

The Obsessive Character and Impulsions

This section deals primarily with neurotic symptoms and not with the obsessive and compulsive character. The obsessive and compulsive character is based upon the same interplay between external, internal, and interpersonal drives. However, in the neurotic symptom, the internal or external drive breaks through more or less transformed—according to the mechanisms described above—and the ego of the patient continues to defend itself against the drive. When the individual has made peace between the ego and the drives, character trends appear. The obsessive character is the sum total of compromises between the ego, superego, and id. In some of these patients, very far-reaching character deviations may appear. The individuals may be misers, hoarders, cruel moralists, collectors, and so forth. The individual may even be of the opinion that his impulses are all right, and he may follow them more or less openly. Bender and I (1940) have shown that, in children, drives of which the child approves are in the foreground. We have called this particular type of childhood urge an *impulsion,* and have stated that this form is in close relation to the obsessive and compulsive neurosis of adolescents. The interpersonal relations and the superego in children have not led to an organized defense. Of course, therapy may be concerned not only with symptoms but also with character. The relation between the two is continually changing. The fundamental problem is the change in the internal and external drives and the organization of a counterreaction. If this counterreaction is weak, then the picture is that of an impulsion. Then the impulsion may be a symbolic expression of a deeper wish. If the counterorganization is strong enough, it leads to the formation of a symptom, and to varying conflicts between the symptoms and the total personality. The individual may, himself, approve of his impulsions. However, these impulsions will be more symbolic than the impulsions of childhood. If the impulsions can be brought into harmony with interpersonal relations, we speak about obsessive character. The obsessive character may be more or less approved by society. This will reflect indirectly on the attitude of the individual toward his personality and character. There is a complicated play between what the individual allows himself of forbidden drives in symptoms, impulsions, and character trends, and what the ego and superego of the patient demand and forbid. The parts of the personality may vie for domination in the total personality and may try to cheat each other.

In some of the cases it is probable that the difficulty started with a disorganization of the external drives. In another group of cases, the family situation provoked a change in the internal drives. This change may have been facilitated by constitutional elements, although we do not have definite proofs of this. The change in the internal drives will influence the external drives. All drives finally end in motility.

We have reason to believe that the obsessive and compulsive neurotic individual feels attacked by motor forces in the outer world, by aggression and attack from other individuals. This attack from others can originate in their motility or in their poisonous excreta such as sputum, feces, and urine. If the individual is in danger of being pushed into an inferior, dependent position, and if his integrity is threatened, he will answer by aggression of external and internal kinds. Both may be reinforced by constitutional and organic factors.

Therapy

Among the twenty cases utilized in this study, four could not be sufficiently influenced by therapy. Two of these are still under treatment, with no particular chance of success. One other patient left after treatment of four months; he was unimproved. Two other patients left of their own accord without having been helped. Of the remaining sixteen cases, seven are improved so far that one may, for all practical purposes, consider them cured. All the character deviations have not disappeared, but they are either free from symptoms or the symptoms have lost all importance and their adaptation to life is fairly successful. Five of the remaining cases show considerable improvement, and four are moderately improved. These results must be interpreted as very satisfactory, considering the severity of the neuroses treated.

The treatment has to be based upon the insight of the patient into the way in which his external and internal drives have made their appearance in all important life situations and human relations. In order to gain this insight, the full armamentarium of psychoanalytic technique has to be used, and the patient must be shown in every instance in which way the contents of his experiences are the expression of the mechanisms described above. He will be helped if his experiences are brought forward in a group. Individual interviews, however, will be necessary at given phases of treatment. I have found it advantageous to have the patients draw whatever comes into their minds, or to draw their dreams. The analysis of the contents must go hand in hand with the analysis of form. It is of particular importance that the patients understand the relation of their symptoms to their motility and aggression. It is, furthermore, necessary that the patient not conceive of his motor drives as isolated phenomena, but as a part of a total situation between him, his love objects of the past, and society.

CHAPTER SEVEN

The Concept of Hysteria

The modern development of medical psychology and psychotherapy started with studies in hysteria. Bernheim (1889), Charcot (1873), Janet (1894), and Breuer and Freud (1893-1895) derived many of their conclusions from the study of cases of hysteria. Freud's fundamental paper "Fragment of an Analysis of a Case of Hysteria" (1905a) finished this epoch. Toward the beginning of this century, the interest in other forms of neuroses increased, whereas interest in the psychology of hysteria diminished. This interest was revived during and after World War I, but quickly subsided again. Parallel to the decline of medical interest in hysteria went a change in the symptomatology which has been noted by many observers, for example, Wilder (1935).

Pisk (1936) found among the 3,840 cases of hysteria he observed in the Viennese Clinic over a ten-year period (1925-1935) many instances with striking signs of major hysteria, but the "grand attacks" were missing. The greatest number were women, but the number of psychopaths was greater among men. This dramatic picture has become rare, and the symptomatology of hysteria has become more modest. Even when there is a "grand attack," it is less spectacular, and the fantastic somnambulistic states have been superseded by less dramatic amnesias of shorter duration. Hysteria now often appears combined with the picture

---

Appeared originally in *The American Journal of Psychiatry*, 95:1389-1413, 1939.

of an organic disease, with and without physiological and anatomical changes. But since hysteria still remains a fundamental problem—not only for medical psychology but for medicine in general—it seems advisable to try again to discuss the concept.

The number of cases diagnosed as hysteria in a large admission such as at the Psychiatric Division of Bellevue Hospital is considerable. Among the 25,260 admissions in the year 1937, for example, 219 cases were listed as hysteria for primary diagnosis. These 219 cases were distributed into the subgroups of the official classification in the following way:

	Male	Female
Anxiety hysteria	21	23
Conversion hysteria	23	30
Anesthetic type	2	2
Paresthetic type	3	0
Hyperkinetic type	9	8
Amnesic type	46	32
Mixed hysteria	12	8

At the same time there were in the hospital 385 reactive depressions among men and 393 among women. In the classification of The American Psychiatric Association the reactive depressions are not listed among hysterias, although in their structure they belong to hysteria.

The total number of psychoneuroses listed was 1,321. Even this number does not give a definite idea of the problem, since in many other cases hysteria was listed as secondary diagnosis.

Furthermore, we have to take into consideration that the revival of interest in psychosomatic diseases and the psychogenesis of organic symptoms is historically closely related to the study of the problem of hysteria.

It is difficult to give a halfway complete enumeration of hysterical symptoms. They may be roughly divided into psychic, motor, sensory, and vegetative symptoms. In the motor sphere we find paralyses of varying types, motor fits with or without loss of consciousness, and, finally, chronic hyperkinesias. In the sensory sphere we find anesthesias, paresthesias, and hyperesthesias in all senses. In the vegetative sphere we find vasomotor phenomena more or less outspoken, changes in the pulse rate, and all kinds of changes in the secretion and in the motility of the gastrointestinal tract. The phenomena in the vegetative sphere very often have a more or less outstanding organic character. Somatic functions are really impaired. In the comparatively rare hysterical impotency, we obviously deal with a real change in the vegetative function, and in hysterical vaginal anesthesia the lack of secretion is most evident. By inference we may say that in hysterical motor, sensory, and psychic phenomena, as well, something is happening in the body. This becomes more apparent since, after all, the separation of these four spheres is more or less artificial. The unit of behavior is a sensory-motor-vegetative one in relation to a specific situation in the field of consciousness; we find a clouding which always remains superficial, confusions of the same type, and hallucinations of more or less dramatic character. Since we deal with a person who acts, we must of necessity think that changes in behavior are closely associated with changes in consciousness.

Organic changes provoked by the attitude of the hysterical patient do not arouse merely passing symptoms in the organic function. The disturbance may go further and excite a lasting functional change of an organ (organ neurosis) and even an anatomical change (organic disease in the narrower sense).

A great part of hysterical symptomatology consists in physical suffering. The hysterical patient seems to be afflicted with disease. However, in the majority of cases, this disease is not accompanied by disturbances of the organic function and structure. It remains an open question whether this formulation is not merely conventional, since we do not generally regard organic disease as the simple consequence of psychological attitudes. I define as hysteria, psychological processes that lead to symptoms of physical suffering which are not accompanied by physiological and organic changes. However, we must also include in a definition of hysteria the psychological symptoms of the fugue state and the hallucinations. These are to be differentiated from similar occurrences in psychoses in the narrower sense by the fact that the psychic symptomatology of hysteria is not connected with a definite disturbance in the biological orientation. The pseudologia phantastica on a hysterical basis is, in this respect, clearly differentiated from hallucinations and confabulations and delusions. As far as anxiety occurs in hysteria it is less persistent and less rigid than in an anxiety neurosis or in psychoses.

In the definition of hysteria one has to place emphasis on the absence of severe physiological and organic changes (in relation to the physical complaint) and also on the absence of a deeper biological adaptation disturbance (in the psychological sphere). The hysterical complaint is fundamentally different from the hypochondriacal complaint, which is much more absorbing and a sign of a deeper difficulty in psychological adaptation. Hysteria can be considered a well-defined symptomatological unit.

Hysteria is not the only psychogenic sequence which leads to a symptomatology of physical illness. Since I do not believe in anything but sensory-motor-vegetative behavior units, one has to expect that every type of neurosis will have a specific physical side. There is no doubt that this expectation is amply proven by experience. Obsessional neuroses, for instance, very often have outspoken gastrointestinal symptomatology. The organic phenomena in depressions such as changes in blood pressure and in gastrointestinal function should be mentioned. I once tabulated hysterical conversion symptoms in comparison with neurasthenic conversion symptoms [see Table 1, p. 58, above]. Also, neurasthenia is a well-circumscribed type of neurosis. One has frequently spoken about the riddle of conversion. According to my opinion it would be a riddle if psychic processes which have no somatic expression should suddenly appear. The problem of hysterical conversion is, therefore, not why the physical symptomatology appears, but merely why these particular physical symptoms make their appearance.

In order to understand these physical symptoms we have to ask which kind of human being the hysterical person is. On which basis does this particular symptomatology which is psychophysiological appear? We are here not so much interested in the question of constitution and heredity. The data on this point are not only incomplete but also exposed to doubts since the seeming heredity might be based on identifications taking place in the family, especially in early childhood. Kraulis (1931) and Szondi (1936) find many such cases of hysteria among the siblings, children, parents, and their siblings. There are also a great number of epileptics and criminals among the blood relations of hysteria cases. Weygandt (1936) found many schizophrenics in the families of cases of hysteria.

One should not overrate the difference between human beings. Although human beings show specific patterns from early childhood, they also have all the other patterns and tendencies latent in themselves, and they make use of them under situations which are particularly favorable to bring out these patterns. Hysteria is a pattern which corresponds to a definite early situation, as we shall later see. However, such a pattern might be given up, and under the stress of circumstances other neurotic or characterological designs may appear. For various reasons, to be discussed later, we suppose that the hysterical pattern has to be developed in the majority of human beings. Such a pattern may be stressed either habitually or under the strain of particular situations.

The hysterical pattern may be more or less in readiness and may be more in the foreground or in the background of the personality structure. In the first case we speak about the psychoneurosis hysteria with which the connotation of the hysterical character is intimately correlated. In the second case we speak about hysterical symptoms in a hysterical reaction. It is obvious that such a differentiation cannot be absolute, but the fact that one has not kept these differentiations clearly in mind has caused much confusion in psychiatric literature. Immediately after World War I, inappropriate conclusions were drawn from acute hysterical reactions; one thought that a simple way had been found to explain the psychoneurosis hysteria. Even Kretschmer (1923) was not free from this mistake. Every individual who has access to reality prefers under certain circumstances to forget this reality and tries to find a simple way out. Such simple escape reactions can be found in a war neurosis, in the hysteriform reactions of prisoners which are more or less near to malingering (the Ganser syndrome in its various expressions), and in the amnesias in criminal cases. The amnesia in noncriminal cases usually has a more complicated structure (Abeles and Schilder, 1935). Even in the simplest escape reactions the personality problem is at least of some importance, as, for instance, was shown in the investigations of Simmel (1919) concerning war neuroses. Even so, there is a wide difference between the psychoneurosis hysteria and the hysterical symptom which chiefly serves as an escape from a difficult situation.

In order to understand hysterical symptoms one has to understand the psychoneurosis hysteria. Freud's (1905a) classical analysis of Dora still gives the best insight into the deeper mechanisms of hysteria. Here is found a deep attachment to the parent of the other sex. The attachment was principally a genital one, although pregenital elements were present. The affection for the father was partially expressed in urinary symptoms (enuresis). The main symptom was coughing. It was based on oral tendencies (penilingus). Freud attributes the incompleteness of the results attained to his neglect in analyzing the homosexual components in the case. The girl was deeply engrossed in admiration of the body of the father's sweetheart. Positive transference was easily obtained. However, the positive transference was soon followed by a negative one, which led to the interruption of the treatment. Dora's coughing was based on a real organic ailment, a slight catarrh. The sick organ became the nucleus of conversion (organic compliance).

I shall now illustrate some of these mechanisms with my own observations.

Ethel is a 25-year-old girl who suffers from hysterical attacks in which she gets sleepy, has to lie down, cries loudly, shouts, and makes wild movements, using her whole body. The attacks have become so severe that she has had to give up her work and now lives with her father and stepmother who have a child of about one year for whom the patient has to care as, otherwise, it would be completely neglected by its mother. The patient hates the stepmother to whom her father has been married about a year and a half. The stepmother is irritable and shouts at her husband, who is amiable but weak. The patient is deeply attached to her father who, according to her opinion, is a very kind person. She cannot remember any particular caresses by her father in early childhood and no definite material has come out so far in this respect. The patient's mother had started an affair with another man when the girl was about ten years old; she finally lived with him, and divorce resulted. After this divorce from the patient's mother, the father wanted to live with another woman, but was prevented from doing so by the patient. The marriage to the stepmother was necessitated by her pregnancy.

The girl's own mother was very good to her while she was small, although she did beat her unmercifully for minor transgressions. The patient surmises that the mother was frigid, although her extramarital affairs probably started when the girl was quite young. Since her fifth year she has felt neglected by her mother and professes that she wanted to kill her. She has a sister two years older who she felt was always preferred to her by everybody. Everyone praised the sister for her beauty, whereas the patient was always considered ugly. Remarks were made especially concerning her deep-set eyes. Patient considers herself ugly. At the age between fourteen and sixteen she had a close friendship with a boy. She never had any sexual feelings, does not feel any particular sensations in her sex parts, and broke off with the boy when he wanted to caress her. At the age of twelve when she felt still more neglected by her mother, she started to complain about a pain in her abdomen, but the mother gave no attention to it. Finally, two years later, the patient had to be operated on for appendicitis. She considers this a sign that she was neglected by her mother. The patient has a psoriasis. According to her it could have been prevented if the mother had listened to her first complaints. The first outstanding symptoms occurred around the eyes. This condition improved during the psychoanalysis when the mother showed friendliness to the patient.

There was no conclusive material brought forward that strong sex wishes of the patient existed concerning the father. It is only by inference that one has to suppose they were present. Her admiration for her mother's beauty was outspoken. The tendency to take her place or the place of the stepmother appeared in no uncertain terms. The jealousy against her sister was obvious. There was an unmistakable tendency to depreciate the human body, due to the attitude of her parents. One may suspect that her psoriasis was facilitated by attitudes of this kind. Her lack of interest in sex was an attempt to deny sexuality not merely to herself but also to her mother, and at the same time to take the place of her mother who was supposedly frigid. Her appendicitis and psoriasis apparently had long latency periods in which she demanded but did not receive attention from her mother. By taking care of her newly married sister's child, and also the child of her stepmother she expressed the wish to take their places. She was very bitter in her condemnation of her mother's extramarital experiences and entertained no hope that a man might marry her because of the handicap of her psoriasis.

There was a strong attachment to the father as well as to the mother, although the deeper roots of this attachment were not revealed. There was, further, a tendency to depreciate her own body and a heroic fight against her sexuality which seemed to have completely disappeared. The hysterical attack was not only a return of the sexuality as love of the father but also imitated the screaming and struggling that occurred when she was beaten by her mother. Whatever may have been the causal factors for her appendicitis and psoriasis, in the final analysis they fit completely the psychological character of the situation. In other words, there were at least elements of conversion in these organic diseases, and they were used by the personality once they had occurred. It is worth while mentioning that the patient made a suicidal attempt in the beginning of her illness by drinking some of her father's eye drops. She immediately called for help, and nothing serious happened. The symbolic significance of this suicidal attempt needs no further comments.

The next case is more simple in its structure. Anna C., a 25-year-old woman, was admitted to the hospital on May 29, having been referred from the mental hygiene clinic which she had been attending since February 16, 1937. She complained that for one and a half years she had been having attacks in which she saw almost blinding flashes and zigzag lines of light which were mostly limited to the right half of the field of vision. Headaches in the right occipital region occasionally accompanied the attacks, but these were not a very prominent feature. At first she was nauseated and sometimes would vomit during an attack, but nausea later became a less frequent symptom. The flashes of light appeared at variable intervals of days or weeks, whenever she was worried, upset, depressed, or when her feelings had been hurt, and lasted a few minutes. At such times she would be very apprehensive lest her heart stop beating, and so she would sit holding her pulse. Between the attacks she experienced a feeling of strangeness which she found difficult to describe but in which she felt she was in a fog and that the world about her was distant and far off. She felt that she had lost her personality, that she could not talk to people as she formerly did, that they noticed something strange about her; she feared that she was going insane.

Because the patient was inaccessible otherwise, we resorted to hypnosis with sodium amytal. It was revealed that the symptoms were in immediate relation to an outward situation of extramarital intercourse in which a flashlight was used. The flashlight was a symbol for the penis of her lover whom she hated because he did not want to marry her. The lover concentrated his caresses on the right side of the patient's body which became hyperesthetic at the time of the neurosis. It was also this side of the body with which she had sometimes touched the body of her father, with whom she slept in the same bed up to the time of her adolescence. Her mother had been rejected by a previous lover and had rejected her own husband whom she considered coarse. The patient's lover corresponded to the mother's lover and to her husband. The patient identified herself with her mother; in early childhood she had a deep attachment to her beautiful mother. She was also unsuccessful in this relation and tried, at three years of age, to jump out of the window because her mother refused to let her wear the dress of her choice; the mother also used to beat her unmercifully. The migraine appeared as a distorted intercourse equivalent. The feeling of being in a fog imitated the narrowing of consciousness during sexual excitement.

One doubtless could go deeper into the explanation of such conversion symptoms, such as coughing as has been done by Wilson (1935). Wilson (1934) also reported the analysis of a case of acute laryngitis occurring as a conversion symptom. The case was one of sleepwalking and psychic impotence. The patient also suffered from severe nightmares. Wulff (1933) tried to prove that the hysterical attack was a repetition of infantile movements, but did not offer very convincing material. His patient's fits were a repetition of actual scenes of being beaten in childhood.

A 30-year-old Negro woman with an I.Q. of 63 who was always striving to improve her mental status, felt continually mistreated by her father to whom she otherwise had a deep attachment. She complained about bleeding from the gums and from the nose, headaches, indigestion, gas in the stomach, weakness on the left side of her body, and bleeding from the nipple of the left breast (which was due to cystic change in the breast). She was completely frigid, but had three children. She had intercourse and married merely because she had hoped that in this way she might recover from her various ailments. In her eagerness for education, she tried to imitate her mother. From earliest childhood she had a disgust for male genitals. The father beat not only the children but the mother as well, and the children were continually hungry. The father ran away from home when the patient was seven years old, and she went to a Catholic school where she worked for two years. She never had the affection she wanted, and this continued throughout her whole life.

One often sees that hysterical phenomena are particularly severe in persons with limited intellectual endowment. In this case it is remarkable that finally an organic ailment developed in the breast, which had given her vicarious satisfaction, inasmuch as all her neurotic troubles had disappeared when she had nursed her last child.

Twenty-eight-year-old Gene lost her father when she was two years old, and after that, like her mother, was afraid of the dark. She was afraid that dead people might come and take her away. She used to sleep in the same bed with her mother until she was seventeen, and afterward, too, whenever she was afraid. Her sex relations with her husband were generally satisfactory, but lately had not been good. And at the time of treatment her husband was sorry about that. She had heard that one becomes pregnant only when there was an orgasm, so she had tried to suppress her orgasms because she did not want any more children. She collapsed, felt weak, could not breathe or talk.

Her attacks usually followed superficial conflicts, once when she saw a fight between two men, and again when she was threatened with dispossession. Our material contains numerous instances of similar type.

One of our cases, a twenty-year-old girl, had fainting spells preceded by palpitations which came after quarrels with her numerous boy friends with whom sex relations were always unsatisfactory. Her first memory was that of seeing her dead brother lying in a coffin when she was four years old. She remembered that her father, who often was drunk, had had similar spells. Her father was a strong man. He left the home when the patient was about eight, and divorced the mother. At that time he repeatedly forced her to have intercourse with him. The patient said: "I have terrible nightmares about animals." (What kind of animals?) "Mice and monkeys." (What do the monkeys want to do to you?) "They just want to kill me or something. The mice—I look at them and I want to get out of the room and I can't; they're all around me. They don't crawl into my sex parts. . . . Oh yes, I am otherwise afraid of mice. They come up my legs." (Do you have sexual feelings when you have these dreams?) "Yes." (It is stronger than the sexual feeling you have when you masturbate?) "Yes. . . . My boy friend is very strong and I like very strong men. I like my boy friend to weigh between 150 and 175 pounds. My boy friend weighs 160 pounds."

In a 44-year-old patient with repeated amnesia attacks and also loss of consciousness, one of the attacks (which was analyzed) occurred when she wanted to bring roses for her father's grave. She was deeply attached to her father and frequently dreamed of him. Under hypnosis she brought out the following material: She was the middle child of three living daughters in a family of five children. For as long as she could remember—up to the time she was married at the age of nineteen—she slept with her father while her mother slept on chairs nearby. Each of the other sisters had a bed of her own. She never remembered her mother sleeping in her father's bed in all those nineteen years. She denied any sex relations with her father, although on one occasion she did say that she would be crucified before she would admit it. She was married at the age of nineteen only because she felt it was wrong to be sleeping with her father at so advanced an age, and then she chose a man who resembled her father and whom she called "Daddy." With this man she has always been frigid in her sex relations. At five years of age she was in an auto accident in which she suffered concussion of the brain and was unconscious for a few minutes, but was not taken to a hospital.

This case increases our knowledge, in so far as we can see, that an early childhood accident is used as a pattern by which she expresses her erotic attitudes toward her father. This case was not deeply enough analyzed; otherwise it would have been found that the patient not only strove for recognition and affection by her father but also for the affection of her mother.

In a fifteen-year-old Negro girl with outspoken homosexual tendencies, an attachment to an aunt played an important part. Her wishes were to be strong, athletic, and at the same time to prove that Negro girls could be as good as white girls. She had an amnestic attack with a hallucination of her dead mother.

A patient who has been observed for years, had innumerable operations on her tonsils, abdomen, and genitals, suffered from asthma and hay fever, and had attacks of fear that she might die suddenly. It was a deep-seated character disorder in which early fears concerning her mother and father played the most prominent part. She was intensely attached to both of them. She was particularly gifted in acquiring new diseases and, if there were no other possibilities, she had an abortion. Although she was not frigid, she was usually hindered by one or the other of her pains or spasms from enjoying sex relations.

In the hysterical character there is a tendency to build up a strong attachment to both parents. The attachment to the parent of the opposite sex prevails (see Fenichel, 1934). This attachment is connected with decided genital sensations or genital activity. In many of our cases, more or less close actual contact of the girl with the father had been reported, and in one instance there was a report of early sex relations with the father. The actual conflict obviously recalls the previous attitudes, which later on are transferred into the symptom by the mechanism of conversion. The conversion is based on either an actual scene experienced in childhood, a disease observed in another, or a previous organic disease. There is always a real event at the basis of conversion. In this event the body image of one's own somatic experience or that of others always plays the most important part. The conversion is based upon childhood experiences, but the later organic trauma may be the nucleus and pattern for the final formation of the symptoms. Amnesia and memory disturbances, for instance, often occur in patients who have suffered from an organic unconsciousness due to either trauma or carbon monoxide poisoning. Erickson (1937) reports that by hypnosis he had prevented such a subsequent organic unconsciousness.

In all cases of true hysteria, the psychogenic problem remains paramount. However, there are all kinds of variations of interaction between psychological attitudes as described, pictures in which the organic problem is in the foreground, and those in which the particular hysterical attitude becomes less and less important. Hysterical attitudes may prevail when the organic disease is either not so severe, or in its beginning, or at its decline. If the organic disease is severe, attitudes come into appearance which try to neglect the organic disease as akin to hysteria. At any rate, the indifference which one has so often observed in the hysterical patient concerning his or her symptoms has a close relation to the attitude of the organic case.

Most of the cases thus far discussed have been women. But there are just as many men suffering from hysteria. A comparatively large number of these are cases of amnesias, which are the most common subgroup of hysteria in our statistics. In women, conversion hysteria seems to be more frequent. Reactive depression is listed separately in the statistics of The American Psychiatric Association, and in the year 1937 there were in Bellevue Hospital 385 cases in men and 393 cases in women. The reactive depressions are, according to their structure, hysterias in which the present situation plays an outstanding part. It is true that as my own investigations and those of Feigenbaum (1926) have shown, particular pregenital components are present in this group. Furthermore, a large number of hysteriform reactions are to be seen in prisoners where the differentiation from malingering may sometimes be difficult.

Our material shows that there is no fundamental difference in the basic structure of the hysterical symptoms in men and women. However, in the cases of male hysteria with severe conversion symptoms, as far as they were accessible to psychological approach, social factors played a particularly important part. Very often the hysterical character change appeared after more or less serious social reversals, as in a 60-year-old Armenian who developed a severe hysterical paralysis which persisted for several years. He also had a hysterical mutism. His hysterical symptoms did not hinder him from embezzling, and at the time of the observation he was a prisoner. He was characterized by particular religiousness, was very mild and pleasant in his whole attitude, and was completely contented in spite of his hysterical symptoms which, as has been mentioned, were present before his offense was committed.

Another of our patients with a similar symptomatology who could be interviewed only under sodium amytal, had scruples concerning smoking; feelings of guilt connected with it offered the superficial motivation concerning his hysterical symptoms. He also had worried about his participation in the C.I.O.

In a number of cases, accidents preceded the hysterical symptomatology. Some of these accidents were head injuries followed by unconsciousness and even organic signs of a lesion of the central nervous system. In some of these cases the accident merely furnished the pattern for the later psychogenic structure. In other instances, organic symptoms remained which were the nucleus around which the psychogenic structure was built up.

Fred L., 21 years old, had a skull fracture at the age of six. For eleven years he has had dizzy spells. He then cries out, "Hold me, hold me." He groans and seeks support and feels his body getting lighter. He can see only one object. He sees spots of different colors; faces become blurred; everything seems to become very large, comes nearer to him, and he himself feels small. He is afraid to go on a bridge because this would provoke a dizzy spell. Anything that goes around or is off the ground makes him dizzy. Dizzy attacks could be produced when he was ordered to close his eyes and stretch out his hand. Whenever such a spell comes on, he grabs for support. The patient has given up all ambitions in life. He has no interest in sex; he often dreams that he is in the middle of the ocean and drowning. He also has wet dreams.

It is probable that the head injury has left minor organic changes which serve as the nucleus of the psychogenic symptom formation. There is an organic compliance, and it is to be expected that the psychogenic mechanisms not only bring the organic disturbance to a clearer focus but also increase the physiological dysfuncton. At the time of the examination, the patient still had a bilateral Hoffman sign and slight tremor in both hands. An unquestionable Babinski occasionally appeared on the left side.

The 62-year-old R. B. was hit on the head in 1929 and was unconscious for six hours. Since then he has had a weakness on the left side. It is a typical hysterical hemiparesis and hemianesthesia. His chief complaint, however, is a gastric ulcer. Although desperately poor, he is happy and contented. Another patient, 64 years old, has had seizures for the last 35 years following an accident. He has a typical right-sided hysterical hemiparesis.

Our material contains other cases in which hysterical symptoms were present in senile and presenile persons. In one case the hysterical symptoms had developed after severe financial reversals which had led to court action. The hysterical hemiparesis and hemianesthesia had developed on the left side, in which true angina pectoris pains were present. There also were states of psychogenic confusion. Throughout his whole life only moderate alcoholism had been present, but it had increased during the time of financial stress.

Only rarely is it possible in cases like the following to gain deeper insight into the psychological structure:

Charles K., 30 years old, suffers from attacks in which his hand becomes numb and itchy. Sometimes these attacks come on at night. Sometimes convulsions follow if he does not rub his hands sufficiently. He cannot sleep after such an attack, is sleepy during the next day, and falls asleep while he is at work. In 1930 he had had an accident. His cab was struck by another cab. His head was pushed against the rear of the car and he was unconscious for six or seven hours. He obtained compensation, although the amount was small since the taxicab company was failing. Repeated physical examinations, encephalogram included, were completely negative. The analysis at the present time is in the fourth month.

In his early history, his attachment to his mother was outstanding. His father left the family when the patient was two years old. He also had a strong attachment for an older brother. He was often punished by the mother, who hit him over the hands, especially when she caught him masturbating at the age of seven. He has had a great number of accidents on his hands, about which he was much concerned, and he has always had a particular interest in his hands. At the age of twenty he had a severe accident in which he broke his nose when falling from a scaffold. He fell on his hands and hurt them considerably. He always was interested in his body and felt bad that he was disfigured after the accident. His heterosexual development was rather uneventful. He had his first intercourse at fourteen and many casual contacts after that. He has been married for several years without caring particularly for his wife.

There were serious doubts whether the case did not have organic components. Protracted observation, however, makes the psychogenesis almost certain. The case shows his tendency to accidents, especially concerning the organ which was given prominence by the action of a beloved person. However, the last accident cannot be brought into connection with the patient's psychological attitudes. The case also shows the importance of social conflict in male hysterias.

Hysterical phenomena in children show with marked clarity the continuous interaction between the attitudes of the patient and of the parents. In the case of Jenny, all the fears of her childhood were closely related to the attitude of the beloved mother. I now report an instructive observation which L. Bender has made on the Children's Ward of Bellevue Hospital.

Jenny, who is thirteen years old, closely resembles her mother, and the mother has limited intelligence and some dramatic hysterical phenomena, which Jennie's behavior closely resembles. The older sister, Salvina, born of a former marriage of the mother, is now sixteen years old and has spent a period in a psychiatric institute as a child for "seeing things." The family history is filled with sickness and operations. The mother and three children have been receiving antiluetic treatment. The infection had probably come from her first husband. The present husband is said to be an alcoholic.

The history of Jennie is that she was a colicky baby and that at the age of three, after a slight cold, the mother noticed a slight strabismus which she felt had developed at that time. She claims that she has been nervous ever since then. In October, 1937, she had an operation for the strabismus, since which she has been more or less hysterical. She had also had measles, whooping cough, chicken pox, and mumps. Jennie's hysterical phenomena all relate to her body sensations. She has periods when she feels as if she is shrinking, other times when she is dizzy and going around, and sometimes she feels hot all over and gets pins and needles and pains all over. She is sometimes afraid of death and states that she is dead. Other times she has optic phenomena with blurring, seeing double, or blindness. On other occasions she cannot hear well. Almost all these phenomena have, in one way or another, been suggested by the mother. We have observed them on the ward, especially after the mother has visited. She also has periods when she is suspicious of the environment. For two days she refused to eat because she was afraid the nurses would poison her. This was the outgrowth of a hysterical excitement which the mother demonstrated on the ward, saying that she was afraid the nurses would get even by poisoning the child. These phenomena are all very superficial. The child can be quickly relieved of them and then settled down to a fairly normal adjustment until she is again disturbed by her mother.

The child is poorly developed, and although of good height, is of asthenic build; there is no evidence of approaching puberty. Blood Wassermann is negative and complete serological examination of the spinal fluid also is negative. There is a refractive error of vision as well as an alternating convergent strabismus. Hearing tests show a hearing loss of 22 percent in the right ear and 19 percent in the left ear. Hysterical phenomena cannot be entirely ruled out. Neurological examination is otherwise negative.

Our psychological tests showed that her I.Q. ranged from 63 to 69 on three tests. Her academic achievement tests were third grade in reading and spelling and fifth grade in arithmetic. She was classified as high-grade defective.

In this case, as well as in others, the low I.Q. facilitates the hysterical fixation. However, since the conflict in such cases more easily provokes the hysterical symptomatology, it is also easier to persuade the individuals to give up the symptoms. In children, an accident may play an important part in the genesis of the neurosis, as in the case of ten-year-old Oliver who showed a similar symptomatology after being hit by a truck. In such cases one can easily show that the car or truck which caused the accident symbolizes the forceful father who pushes the child into an infantile, masochistic, and dependent position.

The following conclusions can be drawn: Individuals who develop hysterical symptoms show a very close attachment to their early love object. This relation is generally stronger toward the parent of the opposite sex; however, the relations to the parent of the same sex are also very strong. These relations have a genital background. The patients have a tendency to deep inner dependence which acknowledges the superiority of the love object. One may formulate that masochistic components are of importance. The aggressiveness is mostly directed against the rival in relation to the love object. The attitude toward the rival is directed at him as a total person and is mitigated by the fact that the rival (the other parent) also is at least a potential love object. In connection with the rather deep genital relations to love objects is a lively interest in the world and a deep sense for the reality of objects. Since the early love relation does not lead to complete satisfaction, tendencies to identification with love objects of both sexes play an important part, which later on lead to a tendency to imitation. It is a matter of course that pregenital tendencies of the oral, urethral, and anal spheres are also present, and the symptomatology of hysteria is often determined by the relation between the pregenital and genital drives. However, the genital drives prevail. Since there has been a fairly complete Oedipus complex, a rather strong superego is built up. It is in connection with this strength of the superego that amnesia plays a very important part. One may at least have the suspicion that the importance of the conversion mechanism is so great in hysterical cases for the same reason. When the conversion mechanism provokes hallucinations and confusions, the strong fundamental relation to reality still remains. However, the conversion mechanism has the power to change physiological mechanisms and sooner or later may lead to organic changes.

One generally has the tendency to consider the psychic, motor, and sensory phenomena of hysteria as lying in a purely psychological sphere. However, my own studies have convinced me that they can be very well understood from the point of view of brain physiology. This is especially clear with regard to the sleep mechanism, which is so often severely disturbed in cases of hysteria. (See Kauders and Schilder, 1923). Van Bogaert (1935) has made a thorough study of this problem. (Also compare Malamud, 1934.)

Conclusions

Early disappointment in the relation to the parents plays a leading part in the structure of hysteria. Later traumas bring this early disappointment into the foreground again. In the early relations to parents, organic disease plays a very important part. It makes the individual still more dependent upon the parent. It also concentrates the love of the parent on the child. Organic ailment is, therefore, of fundamental importance for the whole psychology of hysteria. It reinforces the masochistic attitude in the person afflicted. The affinity of the hysterical patient to organic disease and trauma has to be considered from this angle. Hysteria thus becomes the expression of suffering by disease in its human and social aspects. It reflects the helplessness and dependence of the child on the love of the parents. From this angle it becomes understandable that the actual cause of the hysterical difficulties in women is often to be found in erotic disappointments, whereas in men the social conflict and an accident play the most important part. At any rate, the person afflicted with hysteria addresses himself to a highly organized social structure. The hysterical patient acknowledges reality, but he cannot get a definite hold on it. Therefore, he is curious, eager, and full of interest in human beings.

The transient hysterical symptom is thus based upon the same mechanism as the chronic hysterical symptom and the hysterical personality. However, even the transient hysterical symptom is only possible when the individual has reached the level of the Oedipus complex and also the level of a lively interest in the outer world. The individual takes refuge in the symptom when the erotic or social situation becomes too prohibitive.

On the basis of this discussion, it becomes obvious that attitudes which lead to hysterical symptoms are facilitated by organic disease. However, it is of fundamental importance to note that such attitudes asking for erotic and social help are present only in those organic diseases which are not too severe. In general, it will be found in chronic diseases or at the beginning or the decline of an acute disease. If the organic disease is at its height or completely incapacitating, the individual will get full social recognition for it without hysterical symptoms.

Our material contains a great number of cases of organic disease with hysterical symptoms. But one should not speak of hysteria when the patient merely has an attitude of neglect toward organic symptoms as is true of many organic cases, or where the individual does not make a fight to live in face of organic disease. One should adhere to the definition that hysterical symptoms are the expression of the attitude of love toward the parents in a symbolic form. As with all products of unconscious thinking, many tendencies are condensed in the hysterical symptom. Whatever the share of pregenital and destructive tendencies in the hysterical symptom may be, it is less than the share of the tendencies in immediate connection with the Oedipus complex. This is, after all, the definition of hysteria.

It is difficult to decide when the Oedipus complex makes its appearance. Many analysts believe that genitality and the Oedipus complex make their appearance before the third year, and my own observations point in the same direction. Hysteriform phenomena have been observed in children at the age of one and a half years. However, it seems to me that the structure of these cases is not identical with the structure of cases of hysteria. They probably represent comparatively simple emotional outbursts in which aggressive and destructive impulses prevail. The conversion connected with their outbursts is different in its mechanism from one of strictly hysterical type (see Friedjung, 1925).

We speak of the hysterical character in individuals who easily develop hysterical attitudes or who retain such symptoms through a longer span of their lives. I have also observed hysterical symptoms in schizophrenias; however, they were merely in connection with those parts of the personality which have obtained a fuller adaptation to reality. One finds, accordingly, hysterical phenomena in almost every type of neurosis and psychosis.

I want again to emphasize that the hysterical conversion is not the only expression of psychological problems of the body. Neuresthenic, obsessive, depressive, and schizophrenic conversions also exist. Every level of psychological adaptation has its own way of expressing itself in the body. It should be emphasized not only that the conversion symptom is an expression of psychological tendencies, but also that the conversion symptom often uses as a pattern physiological and anatomical sequelae of organic diseases. The organism not only has a life dependent on the psyche, it also has one of its own. Every organic disease has an influence on, and brings into the foreground, specific behavior patterns and tendencies. The unity of the psychophysiological organism is dependent on both the soma and the psyche.

Finally, the structure of the conversion symptoms cannot be understood unless we get a clear insight of what individuals know about their bodies, and in what specific parts of their bodies they have particular pride. The image of their body which they have is dependent upon how much attention their bodies as a whole, as well as specific parts of their bodies, receive from other persons, especially parents. In hysteria, where the social and human relations with other human beings are so outspoken, this becomes especially evident. The body image of the hysterical case has been built up in its love relationships with the parents. Organic disease modifies it, depending upon the attitudes of the parents to the organic disease, in addition to the immediate changes which are provoked by the organic disease itself.

In order to treat any case of hysteria and, for that matter, any case of organic disease, it is necessary to have insight into the fundamental problems of hysteria. If one understands these, it is not difficult, in many cases, to show the problems to the patient and to help him to a better adaptation in his situation (compare Yaskin, 1936). The problem of hysteria is fundamentally one of social contact with other human beings under the aspect of suffering. It is not sufficient to study the psychosexual development of the hysteria case; one has to widen the problem into that of interhuman relations. If there has been a basic difficulty in the family relationships during childhood, long, continued psychoanalysis or group psychotherapy will become necessary. In other cases, the correct attitude of the physician will help the patient to regain full adaptations to his love objects and to the society he has abandoned under the stress of a situation in the present which revived difficulties encountered in childhood.

Physicians often have misjudged the depth of suffering of the patient afflicted with hysteria. They have seen in such a patient a helpless individual who, like a child, leans upon a stronger person. They have blamed the patient for his struggle for love and his tendencies to imitation. These mistakes have found a classical expression in the theories of Babinski (1934) who made an artificial separation between the hysteria which is purely of the suggestible type and the so-called physiogenic or organic disturbances.

Hysteria is a form of human suffering which affects the psychophysiological person. It is only when we understand the seriousness of the problem that we can help the hysterical patient to the fuller social adaptation for which he struggles. Hysterical symptoms, organ neuroses, and organic diseases are forms of human suffering closely related to each other.

CHAPTER EIGHT

Types of Anxiety Neuroses

It was a great step forward when Freud (1926) stated that anxiety is a reaction to danger.[1] That danger may be an external or an internal one. According to Freud, anxiety is a danger signal on the part of the ego, which initiates repression. The internal danger, in his view, is a perception of rising sexual impulses in connection with the Oedipus complex. If the patient were to give way to his sexual impulses he would be in danger of being punished: the love of either parent might be withdrawn from him. Furthermore, the boy might suffer castration, mutilation, and dismemberment. These formulations go beyond the Freudian insofar as Freud considers only castration the final threat. As usual, he considers mainly the boy's castration fear and thinks of the structure of the girl's castration fear as equivalent to that of the boy. I have repeatedly stated that, in my view, the castration complex of the girl differs fundamentally from that of the boy. The girl is afraid that her sexual organ may be occluded; and beyond this, she has a fear of losing the receptacles within her body and of having no organs in which she could receive and hold either a male sexual organ or a child.

The external danger is, for the most part, incompletely de-

Appeared originally in *The International Journal of Psycho-Analysis*, 22:209-228, 1941.

[1]Compare with my formulations in *Medical Psychology* (1924), which was published before Freud's book.

scribed in psychoanalytical literature. If a child loses the love of his parents, he is threatened not only with lack of love but also with lack of food and loss of equilibrium. There is, furthermore, a danger of mutilation and dismemberment. The final fear of death summarizes all these dangers and, moreover, includes a fear of being deprived of the power of movement.

Melanie Klein (1932) has justly pointed to another fundamental fear, namely, the fear of being deprived of the inside of the body. I have already mentioned that the girl may be afraid of losing the genitals as receptacles. There is, however, a further fear of being deprived of the gastrointestinal tract and of the whole inside of the body—a fear which is, of course, common to both boys and girls. Experiences with schizophrenics have shown me that the patient may also be afraid of being deprived of the food he has ingested and of his feces. This fear is linked with the fear of being deprived of food, since in our "unconscious" the infantile idea is still alive that the inside of the body consists of the food which has been ingested into the body (Schilder and Wechsler, 1935). Bromberg and I (1933b) have shown that fears of castration and dismemberment form the main content of the picture in alcoholic hallucinosis. I have seen these fears reach a peak in a patient suffering from alcoholic hallucinosis who was threatened by voices declaring that everything would be taken out of his body so that he would consist only of bones and the skin drawn over them; he finally experienced this process in fantasy.

Further, Melanie Klein is right when she states that the child regards as his weapons of aggression not only his striped muscles in motor action, but also his feces and urine, which may burn and eat away parts of the body.

It is to be expected that an individual threatened with the dangers we have enumerated will not, and can not, react to these dangers merely by giving in and by suffering this terrible punishment. Furthermore, he will experience more aggression from others the more aggression there is in himself. In other words, the aggressiveness which is feared from other people is in part the projection of one's own aggressiveness. It has also to be considered that the sexual instinct is in itself combined with aggressiveness, and that an overwhelming sexual impulse will be experienced as colossal aggressiveness. We may thus expect that the individual will be more afraid of the consequences of his sexual impulses the more those impulses are coupled with aggressiveness. The fear of punishment may be followed by a sense of guilt and by an impulse toward self-punishment. Helene Deutsch (1928) has shown that a patient suffering from anxiety neurosis (agoraphobia) has hostile impulses against his incestuous love objects, while at the same time he identifies himself with them. Aggressive impulses in cases of anxiety neurosis have also been found by Bergler (1935) and Hitschmann (1937).

My own studies have confirmed the importance of aggressiveness in the psychological structure of cases of anxiety neurosis. One can go even further and classify the different types of anxiety neuroses according to the quality and structure of their aggressiveness.

In the first group of cases, the aggressiveness is directed against the love object as a whole. There is a tendency to wish the loved and hated person dead, but no impulse to dismember him. Cases of this type may be agoraphobic or may suffer from a fear of sudden death. The fear of going insane is not in the foreground. Space is measured as the distance from the love object or from the place which symbolizes the love object. Pregenital sexuality does not play an outstanding part. The hostility toward the love object is very often not fully conscious.

In the second group of cases, the hostility is not directed merely toward the removal of the love object, but seeks a more far-reaching destruction. The anxiety attacks lead to a fear of being dismembered. The love object appears as someone who threatens to put the patient into an inferior position. Pregenital sexuality becomes more important. Obsessional trends are more pronounced. Claustrophobic elements may also be present. There are more severe distortions of space. The fear of going insane may become more important.

The third and final group puts the theme of dismemberment in the foreground. There are severe distortions of space. Violent impulses are more outspoken; pregenital sexuality plays a still more important part. It may sometimes be difficult to differentiate cases of this type from cases of obsessional neurosis and compulsions. Depressive features may be added to the picture.

Classifications of this kind are, of course, to some extent arbitrary. But it is important to keep in mind the fact that anxiety neurotics differ in their attitude to their love object and in the quality of their aggressiveness. Moreover, the relation of the anxiety neurotic to space becomes different when his aggressiveness is directed not merely toward the removal of his love object but toward its more or less complete destruction and dismemberment.

I base these opinions on the prolonged analysis of eleven cases. Some of these have been in analysis for more than five years, and some have come to me after having been analyzed for years by others. In some of the cases the analysis was of the usual type, while the majority of the cases have been treated at one time or another in group analysis.

I start with a discussion of cases of the first group. Rose was a woman of about 40 years of age who had been in analysis with other analysts for more than four years. Her most outstanding symptom was an inability to walk alone in the street. Between the fifteenth and thirtieth years of her life she was hardly able to leave the house. She then married a man whom she considered her inferior. She had one child. During her first analysis she developed an enormous positive transference. She wrote love poems, insisted that she wanted to marry the analyst, and, after two years, was so incensed at his failure to marry her that she left him. Similar transferences developed to two subsequent analysts. She made attempts with two women analysts, but soon developed hostility toward them. There were short periods in which she could walk alone for short distances. When she came to me for treatment, however, she could not leave the house alone and even when accompanied had difficulties in traveling long distances. Once more she returned to the analysis with a strong positive transference. She insisted that she should marry the analyst and had orgasms with her husband only when she imagined the analyst during intercourse. It was easy to show that there was great hostility toward the analyst. This hostility was derived from hostility toward her mother, father, and stepfather. She lost her father when she was four years old. Prior to that time he had been absent for a long period, and it may be assumed that she never got over the feeling of having been deserted by him. At six she wanted her stepfather to give her some bread first at table, but he gave it to the others first. The indications are that her genital attitude was outspoken at this time. Between six and eight she managed twice to get older men to play with her genitals. Outwardly she was deeply attached to her mother, slept with her, and kept her breast in her hand. She was conscious that she wanted to sleep with her mother in order to prevent sexual relations between her and her stepfather. Death wishes against her mother and stepfather were manifest. In the transference situation the underlying hostility toward the analyst often came to the surface. She indulged in fantasies of harming him and his wife, especially at times when he went on vacation. She even thought of inducing her husband to kill the analyst, and also had fantasies of putting a banana peel in his wife's path when she was pregnant so that she would fall and have an abortion. She also thought of stealing the analyst's charts and destroying them in order to hurt him. During the treatment she repeatedly went to the woman analyst who had analyzed her last in order to complain about the analyst.

The patient was convinced of the value of a restrictive diet, which she imposed upon her son and her husband. She had a conviction that the analyst, who did not keep to these dietary rules, would die early unless she saved him.

At the time when she was unable to walk, she wanted to be near her husband or in the house. There were grounds for complaint against her husband, who was unreliable, lazy, and not entirely honest. She was occasionally treated in a group, but was so wrapped up in her own problems that she hardly ever participated in the problems of others.

The death wish against the patient's mother and father were obvious in this case. The death wish was stronger against her mother. Death wishes against her mother were more or less on a conscious level from her earliest childhood onward. There was never any fear of insanity. The anxiety was a fear of being removed from her love object, especially her father. Her impulse to self-punishment was not derived from an identification with her mother. She felt keenly that her love object attacked her by withholding food and love from her. She planned revenge and was afraid that she might be punished for the revenge. There was fear of aggression on the part of her love object, the most important part of it being a fear of desertion.

Active therapy succeeded in making her go out alone and even cross bridges—which she had particularly feared before, even when accompanied. Every active step brought new waves of hostility. She finally regained complete freedom of movement. She insisted, however, that she could not live without the analyst, and complained of bitter pains while thinking of him. At the present time, after about two years of treatment, she has been sent to a woman analyst since it was not possible to break the positive transference.

The second case of this group was a comparatively young man, 23 years old, who came into analysis a few months after his symptoms had started. He was at that time a student in law school and had begun to serve subpoenas for lawyers. When he had to go at all far away from the district in which he lived he felt weak, his heart would beat fast, and he was afraid he was going to faint and die. Only occasionally was he afraid of going out of his mind; and this meant for him merely that he would get confused, not know what to do, and would be in the center of public attention. Finally, he had to be accompanied on his way to school and work.

He lived with his mother and a brother two years older than himself. He was afraid to stay alone in the house, but he also felt ill at ease when his elder brother was out and he was alone with his mother. He thought his mother might suddenly get ill and die and he would then not be able to do anything. The brother, coming home, would find them dead and kill himself. He was also afraid that the brother might die in an accident. Then the mother might die from excitement, and he would die too.

The patient's father died of tuberculosis when the patient was four years of age. The life of the family was overshadowed by the fear of tuberculosis. The patient also had a sister one year younger than himself. There was sexual play between him and his sister, with very strong feelings of guilt, starting at the age of four. His sister died at the age of eleven as a result of a tuberculous hemmorhage. The patient felt relieved because he thought that his sister might have become a prostitute owing to the early sexual play, and he would have been responsible for it. Around this same time, his brother forced him to anal intercourse. The patient was very tall; he had been very thin in his childhood, and his mother warned him continually that he must eat more or otherwise he would die. After the death of his sister, he began to suffer from nosebleeds, which he considered a sign of impending death. He must have felt responsible for his sister's death in consequence of their sexual play, and he identified himself with his sister as a punishment for his sexual activity. The feeling of relief after his sister's death was merely an overcompensation. It is furthermore probable that he considered any hemmorhage a consequence of the passive sexual role in sexuality, which had been imposed on him. He felt pushed into this passive role by his brother, not only because of the sexual acts which have been mentioned, but also because of repeated beatings administered by his brother. The following formula was thus formed in his mind: to be weak = to be passive = to bleed = to die.

His mother played a double role in the scheme. She was somewhat aggressive, not very tender, and continually forced him to eat. She had a stationery and candy store, and, as happens under such conditions, never gave her undivided attention to the patient. Occasionally he stole candies. On the other hand, he threw away other food which she tried to force upon him. Later on he developed an enormous hate against his employer, who "bosses him around too much." He had a conscious wish to strangle him. There was also a strong attachment to his mother, although manifest interest in her body never emerged. He was not inclined to give any deep interest to any other woman.

His sexual experiences consisted chiefly of having intercourse with girls he picked up in the street while out with his friends. His attitude was shown by two dreams. In the first he tried to have intercourse into the stem of a pipe which was rather too narrow, and in the second, he had intercourse by putting his penis between the ribs of a radiator, the space being rather too large. In a summer resort he tried to have intercourse with some of the women there, but they all said they were menstruating.

The patient hardly brought any free associations when he was alone with the analyst, but reacted fairly favorably in the group.

His symptoms disappeared after a few months of treatment, and he stopped coming for several months. He came back after a lapse of a year, this time with the fear that he might not be capable of eating. This, however, did not hinder him in his profession as a lawyer. The analysis of the symptom again showed the displacement from the genitals to the mouth, and the fight to protect his openings against something that was being forced into them. His general mode of living was still unsatisfactory. Although he was fully potent, he had no personal relationship at all with the girls with whom he had intercourse. He still wanted to reserve his libido for his mother. The patient never masturbated. He gained his early knowledge of sex on the street. His life in general was very dull.

The patient was also orgastically potent in Reich's (1927) sense of the term. I have seen full orgastic potency comparatively often in severe neurosis. The correlation between the quality of orgasm and the severity of a neurosis, if it exists at all, is not a close one. Reich's statements in this respect are too schematic.

Neurosis is not a disturbance of orgasm, but a disturbance in human relations and in psychosexuality.

The fear in this patient was the fear of being forced into passivity, to which he replied by counteraggression, which, in its turn, increased his fear of punishment. He responded by self-punishment and identified himself with the sister whom he had attacked. It is questionable whether the deaths he wanted to inflict upon his brother and his employer were a further motive for his fear of dying. There is no question that he identified himself with his dead father, whose place he wanted to take in relation to his mother. When he went out with nice girls, he was afraid he might faint and might not be able to protect them. The oral trends were outspoken in this case. He was, furthermore, afraid of being conspicuous because he was tall, did not want to be seen with girls who were not good-looking, and was afraid of attracting attention by fainting. Exhibitionistic and voyeuristic trends are, as is well known, not infrequently found in cases of this type.

Several cases which I have analyzed in previous years and which are not included in this series show similar characteristics. I will only discuss one patient, who at the present time is still under treatment and who came into the hospital after he had been analyzed for six months by another analyst. His symptoms consist in a fear of death, anxiety, painful sensations around his heart, and difficulties in getting his breath. The patient swallows air. The case is almost inaccessible for free associations. He is a 33-year-old physicist, whose symptoms developed at the time when he and his wife had decided to have a child. He was, moreover, about to gain some measure of independence, which he had not so far possessed. He had previously been dependent either on his parents or on his wife, and had only occasionally made money by teaching. He complains that in his relations to his parents he never got a sufficient amount of love, although all his memories are of friendly actions by his parents. His first memory is at the age of four, when he fell in love with a girl of fifteen. His father died when he was sixteen, but this did not make any impression on him. He remembers only once being beaten by his father, at the age of eleven or twelve, to which he reacted with the wish to kill him. Before puberty he tried to attract a girl's attention by throwing stones at her. When, at the age of 27, he fell in love with a girl, he wrote her biting letters, and when he was rejected, he married his present wife whom he did not love. He divorced her after a month, but remarried her after he had found out that she was promiscuous. During the last few years he has lived with his wife and is fully potent. He has no deep affection for her and has used his neurosis in order to separate from her. He is unwilling to give associations, and rejects all interpretations. He is bland and self-satisfied, does not desire any emotions, and complains that nobody wants to help him. It is interesting that as a physicist he is interested in very low temperatures. Though only a preliminary insight is possible in this case, the patient evidently seeks to show by his neurosis that he is deserted (which he feels as aggression on the part of other people), and that he needs help. He wants to gain love by aggression, and, it may be suspected, he wants to be dead (which means cool) like the love object.

In the second group of cases was a woman who suffered from a fear of sudden death and experienced difficulties in breathing. The neurosis dates back many years following a severe infection after an abortion. She married immediately afterward. Her present husband knew of her previous experiences, and she feels hatred and contempt for him. She is, however, dependent on him. When she feels worse, he has to accompany her; she even prevents him from going to work. She is quarrelsome and aggressive in all her personal relations and has severe hostile outbursts against her father and her mother as well as the analyst. Her earliest memories go back to the age of two or three when she broke her teeth in a fall, at which time her grandmother was so frightened that she had a hemiplegia.

There is a history of early outbursts of unmotivated hate against other children, and of breath-holding. On the advice of a physician, her mother gave her a beating, after which these attacks ceased. There is also a history of quarrels between her mother and father going back to a very early age. Her mother very often responded to these quarrels with fainting spells. Moreover, her father suffered from attacks of asthma, to which the patient reacted very early, at about the age of seven. There were scenes of violence between her younger brothers and her mother. The patient identifies herself chiefly with her mother and her fainting spells, but also with her asthmatic father. Her aggressiveness repeats to a great extent the family fights. Her desire to smash things and her open wish to make murderous attacks belong to the same category. She has had a great number of physical illnesses, which were partly due to repeated abortions and subsequent infections, although she also suffered from attacks of asthma and hay fever and has undergone numerous small operations.

In its structure, the case somewhat resembles a hysteria. With favorable experiences in her outward circumstances, the symptoms stop occasionally for a few days and even weeks, until she acquires some minor physical ailment. The therapeutic results in the case have been very meager. The anxiety is an anxiety of identification with her dead mother and her dead father (fainting and asthma) against whom hostile impulses were directed. Though the case does not strictly belong to the group of anxiety neuroses, it is described because it shows so clearly the sources of hostility in children. It is not only the hostility directed against the child, but also the hostility of the parents toward each other that found expression in continual fights and quarrels. Hostility and the death wish are in this case more direct and more destructive than in the cases previously cited.

In a purer case of anxiety neurosis in a 34-year-old woman, the patient suffered from states of anxiety in which she was afraid of going out of her mind, which, for her, meant becoming aggressive and killing somebody. She is afraid that she might jump out of a window, and that her husband might in a rage kill her son who is at the present time twelve years old.

Many of her anxiety attacks are in connection with outbursts against her son, who has great gifts as a violinist but does not practice sufficiently. He has to be continually urged to practice by the patient and her husband, and in the course of these events has become more or less stubborn. The patient is afraid of all kinds of catastrophes, and these fears appear in dreams again and again. She was frigid up to the beginning of treatment. In her earliest childhood she was submitted to many restrictions by her mother, to which she reacted with hate. Her asthma started in connection with pneumonia at the age of fourteen. There were also violent quarrels between her parents, and her father, too, suffered from asthma. She had occasional rheumatic attacks which were at least facilitated by minor conflicts. Her hostility and her anxiety are in very close and obvious relation to each other, and her anxiety occurs as an immediate reaction to her aggressive impulses toward her son and probably also toward her mother. This case and the previous one have many similarities, not least in relation to allergic phenomena. It is of course difficult to establish that these phenomena are due to the psychological conflicts. Indeed, it is more probable that the asthmatic attacks in both cases have at least organic components which furnish the pattern for the anxiety, and that the anxiety may in turn be partly responsible for subsequent attacks. These cases are classified in the second group because of their more open aggressiveness. The pregenital components of sexuality have not as yet gained any particular importance.

The next patient is a homosexual about 40 years of age. The basic fact in this case is his hatred of his sister, who is ten years older. This sister, who was tyrannical, represented for him a bully with a penis. His earliest memory is of being in a perambulator and of being taken downstairs by his sister and of the perambulator being bumped on the staircase. The sister was the dominating figure in the house, and took the side of his mother when his parents quarreled. The superiority of the female element in the family was assured, although his mother was rather feeble. Throughout the patient's entire life can be traced a longing for a mother who would take better care of him. This longing was tinged with a fear of completely losing freedom of movement, and there is a decided fear of closed spaces, of tunnels, and of elevators.

Homosexual experiences started early, between four and five, the other boy being older and taking the lead. In his later homosexual activities he wanted to gain superiority over a stronger man. His interest in the penis was mixed with unconscious identification between the penis and feces. The feces are very often represented in his dreams by greyish brown or yellowish animals which more or less reminded him of his sister; sometimes they were friendly and sometimes hostile. His anxiety centered around a fear of traveling. At bad times he is also afraid when he is alone, and then has an impulse to jump out of the window. He has many dreams of persecution in which the persecutors represent his sister with a penis. In his everyday life he is an unusually kind person. His anxiety is partly the fear of being brutally attacked, and partly the fear of his own violence, which might be answered by an increase in hostility on the part of others. His hostility is primarily directed against his sister and mother, his father not playing any important part in the family. However, there are from time to time hostile impulses against elder brothers. Alcohol and benzedrine give him a feeling that he loves and is loved more by others.

It is remarkable that his insecurities in life started with the experience in the perambulator and the threat to his equilibrium. An early threat to equilibrium is a fundamental point in cases of anxiety neurosis. Such a threat, to which every child is exposed, always gains greater importance in an individual's life when insecurities, such as insufficient love and care by parents, are added to it. The threat to equilibrium is then experienced as hostility coming from outside, which might lead to more or less complete destruction. It is arbitrary to talk here about identification. It is a question, rather, of attack and counterattack. Feelings of guilt, even if they are present, are overshadowed by the fear of attacks.

Similar problems were in the foreground in another case of severe anxiety neurosis who had been analyzed for three years before she came to be treated by me about two years ago. The patient suffers from such severe anxiety that she cannot stay in her apartment alone, and only specific persons, such as her husband and some of her friends, can protect her. When the anxiety comes on, she feels that she may go completely to pieces, scream, become violent or insane. This patient showed clear signs of early insecurity in walking. There were, in addition, early experiences of vomiting in the subway. In this case, too, insecurity concerning equilibrium was reinforced by insecurity in relation to the parents. Her mother was possessive but not demonstrative, and the erotic advances made by the patient to her parents were rejected, especially by her father. Stories about burglars told by a Polish maid, and the violent and cruel behavior of this maid and her mother toward newborn kittens, produced a further sense of insecurity. Early sexual play with her brother added feelings of guilt. She has a definite fear of being dismembered, but she is also afraid that she might be exploded from inside by too big a penis, by a child, by a drug, or by an enema.

She is rather greedy about food, wishes to take in plenty of it and to be stuffed with it. It is of paramount concern to her whether she is empty inside or not. Her actual sexual life is more or less normal. During orgasm she feels her insides turned out. She feels that orgasm is something which she has in herself, and which merely comes out. Only the presence of a love object protects her from internal and external danger. She is less anxious about the love object, although his presence assures her of his well-being, for which she is concerned. The patient's fears are of being alone and of going to pieces. The fear of death does not play an important part. Death, felt as mere removal, obviously belongs to those types of anxiety neurosis in which the subject has less destructive tendencies. This patient, however, sometimes feels during the analytic hour that the analyst is 30 feet or 30 miles away. This is partly an expression of the fear of being separated from the analyst and partly an expression of destructive impulses toward him. The patient is proud of her strength, and feels that she has enough weapons of destruction so that a penis is not necessary for her, although she sometimes uses movements of her toes to express feelings of tension. Masturbation began at the age of eleven, and was linked with feelings of anxiety and guilt. It was connected with a urinary impulse. Masturbation threatened her with the destruction of her sexual parts and with inability to conceive. For a while she felt that her breasts had hardened as a consequence of masturbation. It was an earlier theory of hers that children were carried in, and born from, the breasts. Later on, shortly after marriage, she developed an exophthalmic goiter. It is an interesting fact that there was a family tradition that she was bitten in her neck by her brother, and she even has a feeling that she remembers this event. All through her later life she felt that not only her father and brother but also her mother and elder sister were aggressive. It was necessary for her to become strong, or at least to feel so. She feels that, taken all in all, there are no real men, and in her dreams the famous he-men of the screen are shown up as feminine. She does not want to give food to her guests, and she has no sexual generosity. She does not want to give in to a man unless he gives himself up completely. She is afraid of being trapped and of being restricted in her motility. To be trapped means, for her, to be enclosed in her mother's womb. She strives for power and strength, although she is afraid of them, since they might lead her to destructive acts. Her neurosis started shortly after the death of her father when she heard a story of a gonorrhea infection which reminded her of the dangers of sex and especially of masturbation.

This patient gives us a deeper insight into danger situations. She is afraid of being cut to pieces and mutilated. There is a particular fear that she might be deprived of her insides, of her genitals, and of food. There is also the danger of being stuffed too much, and of being exploded from the inside. She is, moreover, afraid of being robbed of her motility and of her strength. She is afraid of the outside dangers represented by her family and by their maid, and defends herself by adopting their aggressive qualities herself, which in turn increases the danger of counteraggression. The external world threatens her equilibrium, and she is afraid of slippery surfaces, inclined planes, and heights. The presence of the love object reassures her that there is no danger and that she is not being harmed. She really needs love objects who, in spite of everything and in spite of her strength, remain independent. The patient measures distances in the world as distances from the love object, and if the love object is distant the world seems to be enormous. Although in her personal development she has reached genital sexuality and complete love relations, her neurosis is only to a small extent based upon the Oedipus complex. It is based chiefly upon very primitive, cruel, and destructive impulses in herself and in others, and the difficulties of the treatment are connected with the primitiveness and force of her aggressive impulses. Accordingly, she fears death less than destruction. The distortions in space are present but not very outspoken, which may be partly related to the fact that her fears are concentrated on the inside of her body.

In my paper on the psychoanalysis of geometry, arithmetic, and physics (1936b), I reported upon a 23-year-old man without any manifest sexuality and with hostile impulses who at an early age had felt very much threatened by his mother. He had particular fears in connection with space—for instance, with "the middle of the room." Symmetry was a particular danger. When objects were about to lose their balance, he also reacted with anxiety. When he touched anything with his right hand he fell into a state of anxiety which he had to relieve by compulsive movements of his left hand. He also had a particular relation to numbers. His primary fears and anxieties were in connection with a scene in which his mother had washed his sisters' heads with kerosene. The case centered around fears of attack and counterattack. His anxiety attacks were accompanied by severe vasovegetative symptoms: he became extremely pale, almost fainted, and his pulse was almost imperceptible. There were insurmountable difficulties in arriving at deeper material. However, the threat of complete annihilation was in the center of the picture, and spatial qualities constituted one of the threats to which he reacted with anxiety. The compulsive elements in the case were remarkable.

It is very probable that all cases of anxiety neurosis in which obsessional trends are of importance belong to this group. A 36-year-old patient had developed an anxiety in connection with an operation for hernia which thwarted his ambition to become a baseball player. He was very much afraid that the truss might drive germs into him. Besides obsessions, which went to the point of delusions, that everything was infected with germs and that nothing should be touched, he had constant anxieties of being struck by an automobile and of something falling on him. He hated everybody who did not conform with his obsessions. He constantly dreamed of being hurt. The incomplete analysis suggested the probable existence of a strong hostility against his father.

One sees how great the variety of problems are in cases in which the aggression comes more strongly into the foreground. It is obvious that this second group shows a closer relation to obsessional neuroses than does the first group. In at least two of the cases, obsessional and compulsive features were of importance. In two cases a definite relation existed to organic diseases of the asthma type. In another case there was some relation to exophthalmic goiter, and in a further case the vasovegetative phenomena were particularly in evidence. The spatial problems are severe. Identification mechanisms seem to play a less important part than in the previous group, and the anxiety is based less on a fear of death than on a fear of destruction.

In the third and final group the problems of space, numbers, and counting play a still more pronounced part, and the aggressiveness is of a still more destructive character than in the previous cases.

E. G., a rather good-looking woman of 23, rather smallish but proportionately built, suffers from anxiety in connection with the topics of death, crime, sickness, and war. She is particularly afraid of thunderstorms. She is almost obsessionally preoccupied with the idea that the world may come to an end and that the world is too small. She has dreams of time, space, relativity, and other concepts of physics. At intervals, her anxiety increases to panic, especially at the time of her menstrual periods when sexual excitement also increases. On account of her anxiety states, she had to forgo a promising stage career and was reduced to complete poverty. She was never sexually satisfied except by masturbation, though toward the end of treatment she experienced sexual gratification through intercourse. At sixteen she had an affair with an elderly man for a year and a half, but she discontinued it when the man showed no intention of marrying her. There were other affairs which were also unsatisfactory. While she was on the stage she wished to receive advances from another girl who was reputedly homosexual. When she was eighteen, a wealthy publisher offered her money if she would let his mistress practice cunnilingus on her. She was shocked, and refused. Later on she had nightmares that the world was coming to an end and that this man was the only person who could prevent the catastrophe. The infantile situation centered around her father, who died of cardiac asthma when the patient was twelve, his illness having started when she was seven. He was in continuous conflict with her mother, who scolded him for being too generous. The patient has several memories that he took her out and gave her a good time against her mother's wishes. She remembers with pleasure that her father took her out in a thunderstorm when she was three and a half years old. At present, thunderstorms provoke a great amount of anxiety in her. She has no direct memories of having ever observed her father's sexual parts. At about seven or eight she saw a man masturbating in the park. His organ looked extremely big to her. When she got home, she felt ashamed and vomited. She is always afraid that a stiff penis might hurt her sexual parts and would prefer to have a soft penis rubbed against her external organs. She generally has a feeling that the female sexual parts are too small for the enormous stiff male sexual organ. When she was five, an uncle took her on his shoulders, and she was afraid of being torn in the middle. Her mother and sister appear as threatening and interfering agents. At the age of two, her sister, who is two years older, told her there was poison in the water she had been drinking. Between four and five, her sister told her that the police were looking for her. She always considered her older sister better looking and more attractive than herself. The patient was particularly afraid that the girls at school might not like her.

It may be inferred that a strong fantasied heterosexual relation existed between her and her father, which was impaired by the fear that her father and his sexual organ might hurt her. She was furthermore threatened by her mother and sister because of this, and she decided to accept them as love objects.

The patient's dreams show the conflict between homo- and heterosexuality. She dreamed of being in a train full of girls all dressed like men, and the costume was most becoming to herself. She would have liked to stop off to meet an old lover, but the train would not wait, so she decided to continue. The patient had, in fact, wanted to be a boy between her eighth and twelfth years. In another dream she would have liked to ride an imperious horse like her friends, but the horse reared and looked displeased. The following dream is more intelligible: "I dreamed about an Oberammergau Passion Play. I saw Christ. He was nailed to a cross but was transparent and smiling. Little boys were there in medieval costumes which were too big. The boys jumped up and down in them laughing." Christ suffering is a symbol for herself and her tortured genitals. She believed, indeed, that menstruation was due to a lesion of her body. The second part of her dream expresses hope. The costumes stand for the vagina, while the boys jumping up and down are symbolizations of the male sexual organ.

Another dream of Christ ran as follows: "The voice of an explorer delivering a travelogue talked about an island which was shown in black and white on the screen. It seemed to be viewed from an airplane. He said the world was his oyster. The island turned to clay and whirled around until it formed a globe. At this moment a Lesbian friend sitting near me put her hands over her eyes. I did so too, but looked out sideways behind my hand at a very good-looking man sitting next to me. Then I took my hands away from my eyes, and the clay in the picture seemed to form a statue of Christ crucified. The globe was gone; I was frightened and put my hands over my eyes again." The crucified Christ, the small world, and the island symbolize femininity and, more precisely, the female sexual parts: they are at the mercy of men ("the world was his oyster"). However, the awakening of her heterosexuality is indicated by her interest in the good-looking man.

She often dreamed about the world: "A medieval castle in the water; sky and water around; it was supposed to be the world." She gave much thought to the question of how long the world had existed. She felt that it had not been in existence long enough, only a few thousand years. The following dream is remarkable: "A woman friend complained of an unhappy love affair. I said: 'Why do you complain? I have a much more serious condition connected with Einstein and his theory of relativity, and that is not curable.'" The patient is afraid of sudden death. She also thinks that in intercourse she may suffer instantaneous hurt. She has no trust in the stability of the world. "What is holding everything up? I cannot look at the sky; it goes on and on. Sometimes everything looks dreamlike to me. The buildings look so temporary. I think of the changing generations. Mortality casts a shadow on everything." The patient is afraid that the buildings (for instance, the Empire State Building) might fall down. During anxiety attacks, she is not even sure whether the floor will remain horizontal. In one dream she was high up in a tall building when, suddenly, the room seemed to slant and she was in danger of falling out of the window which was close to the floor. She was sitting on a couch with a man; she slipped off, but grabbed an easel. The man seemed to fall out of the window. This was a recurrent nightmare which centered around the fear of falling out of the window. This meant that she was afraid of losing contact with her mother. As a result of her neurosis, she lived with her mother and her sister. Sometimes she felt that her nerves were too big for her body and that they protruded. With the fear of sudden death came feelings of emptiness and pain. These sensations are closely related to her frigidity, through which she denies that there is anything in her genitals. In spite of her fears concerning the male sexual organ, she wants to be in contact with the other person who represents her love object. Her neurosis says: "Look how small and helpless I am in comparison with my towering father (sister and mother)! I am in danger of being annihilated. I am small as a whole, but my genitals are small too."

The anxiety in this case expresses itself in relation to the problem of size, stability, and extension in space and time. Furthermore, the anxiety also changes spatial directions and exposes her more to gravitational forces. Her fear of death is primarily a fear of torture and annihilation. The fear of being separated from her love object plays a less important part. As has been mentioned, the patient has strong homosexual trends. The woman she desires is a man with a softer penis. Indeed, she had a dream in which a woman with a penis had intercourse with her. Her passive and masochistic trends are due to her relation to her sister and mother. The male penis, however, appears as a particularly dangerous weapon. Moreover, she is subject to a general threat of annihilation.

In my paper on the psychoanalysis of geometry and physics (1936b) I reported on a patient with severe fears of dismemberment. This patient had violent fantasies of attacking and dismembering women, coupled with cannibalistic impulses. He had an obsession for counting, connected with impulses to divide objects into small particles and to tear them to pieces. Problems of arithmetic and geometry are primarily problems of the ego, but the libidinal situation also plays a part in deciding to what extent arithmetic and geometry will be efficient. Threats made by physical forces are also threats made by the father. And the anxiety that supervenes is a dread of the uncanny forces of the external world, which throw one down and break one to pieces, and is also a dread of the father, who dismembers and castrates.

Anxiety is a phenomenon which may originate from experiences of very different types. In the earliest stages of its development the child is threatened particularly by the loss of equilibrium and by the physical forces of gravitation. Only gradually does it learn to orient itself in space and to appreciate the definite importance of the vertical and horizontal directions. It is very probable that at this stage of development the love object represents among other things an insurance against the danger of falling. I have described (1937) the love object in this respect as a supporting figure, *Stützfigur*. However, the child also reacts with anxiety when its supply of food is not assured. For the child, moreover, food means the inside of its body, since, according to the notions of young children, the inside of the body consists of the food which has been ingested. Direct threats against the integrity of the body are probably experienced only at a later stage. They are closely related to the child's aggressive impulses directed against the bodies of other people. At this level, fear of dismemberment in general will become important, and later on, with the awakening of genitality, this will culminate in the theme of castration. During this whole course of development, the love object will offer protection against deprivations and will, on the other hand, be feared as a possible aggressor. The fear of losing the love object will come into the foreground when sexual development has reached a higher level. When there are hostile impulses toward the love object, they will be reacted to with feelings of guilt. At the earlier levels there will be fears of counteraggression on the part of the love object; at the higher levels there will be identification with the love object, which is also hated, and the insecurity connected with the dread of its loss will be increased by the guilty feeling which forces the subject to identify himself with the person he has killed in fantasy.

If we consider the variety of the situations which, in the course of development, provoke anxieties, we shall not be astonished at finding a great variety in the types of anxiety neurosis which revive the various types of developmental anxieties. We must further take into consideration the fact that any anxiety will contain all the possible anxieties, though in various degrees and proportions. It must also be remembered that, in spite of the deep regressions which we have described, the typical case of anxiety neurosis has reached a level of heterosexual adjustment, in the sense of the Oedipus complex, and that it has one point of fixation in the genital relation to the parents. From the clinical standpoint, this distinguishes a case of anxiety neurosis with regressions going to fairly primitive levels from cases of obsessional neurosis, although cases with space distortions very often show obsessional trends. It is characteristic of neurotic anxiety, in contrast to psychotic anxiety, that the former is always accompanied by some appreciation of the love object.

The various types of anxiety are connected with different attitudes toward death. In a case of anxiety neurosis with only a moderate degree of aggressiveness, a type of death will be pictured which means merely separation from the love object. When the regression goes deeper, a fear of death may be replaced by a fear of dismemberment and annihilation, and the idea of death will be colored by these ideas. Bromberg and I (1933a) have shown that various types of concepts of death exist, and that the idea of death changed with the type of neurosis and with the type and degree of regression.

I think that an insight into the problems which have been discussed here is of fundamental importance to a deep analysis of cases of anxiety neurosis. It should be understood that the fundamental trends discussed in the various types of cases must find a reflection in the type of transference and in the analysis of the transference.

CHAPTER NINE

The Social Neurosis

I speak of a social neurosis when the clinical picture of a neurosis is dominated by suffering in social contacts. Patients of this type can be comparatively happy when they are alone or together with their families. They feel severely incapacitated when they meet other people. They feel particularly bad when confronted with groups; they are unable to enjoy themselves in such situations, and they are unable to function according to their abilities. Shyness is therefore the central symptom of this group of cases. The shyness is experienced by the individual as such and may not become obvious to others. However, the person cannot talk freely and functions mostly below his potential intellectual and emotional level. In many cases the shyness leads to a more or less complete blocking. The patient may be unable to clearly formulate any thoughts and may remain silent against his will. He may also prefer to remain silent instead of saying banal and unimportant things. In severe cases the social conduct becomes severely impaired. In some cases this impairment manifests itself in the discharge of professional as well as social duties. In other cases the difficulty remains restricted to the one or the other sphere. The disturbance becomes more severe when the situation is exacting or important. It may occur only in the presence of specific persons who are socially or professionally superior. The individuals I am describing usually derive feelings of inferiority

---

Appeared originally in the *Psychoanalytic Review*, 25:1-19, 1938.

from their inadequacy. They may consider themselves intellectually inferior, or they may consider their physical appearance and behavior unattractive. They may blame themselves for the insufficient care they have given to their intellectual and emotional and physical development. The complaint of fatigue is very common. Some complain about sleepiness.

The shyness also expresses itself in physical symptoms. The patient is not sure of his voice. He cannot talk loudly. His voice becomes flat. Stammering may occur. In general, it may be said that stammering can be considered a subgroup of social neurosis in its wider sense. In this discussion, however, the term "social neurosis" will be used only for those cases in which the physical symptoms are not paramount. During psychic stress the patients may become stiff and awkward in their motility, and some start to shake. In the vegetative sphere sweating and blushing are common. Severe cases of erythrophobia—flushing and fear of flushing—stand in a similar relation to the social neurosis as does stammering. The urge to urinate and to defecate may occasionally occur in trying situations. Difficulties in potency may occur, but are not especially prominent. These individuals by their shyness are much more hindered in their approach to sexual objects.

Symptoms of this type are very common. One should speak of a social neurosis only when they are a prominent part of the clinical picture. The literature on the subject is meager in spite of its great practical importance. F. G. von Stockert (1929) has spoken of contact neurosis in which he includes erythrophobia and stammering. The psychoanalytic literature has not given special attention to social shyness. J. Hoffman (1931) has described a case of social anxiety. The patient reacted to social situations with a high degree of anxiety which made him avoid all situations in which he had to meet other persons and especially groups. The literature of Adlerian individual psychology stresses the symptoms of social neurosis under the general heading of inferiority feelings, but contains very little specific material (see Adler, 1907).

Some of the patients I observed drank alcohol excessively in order to escape their social difficulties. There is obviously a relation between some types of alcoholism and social neurosis, although, in spite of their inner relations, the two have a different psychology. [This subject is discussed in Ch. 17.]

I have observed eighteen cases of this type during three years. All these cases were treated by me, some of them with a strictly psychoanalytic technique; the majority were treated in group psychotherapy, the treatment lasting from a few weeks to more than a year. The following reports are given of cases in which a deep psychological insight was gained.

Hugh S. was 30 years of age, tall, rather good-looking. He complained of extreme shyness when in the company of other people. He felt shaky and could hardly talk. He had to drink in order to feel better. He was terribly afraid that people might realize his difficulties and therefore avoid his company. He was particularly afraid of parties where women were present and feared persons most who were socially at ease. When he was shy, he felt as if his body had no substance and no inside. He felt like an empty shell. He felt continually tired. The fatigue was sometimes so extreme that he stayed in bed and did not go to his office. He had difficulties in falling asleep and also in potency.

From his early history the following data were of importance. He was brought up with a sister B., two and one half years older, and a girl cousin R., about the same age as the sister. He did not play with boys. A little later he also played with the daughters of the gardener. He was weaker than the girls. He liked to wrestle with R. and was glad when she proved superior, especially when she kneeled over him, her thighs touching his body. Sometimes he let her win in order to enjoy this situation. Once he also played with a girl called Mickey. From this play originated a strong influence on his life. A great part of his early life concentrated around a pillow which he especially liked. It was called Kissen, and he started to call it Kiss Me. He did not want to have this pillow badly treated—for example, beaten by his sister. Serious quarrels with his sister followed when she either did something to the pillow or threatened to. He was also afraid that Kiss Me might feel cold, but he played a game stamping on this pillow and imagining that he was the pillow and was stepped on by Mickey. He then said "Mean Mickey" to himself. Still earlier he liked a toy bear. After much urging, he once lent it to another boy who brought it back disheveled, which grieved him very much.

His mother displayed an aggressive love toward him. According to what she later told the patient, she loved to bathe and powder him. She fondled him very much and gave him all kinds of endearing names like "little bean," "baby face," etc. The mother was always tired and suffering. She always thought that the children were tired and should rest. Her relation to her husband was never good. When the patient was ten or eleven years old his father complained that the mother did not love him. The patient's father was a rather energetic but tactless man. He was very strict in the education of the children, insisted upon their rest hours, and restricted their freedom considerably.

During the analysis, the patient dreamed repeatedly about his father having hermaphroditic genitals. The patient attempted, in his dreams, to have intercourse with his father. At the age of six the children showed their sex parts to each other. He was particularly interested in the buttocks of his sister and cousin and was astonished that their interest was concentrated on his front parts. They often played at spying on other persons. He was an obedient child, but lively, was a good student in school, and was in many respects a leader in school activities. He was editor of the school journal and wrote a long detective story for it. At sixteen, an acne broke out which disturbed him severely. He felt disfigured, and all his difficulties started. His neurosis never left him after this. At fifteen or sixteen he admired a cousin who boasted about his sexual adventures. Masturbation started at seventeen, after an educational talk which made him curious. At seventeen he came in close relation to a girl with whom he was very much infatuated. He felt that he suffered and that he made the girl suffer. Coitus was not attempted. A similar relation took place when he was 21 to 22 years old. There were casual erotic relations with girls for whom he did not care. Since the age of 25 he had been erotically rather active. It started with a girl, D., whom he later married against his will because she insisted. A year later he divorced her. He was particularly attracted by her smallness and helplessness. He could not stand to see her suffering. She complained continually about some kind of ailment or suffering. Immediately after the marriage she had a gastric ulcer. He did not have any potency difficulties with her. There were occasional difficulties in his rather numerous other affairs. After the divorce, in addition to numerous more casual contacts, he had two rather serious love affairs. Although the two girls were of different character, the two affairs, which followed each other, ran a very similar course. After a period in which he was chiefly interested in the conquest, he became deeply dependent, thinking continually that the girls might suffer when he deserted them, since he did not intend to marry them. There were occasional lively outbursts of jealousy, although he did not suspect that they were unfaithful to him. He merely felt neglected and badly treated. In endless discussions he tried to convince them how wrongly they had acted. He felt that because of his deep suffering, his fatigue, and his shyness, he deserved special consideration. He wanted to be loved deeply. They, however, should be able to give up the relation any time he felt like it. He resented his own dependence and often felt that he would like to cut the girls off like an infected arm. He often felt that he was driving them into neurotic states. He would have like them to have beaten him, but never attempted to transform this wish into reality. He had developed a specific although consciously unformulated ideology about sex. He felt that women should not hesitate about sex relations, especially with him. They should have relations without demanding love and attachment. He should be free to leave them any time he felt like it. However, he expected that they should give him deep love and should admire him. They should not be too much hurt when he left them. A direct fear of castration existed. It came out openly in dreams. He was also particularly squeamish about his eyes. There were slight obsessional trends.

The outstanding feature in this case is the masochism, which culminates in the Kiss Me scene in which he was the mistreated pillow. He wished to be mistreated by the gardener's daughters, by his mother through her aggressive tenderness, by his sister, by his cousin R., and finally by the women whom he loved and by whom he felt mistreated. With the exception of fleeting wishes to be mistreated by an instructor in camp before puberty and some wrestling games in which he let the weaker boy win, there were no passive masochistic trends in relation to men. However, he sometimes felt badly treated by his father. He also wanted to play the part of the person who was superior. He wanted to punish the women he loved when they were not completely subservient. He was also the person who stamped on the pillow. There was otherwise remarkably little aggressiveness. It came out occasionally in relation to the analyst, whom he blamed bitterly when he did not feel improved. His mother's aggressive love and his father's strictness had forced him into a passive situation. The aggressiveness came out in an indirect way. He chose, preferably, weak love objects. He was their protector who made them suffer. He played, therefore, the double role of the protector and the torturer and added to these two other roles of being protected and being tortured. For his suffering he expected to be compensated with care and love, freedom and sex pleasure, financial and economic security, freedom from struggle, and independence from bonds.

This general problem found the following expression in experiences of his body: a love for his body and great distress about everything which might encroach on it; a wish for beauty and fear of an impairment of attractiveness—a narcissism of high degree. He also had a wish for knowledge, for sexual knowledge, and a wish for intelligence. These were probably safeguards against a too dangerous submission and masochism. To this was added a great fear that the suffering might lead to castration or disease of his eyes. He had a strong interest in the buttocks and the thighs.

In his relation to others he wanted their love and their admiration for his physical and mental qualities. His shyness and fatigue protected him against failure and kept him independent. At the same time they increased and intensified his relations to other human beings. His difficulties started with an acne which might have been partially determined by psychogenic factors. He perspired excessively. The skin is particularly important from the point of view of relations to other human beings. The shyness of his mother was a pattern which he imitated. His fatigue made action, aggression, and sadism impossible. This was patterned after his mother. Since his father was aggressive and active and was not liked by the mother, he avoided this danger by fatigue and inactivity. This was obviously a reversal of the activity which he displayed before puberty. His ideology centered around the problem of suffering, which he saw everywhere.

Shyness and social neurosis thus appear as self-inflicted suffering closely related to passive attitudes which were enforced through the family situation. In this case the mother played a much more important role than the father.

In the following case the relation to the father played the most important part.

Dave B. was 24 years old, good-looking and well dressed, and had above average intelligence. He complained that he was continually drowsy, that he was in a haze, that he could not think clearly, and that his social contacts were severely impaired. He could not talk freely or make conversation, and he was afraid that people might consider him mentally inferior. In the later course of the treatment it turned out that he was very much afraid of being thought to be "queer"—that is, a homosexual. He could not work because he was too drowsy and forgot everything. He had an enormous desire to sleep and fell asleep often during the day. At times the picture resembled narcolepsy.

The patient was the second child of parents who had been separated for seven years. The patient described his father as an unreliable "show-off." His memories of his father went back to his third year, when his father was very good to him. He would take him out and buy him things. His father often beat him. He was particularly afraid of being struck with the father's belt, and was terrified when the father tightened his belt at the table. As he grew older, the father liked to show off with him. He ordered the boy to swear before his friends and whipped him if he refused. At the age of seven he saw his father's penis, which looked enormous. When the patient once stole a dollar and was found out, his father held him outside a seventh-story window and threatened to drop him. Two or three times he wanted to kill his father. For ten years he had seen little of his father and was full of anger that the father had deserted him and his mother so completely. In his dreams he showed love and longing for his father and the fear of being neglected by him. There were strong castration fears in relation to his father, expressed especially in dreams.

From earliest childhood he had dreams in which he was being chased by animals or men, with whom he fought. One of his earliest remembrances was of being bitten on the lip by a large dog when he tried to kiss it. He loved dogs. He had been bitten twice by animals thereafter, once by a horse.

The patient was very much attached to his mother, who worked and supported him. However, early memories about her were scanty. She intervened when his father tried to beat him. He always turned to her for sympathy. At thirteen, while sleeping with her, he rubbed his penis against her buttocks. His mother hardly ever appeared in his dreams. When he was fifteen he tried to see his mother undress and often had fantasies about her clothes.

His brother, two years older, had always been stronger. They were always fighting. Between five and six, the patient and his brother stayed at a farm where there were two other boys. At that time they had lively sexual play with each other. They put their penises into each other's mouths and also had anal intercourse. When he was seven, a man tried to have anal intercourse with him. This hurt him so much that he ran away screaming. There were occasional other homosexual contacts in his early puberty. When he was seven a little girl showed him her genitals, and he reciprocated.

Up to the age of thirteen, he often wet his bed. He even fell asleep during the day and wet himself. The material brought forward by the patient suggested that the enuresis was an expression of a passive homosexual wish concerning the father. He was scolded and beaten for this enuresis. He had to urinate very often.

Masturbation started at eleven and was actively continued for a long time. The patient also tried to take his penis into his mouth and used suction by a milk bottle and other variations. He not only had a severe feeling of guilt in connection with these experiences, but also thought that he had harmed himself by the masturbation. There was an inexhaustible wealth of hypochondriacal ideas concerning his penis. He was contented with neither its shape nor its posture, complaining that his erect penis pointed down too much because he had squeezed it between his legs when masturbating. He worried a lot about a discharge from the penis when he was sexually excited or merely talked with girls. He was always very curious about sex and urination. At puberty he tried to see women undressing or going to the toilet. His curiosity concerning his own body was even greater. He looked at his penis and at his anus with the help of mirror arrangements. He was afraid that his hair might become too thin and fall out. He was very self-conscious about his appearance and gestures and was continually haunted by the fear that he might appear homosexual. He felt that people stared at him. When in a public toilet he thought that people looked at his penis and was afraid he might show an interest in theirs. In order to see whether he liked it, he stuck a piece of soap into his rectum. He pondered over the idea whether he should not have homosexual relations in order to find out whether he was a homosexual or not.

His first attempt at coitus occurred when he was fifteen. He often had difficulties in potency, which he attributed to his masturbation and to his homosexual leanings. The patient had many erotic contacts and two longer affairs. He was afraid of becoming too dependent and gave up the relationships. During the treatment the patient had a period of three months in which he worked steadily and was able to suppress all erotic thoughts. The drowsiness disappeared at this time too. He relapsed when his sex urge returned during treatment, for which he blamed the analyst severely. He complained that fear of impotency and homosexuality marred his sex life.

The patient wanted to impress others by his intelligence and by his appearance. He was vain in that he wanted continual praise and affection from everybody. Since he felt unable to get what he wanted, he escaped into drowsiness and social inhibitions. He felt then that others were hostile to him and looked down on him. His striving for love and recognition derived from his early attachment to his father. He wanted to be the passive homosexual love object and at the same time protested against it. His passivity was enforced by his father's aggressiveness. His older brother played some part in this development. His overwhelming interest in the father had made heterosexual adaptation difficult. In the relationship to his father, peeping and exhibitionistic and urinary tendencies were paramount. He offered himself as a love object to his father, and when rejected he offered himself to everybody. He was concerned with his mental and physical endowment, and vanity and self-consciousness were the result.

In therapy the transference situation was stormy. Attempts to gain the love of the analyst by complete submission and violent outbursts of rage against the analyst followed each other; the analyst was accused of making him a homosexual. The negative transference was particularly strong when the analyst insisted on work, social contacts, and heterosexual adaptation. But nevertheless, he improved steadily.

This case was chosen as an instance of a social neurosis based upon the relation to the father. From the point of view of symptomatology, the drowsiness was remarkable. Both this patient and the preceding one had been forced into passive and dependent positions by early experiences with one parent. It did not matter whether the parent was of the same sex or not. This passivity was enforced not merely by violence but also by love. It was also of importance that both patients, as children, received a great amount of admiration. This admiration pertained to their physical as well as to their mental qualities. The passivity was not merely sexual, although it was expressed through infantile sexuality, in anal and urethral trends. Sleepiness, drowsiness, weakness became methods of expression for this passivity. In order to gain love and admiration, the individual had to display his mental and physical excellence and thereby became narcissistic. He wanted to be able to love himself in the same way as he wished to be loved by the parent and parent substitutes. Even if the beloved parent continued to give the desired attention, others did not do so, and conflicts occurred. Further difficulties arose from the fact that passivity alone became unsatisfactory. Too close a relation to the parent led to difficulties in puberty, and sex relations were either too closely bound to the mother image and masochistically underlined or remained pale because of the unresolved attachment to the father image. In the manifest symptoms of the neurosis the shyness stressed the passivity and checked the counteraggression which the patient did not dare to display, bound either by fear or by love or by both. By his shyness and the symptoms connected with it the patient came into a close relation to everybody, a relation which resembled a relation to the beloved parent.

The conflict almost never remained in the psychic sphere alone. Our first patient trembled and sweated, and our second patient became drowsy in a difficult situation. Alcohol was sought as relief by the first patient. Finally, the patient may want to withdraw completely, to give up all social contacts, and an attempt at suicide may symbolize this desire.

In another of my cases the patient had a similar attitude to his mother, and his neurosis led him to a complete withdrawal from social contacts. He felt that his face resembled a Mongolian type, and he complained bitterly that his nose was too small. He was Jewish. Severe impotence complicated the picture. He, as well as another of my patients, complained that his voice was low and uncultivated and that his speech was without modulation.

The same basic motives repeated themselves in an almost monotonous way in the majority of the cases I observed. Another patient retreated into abnormal gorging with food when he felt rejected. His basic conflict was a conflict with the mother, who preferred his twin brother. He was brought up by foster parents who spoiled him and gave him a great amount of food. His first sex experience occurred at five, when he threw pebbles at a buxom woman and exposed his erect penis to her after he had caught her attention. His favorite fantasy from earliest childhood consisted of having large women punished by having a penis as big as a horse's inserted in their anuses.

Another case was not quite typical in the symptomatology. In his striving for social and sexual recognition by a woman cousin, the patient developed queer and ticlike movements consisting of bending the hip while walking and making a large circle with his outstretched leg. The material from the analysis showed a close connection between these movements and his attempt to be like his father, whom he had observed having intercourse with his mother. The leg symbolized the penis and the whole procedure was an exhibitionistic act in the attempt to gain recognition.

Two of my cases showed an astonishing lack of sex urges. In one case the social neurosis followed rejection by the father. It was complicated by enuresis. The other case, with hypothyroid disease, complained that he was too slow, inefficient, and could not fulfill tasks. He had a hypochondriacal attitude concerning his bowel movements. In long, drawn out treatment, the psychogenic material brought forward was negligible. No definite psychic etiology could be established. The treatment had to remain on the level of the discussion of ideologies and of group discussions. His general understanding of sex problems remained on a superficial level. Complete recovery was achieved.

Fifteen of the patients observed were men. I have, however, observed three female patients in which the same basic problems were present. All of them held social and professional positions which made great demands upon them. One of these patients, for instance, with artistic achievements, complained about severe feelings of inferiority. She felt that she was not good company, especially with women. She thought she had no real inner life and no real memories. She felt unable to live up to the expectations of her second husband. She felt inhibited in her art work. Unusually attractive, she felt that she was losing her looks. There was a masochistic trend acquired by the relation to the father, who was rough and tyrannical and expected as much in physical endurance from his two daughters as from his sons. The patient had the ideal of suffering gloriously and silently and demanded from herself complete submission to her second husband. The father had beaten her repeatedly. Nearsightedness increased her feelings of insecurity. She put extremely high demands on herself in her art and in her life. The more acute pressure by the father, who was the most important figure in her life, was augmented by a steady repression by the mother. Both parents had expected complete perfection from the child.

Another of my female patients with severe feelings of social incapacity was an overt homosexual with strong masochistic tendencies. However, the features of social neurosis in this case were overshadowed by a manifest sex difficulty and alcoholism, so that the case was not included in the group.

In this group of eighteen cases, one made a suicidal attempt, two had a tendency to drink alcohol, three were bedwetters, one had a hysteriform tic, two had unusually low sex urges, one had severe difficulties in potency, and four had minor potency problems. As mentioned, almost every case had one or another physical symptom, such as occasional sweating, blushing, stammering, and shaking. The obvious cases of stammering or blushing, although they have a very close relation to this group, are not included. It is impossible to give a detailed discussion of the psychological differences between social neurosis in the specific sense and erythrophobia and stammering. However, in erythrophobia, the voyeuristic and exhibitionistic elements are more outspoken. The fear of being seen and observed plays a still greater part, and paranoid attitudes, which are not uncommon in the other cases, are of greater importance in cases in which blushing is an outstanding symptom. In an analyzed case of erythrophobia, the fear of the threatening look of the father was paramount. The paranoid attitudes concerning the father were most prominent.

In stammering, the patient's counteraggression especially in the oral sphere, comes into the foreground. Speech becomes the weapon which the patient would like to use. The narcissism, of paramount importance in all social neuroses, concentrates in the oral region. Vocal counteraggression plays a greater part in stammering than in the other types of social neurosis.

It is difficult to describe the emotions occurring in the social-neurosis patient when he comes into a difficult situation. It is not anxiety but discomfort. One may consider this discomfort, which is expressed in blushing, sweating, dryness of the mouth, and shaking, related to anxiety. The danger which is feared by the social-neurosis case is not as acute as the danger experienced in anxiety.

In every type of social neurosis, the patient blames himself more than he blames others. When outspoken paranoia occurs and the patient is sure of the hostility of others, the symptoms of social anxiety and social neurosis disappear.

There are no outspoken feelings of guilt in the social-neurosis case. He merely suffers. In a case of atypical depression I have previously published (1934b), symptoms of shyness and sweating in the presence of others were present, and the patient insisted that he should get the same exaggerated admiration from himself and others that he received from his parents. The patient complained more than usual that he was not able to gain the affection of others.

Every child receives from its parents a certain measure of reassurance and admiration. The love and appreciation the child gets from its surroundings builds up the consciousness of self. What we call self-love is to a great extent love which the child has received primarily from its parents and continues to give to himself. If the child has received a great number of such erotic gifts from outside it will continue in self-admiration and self-love. If infantile experiences have heightened the demands for self-appreciation, the amount of appreciation offered in social contacts will become insufficient. The individual will not be capable of maintaining the level of self-appreciation, and social insecurity will follow. Admiration and appreciation may be bestowed on the child's physical appearance or on his mental and emotional capacities. The influx of appreciation will be directed especially to those children who have a special place in the family. The first-born child, the only son, the youngest child, the child particularly good-looking or particularly brilliant, is liable to attract greater attention from the parents. The social difficulties will appear later on in the sphere of experience which attracted particular praise from parents and parent substitutes.

One may talk about the increase in narcissistic libido, but it should not be forgotten that this is the consequence of object libido invested in the child by the parents. The child is passive or comparatively passive in this process. It seems that the passivity in the social relations which follow the pattern laid down by the parents is an outstanding trend in all cases of neurotic difficulties in social contacts. It is necessary for the development of the social neurosis that the passivity be reinforced from other sources. The parents' strictness and aggressiveness play the important part here. Aggressive tenderness and aggressive fondling have the same importance. In consequence of this, the child is forced into a passive position in which sexual elements are emphasized. When a child is severely beaten he assumes a masochistic attitude, since the beating almost invariably provokes sexual sensations. Beating on the buttocks, especially on the bare buttocks, has a particular consequence in this respect. The sexuality provoked in this way is almost invariably of anal character. However, aggressive tenderness may lead to genital stimulation; even then the enforced passive role overemphasizes the anal zone. If the main pressure comes from the father to the son, anal homosexual tendencies will be combined with a masochistic attitude. If the pressure comes from the parent of the other sex, homosexuality will be insignificant. This describes the infantile situation observed in all our cases which have been studied carefully enough. As long as the child is not exposed to particular demands, symptoms do not appear. They may occur for the first time when the individual strives for recognition in particular situations—for instance, reciting before a class.

In the majority of the cases observed, the real difficulty does not start before puberty when the individual demands not only social but also sexual recognition and finds that he cannot get them in full measure. He may feel that his physical appearance prevents such full recognition. He may feel that he is either too tall or too short or that his skin and complexion are not good enough. He may concentrate his feelings of social insufficiency around his hair, his body build, or the distribution of fat, and he may feel that his sexual activities, especially masturbation, are to blame. It is obvious that in the majority of cases the shortcomings in appearance and in physical and intellectual function are merely used as explanations when the exaggerated infantile demands concerning recognition in the widest sense are no longer satisfied.

The individual would not suffer so deeply if the suffering did not remind him of the satisfaction he received from his masochistic experiences in childhood. He now becomes dependent upon the social surroundings which take the place of the parents. However, he no longer dares to openly enjoy the dependency relationship, and his suffering no longer contains any manifest elements of pleasure.

The different somatic symptoms express the various desires in a symbolic way. Blushing is the exhibitionistic demand for sexual appreciation, inviting sexual activity from the partner.

Feeling cold expresses the inability to receive this gratification. Dryness of the mouth and the flattening of the voice deny that oral aggression is intended. Aggressive action also is denied by trembling. In this symptom, as well as in sweating, the superiority of the other person is acknowledged. Even if social contacts are avoided, the patient is continually surrounded by an imaginary society in which he lives intensely. It is characteristic that social contacts are all of the same level. Everybody has an importance. He wants everybody's admiration and appreciation. Sensitiveness and irritability may follow, and harmless remarks may provoke the full impression of complete rejection. A reactive hostility follows in some cases, but this is comparatively rare. The symptoms will multiply in proportion to the number of individuals present. Persons who otherwise do not show symptoms of this type, when faced by an audience may show symptoms of stage fright in which the speech phenomena and forgetting or inability to think clearly are conspicuous. In approaching heterosexual love objects, the symptoms are often present, especially in cases in which the parent of the same sex was the aggressor. In more severe cases, homosexual preoccupations, moral masochism or severe impotency may occur. There was no overt homosexuality in any one of my cases. I have seen only one social neurosis among my homosexual patients, but that may not be representative. In less severe cases, the manifest sex life may be normal, although masochistic trends are very often noticeable. Individuals of this type have the ideal of possessing poise and social grace. They desire to have as many friends as possible. They admire the social lion, the actor, the public orator and, last but not least, the salesman.

Aggressive and sadistic tendencies are never completely absent, but in the majority of cases they do not come out openly even in fantasies. Direct aggressive actions and behavior are rare exceptions.

Feelings of guilt do not belong in the picture, although unconscious feelings of guilt are not completely absent, especially in those cases in which the sadistic tendencies are more outspoken.

The patients not only feel miserable but depreciate themselves and are dominated by feelings of inferiority.

One may wonder that little has been said about castration fear and castration anxiety in these cases. It is true that castration motives can be found in almost every case examined carefully. Their dynamic significance in the picture of social neurosis is of importance only in those cases in which they form a part of a passive homosexual attitude.

From a general psychological point of view it is of importance that the self-appreciation of the individual is dependent upon the appreciation given by early love objects. Self-appreciation can only be sustained when supported by the continuous approval of others. The appreciation of others becomes insufficient in this respect when the individual demands from himself an extraordinarily high degree of self-admiration and self-love. These could be characterized as cases of disappointed vanity. The question could be raised whether on deeper levels the admiration is wanted merely because it is one of the expressions of love.

In severe cases, individual psychoanalysis of long duration may become necessary. In many cases, group psychotherapy in which the patient learns to have contact with other human beings is of particular value (Schilder, 1936a). In shorter treatments, the insight into the basic mechanisms which have been characterized here is of great value. In particularly trying social situations, benzedrine, which intensifies interpersonal relations and gives the feeling of being appreciated and loved, has been useful.[1] The use of alcohol, which has a similar effect in minor degree, is dangerous. The therapeutic results have been satisfactory on the whole. Some of these patients were considered cured, and the majority were improved.

[1] [Benzedrine had only recently been introduced in 1938.—Ed.]

CHAPTER TEN

Neuroses Following Head and Brain Injuries

It seems advisable to define the terms used in this chapter, since various authors do not use the same terminology.

We speak about neurosis when someone develops symptoms in relation to a past or present situation—symptoms which can be understood as the reaction of the individual as a personality. An individual afflicted with a neurosis suffers. The neurotic retains a close relation to social reality even at times when he does not seem to be responsible. The hysteric never denies reality as completely as, for instance, the schizophrenic, and his emotional disturbance never reaches the absoluteness of the emotional disturbance of the manic-depressive. Apparent disturbances in memory and judgment are merely the expressions of emotional attitudes and are not due to a more or less fixed inability. Psychological processes are always psychophysiological processes correlated with structures in the organism and especially in the brain. This must be true, also, of neurotic attitudes. However, neurotic attitudes and their psychogenic sequelae are not produced by structural changes, but from problems of the personality. They are always accompanied by more or less measurable changes in the organism, among which the vasovege-

---

Appeared originally in *Injuries of the Brain and Spinal Cord and Their Coverings*, ed. Samuel Brock. Baltimore: Williams and Wilkins Co., 1940, pp. 298-328. Reprinted by permission of the Publisher.

tative changes are outstanding. These may finally lead to structural changes in the organism or, in other words, to organic disease. The extent to which this is possible and exactly what part psychogenic sequences play in the genesis of organic disease is controversial. Groddeck (1923) and Jelliffe (1933) are inclined to the belief that practically all organic diseases arise in such a way. Most of the others—F. Deutsch (1933), for instance—are more conservative. Nobody denies that structural organic changes, even in a previously healthy organ, can be provoked by psychogenic sequences.

A traumatic neurosis is one which follows an injury to the body. In the case of trauma, one means a comparatively acute influence on the body structure which causes more or less demonstrable effects. One also speaks, in a metaphoric sense, about psychic traumas, meaning, thereby, influences which cause acute disturbance in the life situation. However, the term traumatic neurosis is used merely in the sense of neurosis following a physical trauma. The newer analytical thinking concerning the connotation of trauma is discussed by Fenichel (1945). If one considers the first definition, it is clear that traumatic neurosis cannot be the result of anatomical physiological changes. The physiological consequences of the trauma, especially as they affect function and structure of the brain, do not constitute the neurosis, but offer material for the neurosis as far as the individual is aware of them.

The term traumatic neurosis was first used by Oppenheim (1889) who had the fantastic idea that traumatic neurosis is due to neural changes of palpable or "molecular" character. Whatever the actual merits of such an assumption may be, according to our definition, a "traumatic neurosis" in the sense of Oppenheim would not be a neurosis. Moreover, the assumption of molecular changes neither has a basis in fact nor can it be used as a working hypothesis. Strauss and Savitzky (1934b) have therefore objected to the use of the term traumatic neurosis. In a later study (1937), however, they consider it a convenient designation if it is used only as a generic term to include the wide range of psychogenic reactions to trauma and its sequelae. Wechsler (1935) speaks about traumatic neuroses as different from traumatic hysteria. His description shows that by this term he means anxieties and a neurasthenic-hypochondriacal picture. It does not seem advisable to use the term traumatic neuroses in such a restricted sense. One can also speak about traumatic neurosis after head and brain injuries as Huddleson (1932) has: "A traumatic neurosis may be defined most simply as a psychogenic or a nonstructural nervous disorder, shortly following a physical injury, and complicated or not by structural changes in the central nervous system or elsewhere" (p. 1). This definition correctly points to the fact that the physical trauma in itself provokes physiological and anatomical changes which are either closely related in time to, or are coexistent with, the neurosis. However, these organic changes are not the basis of the neurosis.

Strauss and Savitzky (1934a) have studied the postconcussion syndrome. This symptom complex was originally described by Friedmann (1892) and later by H. Sachs (1909), Pierre Marie (1916), and others. It is characterized by headaches, often of paroxysmal type and dependent upon the position of the head. Various types of dizziness are always present. The patient fatigues quickly and has a tendency to emotional outbursts and irritability. Vasomotor instability is often present. This is an organic syndrome even in its psychological manifestations. Objective signs in the vestibular cerebellar apparatus and in the motor and the sensory fields are frequently present. Encephalographic findings may give further evidence of organic disease. One may object to the term concussion which for some authors includes many definite organic changes, especially small hemorrhages, edema, and vascular abnormalities. However, the term is so widely used that it can hardly be displaced by another at the present time. The postconcussion syndrome is an organic syndrome and cannot be classified as a neurosis. It can be differentiated from the obvious and severe consequences of brain injury only with difficulty. Character changes are found in connection with the postconcussion syndrome comparable to those seen often after brain injuries with more florid symptomatology. It might be better to speak of syndromes due to brain injury, of which the postconcussion syndrome comprises a rather ill-defined group.

The objective impairment and the subjective experiences originating in organic cerebral changes following head injury may become the nucleus for neurotic attitudes. The neurotic attitude is what constitutes a traumatic neurosis and, in this specific instance, the traumatic neurosis following head injury. However, traumatic neurosis following head injury is not necessarily based upon the anatomical consequences (and their psychological reflection), but may be merely related to the psychic experience of the trauma or to psychological attitudes pertaining to injuries of the head in general. Only in the first case might one speak about somatic compliance in the sense in which Freud (1920a) employs it. He used this term in describing the readiness of psychogenic attitudes to express themselves in symptoms referable to a diseased organ or to an organ which has been previously diseased. In the case of the post-traumatic syndrome, attitudes of the personality in connection with life problems may transform the concussion syndrome into a unit, colored by the personality tendencies.

Traumatic neurosis in general, and neurosis after head injuries, may occur in individuals who were neurotic previously or had neurotic tendencies; or it may occur in individuals who were not neurotic, in the commonly accepted sense, before the accident. One must find at least considerable modification of the personality or of a pre-existing neurosis after the trauma before speaking of traumatic neurosis, or one following a head injury.

Human beings do not live as isolated individuals and do not suffer in isolation. They live in a social milieu, and the head injury and its subsequent suffering is a concern of the community. Such sufferers have to be taken care of in some way by the community, especially when they are rendered incapable of working and are entitled to compensation in some form. It is natural that the problem of compensation will enter into the psychogenic sequences evoked by the injury. One may use the designation "compensation neurosis" when the claim for compensation becomes the dominant motive in the creation of the psychogenic sequence which leads to the neurotic symptoms. The problem of compensation has been handled by various authors in different ways, according to their political and social attitudes. One of the German authors (Hauptmann, 1926) gave to one of his papers on this subject the almost hysterical title *War on Traumatic Hysteria*, and Reichardt (1928) and Kleist (1927) speak almost contemptuously about the traumatic neurotic, whose chief aim is supposedly compensation. Attempts are made to separate compensation neurosis from traumatic neurosis in the narrower sense. However, if one considers that human beings live in a social environment, one must be very careful before deciding that neurotic symptoms are due merely to greed and an unwillingness to work.

The question of malingering will have to be considered in relation to traumatic neurosis. Malingering may be defined as the conscious attempt to imitate symptoms, with the idea of bringing either economic or social gain to the individual. It is the general consensus that pure malingering is rare. Wechsler (1935) found only one instance of it in about 100 cases of nervous sequelae following head injuries.

It has been previously stated that the organic consequences of a head injury with their reflection in psychological symptoms have to be considered as a structural syndrome which has no direct bearing on the psychological attitudes we consider neurotic. However, this differentiation should not permit us to overlook the fact that neurotic attitudes are dependent upon the state of the organism. It cannot be denied, for instance, that alcoholism may facilitate psychogenic sequences. The neurotic attitude is, after all, the attitude of the total psychophysiological organization and is not independent of toxic or any other influence that acts on those parts of the central nervous system which are concerned with instinctual drives and the state of consciousness. Huddleson (1932) cites, for example, syphilis of the central nervous system, epidemic encephalitis, malaria, alcoholism and other intoxications, as etiological factors in the provocation of traumatic neurosis. We would particularly stress the fact that the organic concussion syndrome may facilitate attitudes of the personality of a neurotic character.

On other occasions (1933b, 1934a) I have pointed out that insecurity and changes in consciousness connected with dizziness of central or peripheral origin facilitate neurotic attitudes. One must therefore note that cerebral organic syndromes may change functions of the brain in such a way as to provoke neurotic attitudes. One cannot claim similar mechanisms for traumas which afflict other parts of the body. The mechanism described is different from somatic compliance, mentioned above, which merely implies that the experience of organic impairment is used for the expression of neurotic tendencies.

If the assumption of the previous paragraph is correct, one gains the first hint that neurosis after head injuries might have to be differentiated from traumatic neurosis in general. The literature on this point does not make a clear distinction. Neuroses following head injuries are generally not differentiated from other traumatic neuroses. However, Wechsler's paper (1935) seems to be based on the assumption of a specific differentiation. Those authors who give attention to the postconcussion syndrome justly separate it from the traumatic neuroses in general, and Strauss and Savitzky (1934a, 1934b, 1937) occasionally speak of neurotic admixtures to the postconcussion syndrome; but the problem of whether neuroses following head injuries are to be distinguished from other traumatic neuroses remains undiscussed. It seems that besides the predisposing factor to neurotic attitudes connected with brain injuries of specific localization, the additional problem arises of whether an injury to the head is not experienced in a different way, and whether such an injury does not provoke attitudes different from the ones evoked by injuries of other parts of the body. Subsequent discussions will show that this assumption is justified. I differentiate, therefore, neuroses after head injuries from other traumatic neuroses. This separation is based upon the production of changes in cerebral mechanisms facilitating neuroses, and upon the particular psychological value which the individual places upon his head.

It is true that in general the literature neglects these formulations. Kehrer (1924), for instance, basing his discussion of hysteria and neurasthenia on experiences with war neuroses, does not differentiate neuroses after head injuries from those following other injuries. Nor does Huddleson (1932) note any sharp distinction between these two groups. This is not astonishing, since many authors do not even want to commit themselves as to whether traumatic neuroses are different from other neuroses. Sands (1936) seems to be inclined to differentiate conduct disorders following brain injuries from psychogenic behavior disorders. However, he recognizes not only the post-traumatic constitution but also traumatic neurosis and traumatic hysteria. Strauss and Savitzky (1934a, 1934b) state that only terror neurosis is traumatic in the strictest sense of the word. The psychoneuroses precipitated by trauma, according to them, hardly differ in their further course from the usual psychoneurotic syndromes, except for the presence of the compensation problem.

Huddleson (1932) writes: "The symptomatology of traumatic neuroses is that of nontraumatic anxiety neuroses, neurasthenias, hypochondriases, and conversion hysterias, plus more or less of the wound-of-the-head syndrome. Ego neuroses are more characteristic of the group as a whole than are psychosexual conflicts" (p. 87). It seems, therefore, that most of the authors reluctantly agree that, in spite of great similarities to the usual neuroses, traumatic neuroses present definite peculiarities. A casual survey of the literature shows, indeed, that there is a particular psychological attitude evoked by the trauma, such as an acute fear, fright, or terror reaction; and, furthermore, that the sociological reactions in connection with traumatic neuroses differ from those occurring in other neuroses. Differentiation of various types of neuroses presents difficulties. But as far as such distinctions are possible, I would emphasize that traumatic neuroses form a specific group in the realm of neurotic disturbances and, furthermore, that traumatic neuroses following head injuries can be differentiated from neuroses following trauma involving other parts of the body.

I have emphasized on other occasions (1938) that traumatic neuroses in general belong to the group which are generally characterized as "actual neuroses." Freud (1920a) has stressed that the trauma breaks through the *Reizschutz* (protection against stimuli). The organism tries to defend itself by encapsulating itself again and attempts to keep the overwhelming stimulus out or to let it enter the organism only in small quantities. In this way Freud explains the fact that the patient suffering from a traumatic neurosis repeats in his dreams the traumatic scene, again and again. According to psychoanalytic terminology, the protection against overpowering stimuli is one of the problems of the ego and is not a problem of the libido. Kardiner (1932) also states that in the traumatic neuroses the ego problem is paramount. Psychoanalysis, therefore, emphasizes the special character of traumatic neuroses. Thus, I come to the conclusion that we have a right to speak of traumatic neuroses as a separate group.

Innumerable attempts have been made to characterize the different types of traumatic neuroses (Kardiner, 1932; Moorhead, 1931; Buzzard, 1924; Dana, 1920; Osnato and Giliberti, 1927; Bing, 1926; Stier, 1926; Huddleson, 1932; Wechsler, 1935). Most of the authors separate the postconcussion syndrome, which is variously named, from traumatic hysteria, anxiety states, and neurasthenia. From a survey of the literature and my own experience, I would list four types of traumatic neuroses following head injury (according to our definition, the concussion syndrome and other brain-injury syndromes are not to be classified as traumatic neuroses):

1. Reactions of terror and anxiety.
2. Reactions of neurasthenic and hypochondriacal character.
3. Reactions of hysterical type. The conversion symptoms are very often based upon somatic compliance.
4. Reactions to social and compensation problems.

Strauss and Savitzky (1934a, 1934b) report that they have also observed obsessional states. This, however, does not coincide with my observation or that of most other authors.

Although somatic compliance is of greatest importance in group 3, it is also of importance in the other groups.

One may remark that almost all the forms mentioned can occur either acutely, subacutely, or chronically. Naturally, such a classification cannot completely cover the variety of pictures, since the psychogenic pictures can either coincide or be interwoven with organic sequelae of head injuries of either slight or severe degree. The commonly held opinion that psychogenic pictures do not occur in connection with severe head injuries is correctly contradicted by Strauss and Savitzky (1934b). The psychogenic transformations of severe organic pictures are sometimes difficult to analyze (Pötzl, 1917), and the psychogenic mechanisms may be overshadowed by organic personality changes. It is true, however, that the general attitude toward severe organic disease in those suffering from organic brain disorders is not different from the general attitude of patients with organic disease elsewhere who try to maintain their feeling of health by means of psychogenic mechanisms.

This preliminary survey of the problem has led me to the following formulations: The postconcussion syndrome is not a neurosis. A neurosis cannot be considered due to either palpable or molecular changes in the brain structure. However, lesions in specific parts of the brain (producing, especially, changes in consciousness and dizziness) may facilitate neurotic reactions of the total personality. The organic consequences of head injuries may become the nucleus around which neurotic attitudes crystallize (somatic compliance). The organic nucleus may be transformed into that of the neurotic.

Traumatic neuroses taking place in specific social settings are connected with specific social attitudes (compensation, malingering). Traumatic neuroses following head injuries can be differentiated from other traumatic neuroses because of changes produced in the cerebral mechanisms which facilitate psychogenic reactions, and because of a particular psychological value attached to the head. Traumatic neuroses in general and especially following head injuries, can be considered as a comparatively well-defined group of neuroses. The following subgroups can be recognized: (1) Anxiety and terror reactions; (2) Neurasthenia and hypochondria; (3) Hysteria; (4) Social reactions. We are now ready to enter into a discussion of specific material.

Anxiety and Terror Reactions

Some accidents which may lead to head injuries occur because of circumstances, and the individual is simply the passive recipient of the injury. However, it has often been noted (for instance, by Marburg [1936] and others) that a comparatively large number of individuals who suffer accidents have physical ailments and incapacities. Furthermore, it has been noted that those who once have had accidents are inclined to have more accidents and that, statistically, a larger number than expected have experienced several accidents. Alexandra Adler et al. (1931) have studied this problem in detail and are inclined to believe that certain types of personality are more liable to suffer accidents than others. One group is made up of paranoid personalities, and in other groups we find people who always come to grief or run actively into dangerous situations. There are, furthermore, the overanxious and overconfident types. My own observations have led me to similar conclusions. One gets the impression that it is very often a specific attitude of the individual which leads him into an accident, although there are doubtless cases in which the accident occurs without being sought and is merely inflicted upon the person. Observation of children shows that the restless and hyperkinetic type suffers accidents very easily. In other cases, one gets the impression that the accident is sought as a symbol of submission and masochistic self-abandonment to a superior force. Finally, accidents may be sought as self-punishment. The psychological attitude which leads to head injuries does not seem to be different from attitudes which lead to other types of accidents.

In the material of Bellevue Hospital in New York City, head injury frequently follows alcoholic intoxication. In the majority of cases, it was impossible to obtain clear insight into the connection between the alcoholic intoxication and the subsequent accident. The mere fact of the intoxication, with its motor impairment and with the clouding of the sensorium, was sufficient to explain the great frequency of head injuries in alcoholics.

At any rate, in every case one should study the question of whether psychological factors play a part in the genesis of the accident.

Wagner (1932) has studied the hereditary predisposition among those who get compensation by reason of a neurosis. He found a hereditary taint in a much higher percentage than among others. However, his statistics do not deal with head injuries, but were gained from limited material, and in addition, seem to be prejudiced.

It is difficult to come to a clear understanding of what the individual experiences at the moment the accident occurs.

Children look upon the vehicle that runs over them as a symbol of unlimited power and feel that they have to die (Schilder and Wechsler, 1934). It is often difficult to get any description of the experiences at the time of accidents in head injuries, since severe head injuries are almost regularly accompanied by a retrograde amnesia which covers the time of the accident. However, the literature cites many instances of persons who knew what was happening at the time of the accident and even experienced a particularly clear insight into the present and past situation. This happens especially to those who fall down a mountain. At the time, some individuals even noted a definite feeling of happiness. The clinging to the present and the past and the feeling of bliss are obviously defense reactions against the terror of threatened annihilation (Pfister, 1930). It also may be that terror, fright, and anxiety need some time for their development. The terror undeveloped at the time of the accident may appear later on (Sperling, 1929). There can be no doubt that the terror experienced at the time of the accident is not exhausted after the accident has happened. Freud (1920a) has pointed to the fact that the accident may recur in subsequent dreams, and he has based his theory of repetition compulsion upon this fact. Kardiner (1932) has shown that there are not only dreams which repeat the accident, but also dreams which repeat the terror in a more general way. My own observations show that repetition compulsion is not merely a simple repetition, but that it is dependent upon the total psychic situation; moreover, the basic motives might be transformed in various ways. We have no definite proof that the initial terror of the accident is different in cases of head injury from the terror experienced by those sustaining injuries to other parts of the body. However, the part of the body which is hurt plays an important role in the further development of the psychic sequences after injury. Whether there is danger of disfigurement, and whether the individual has any special ideas about the particular accident are also important.

Without doubt, the head has an outstanding part in the body image. It is the carrier of the distance receptors, and everyone knows that it contains the brain, the intactness of which is necessary for proper emotional and intellectual functioning. This was emphasized in the answers to questionnaires I submitted to about twenty persons of average intelligence but without specific medical training. These were persons belonging to the lower economic strata, but some of them had a very good general education. As I myself and Hollós and Ferenczi (1925) have repeatedly emphasized, man is especially anxious to preserve himself as an intelligent and responsible individual. When he has feelings of guilt, he is quite often afraid of being punished by impairment of his mental health. One may also state that head, brain, and mental functioning are invested with a particular amount of narcissistic libido.

I would illustrate these problems by the case history of a social worker who suffered a head injury while on the way to her work. She was sitting in a taxi and was in a great hurry. The taxi ran into a pillar, and she was pushed forward and fell against the front seat of the car. She was only slightly bruised and a trifle dazed. There was no unconsciousness. She continued on her way to the hospital where she was put to rest. She vomited repeatedly. There was no slowing of the pulse. An X-ray was at first interpreted as showing a skull fracture about two inches long in the right temporal region. However, a review of the plates showed that this interpretation was erroneous. No blood was found in the spinal fluid.

There was no reason to believe that the patient had any intent with regard to the accident as such, even though her father had repeatedly warned her against getting up so late and that something might happen while she was rushing to work late. The patient lives with her father, mother, and four brothers in a rather happy family situation. There were no pressing erotic problems at the time of the accident. The patient is gifted and a reliable worker with good psychological understanding. She is allergic. During her stay in the hospital her recovery was rather uneventful, with the exception of one episode to be described. After the discharge from the hospital, the patient gave a detailed report, which was checked on by the observations made during her illness. The following description is taken from this report:

> In my social work I have found that children with head injuries can be recognized very easily. I have always looked upon the skull-fracture group as poor unfortunates. It is difficult to attempt to explain how I felt when the doctor thrust a typewritten report before me. I recall reading, "right temporal, two inches," and immediately I placed the fracture on the left side of my head. To me that was "right temporal" until the day before I was discharged from the hospital. Even today it remains an enigma why I should have made such a gross error. [When the patient arrived at the hospital after the accident she assured the physicians that she felt perfectly well, wanted to go to work immediately, and it was difficult to persuade her to undergo the necessary observation and stay in bed.]
>
> Throughout my stay in the hospital I was careful not to lie on the injured part, and at all times I was very conscious of the area

I thought to be fractured. On one of Dr. S.'s visits, I pointed to a ridge which I thought might be the fracture and asked him if I had located the proper place. I couldn't understand why he pointed to the opposite side of my head and said that the fracture was in this particular region. When I first read the report I disbelieved every word of it. I felt certain that it was due to a fallacy in the X-ray plate and the report belonged to another patient. The doctor seemed indifferent to my inability to accept the news and, without wasting time or words, informed me that he would do a spinal tap. At that moment I felt a rush of blood to my face, followed by terrific pounding in my head. My eyes felt as if hot lead had been poured into them. I grew very weak, and for a moment I seemed to await a great tragedy descending on me. I must have been stunned; my mind was prostrate, cloudy, and heavy. I think I felt as I have on occasions imagined I would feel if someone near or dear to me were to die suddenly. I was to suffer an irretrievable loss. Neither time nor nature could make amends. Gradually the sluggish, dazed feeling left me and my mind picked up momentum. Thoughts crowded in and out of my head in wild confusion. Instantly, all the thoughts I ever had concerning skull fractures became alarmingly significant. Would I change? Would my behavior be impulsive, restive, irrational? Would people look upon me as an old skull-fracture case? Thoughts of this nature presented themselves intermittently and with renewed poignancy during the first twelve days of my stay. Briefly, fear and doubt possessed me interchangeably; fear as to what the outcome would be and doubt as to the authenticity of the fracture report. Whenever a thought tortured me, it was comforting to think that I hadn't a fracture at all. There were times when my mind seemed akin to a beehive. This was probably why I asked for sedatives at night. I was afraid to lie awake and think, and equally afraid to fall asleep and dream. The first nine nights I enjoyed sedatives, but the tenth night I had a reaction to the drug, and thereafter I was denied sleeping aids. [The patient had small amounts of luminal.] I was unable to read because the print jumped.

In the morning and occasionally during the day the walls appeared to be rushing past me. The framework around the doorway seemed very irregular and wobbly and the electrical fixtures "shimmied." Very often I felt heavy throbbings or sensations in my eyes. When I closed them I saw bright jumpy lights in front of them. My back felt restless and squirmish. My knees in particular had quivering sensations around them. I lost all desire for food. At times I felt tremors through my body.

The day after I entered the hospital, the doctor sent a specimen of my blood to the laboratory for a Wassermann. At the time it meant nothing more to me than a part of the routine. Three days later I felt nervous all day. In the evening I saw the nurse inject something into a patient whom I knew to be suffering from a venereal disease. The nurse came directly to me after she had finished with the patient and stuck the needle into me. I immediately decided I had syphilis. The thought obsessed me. I was convinced that the Wassermann had come back positive and that they withheld the information from me but had already started treatment. I was panic-stricken. Every moment I had spent worrying about the fracture suddenly seemed ridiculous as compared with my new big worry. When I awoke the next morning my fear hadn't diminished any. If possible it had become more intense. Evidently Dr. B. sensed that I was upset about something, and when she asked me, I weakened and inquired about my Wassermann. It hadn't been returned. I wanted to believe it, but just couldn't. Later that afternoon the slips were sent to me. They were marked negative. Even then I was somewhat fearful but finally accepted it as the truth. It was strange that all during the scare I looked upon the skull fracture as a strawberry ice cream soda by comparison.

The ninth night I took a sedative and fell asleep as usual. Some time later I awoke to find myself hanging out of the bed, sick to my stomach. I couldn't get any air; there were tremors throughout my body. I felt hot and feverish. Just what happened after that was very hazy. I remember they rolled me out of the room to some place where the lights were bright until they grew dim, and finally I couldn't see or speak. People spoke to me but I couldn't answer. My tongue felt hard, small, and stiff as if paralyzed. I lost complete control of my arms and legs; they felt as if they were tearing wildly through space. I was sure I was dying. I wanted to let the doctors know that my mind was very active, but I couldn't get a message to them. They all seemed hopelessly stupid. I wanted them to tell me what to do to snap out of it, but, instead, they were busy poking at my eyeballs, taking my pulse, hammering my reflexes, and snapping my finger nails. I must have fallen asleep, because I remember waking up the next morning, completely exhausted, drowsy, and dull. When I heard Dr. S. would be down, I was relieved and felt I could hold off the other doctors until he came. I begged them not to do anything without Dr. S.'s consent. They were about to do a spinal tap, but consented to wait.

[The patient was examined at this time. The episode was

considered hysterical. The patient was informed of the psychogenic character of her complaint. No spinal tap was performed.]

Except for some slight speech difficulty during the day, I recovered quickly. I spent most of the day sleeping, and the following day I felt as if burdens had been lifted from my shoulders. It was at that time that I began to look upon the injury somewhat sensibly, and have improved ever since. At present some few things still bother me, namely: 1. Why do I tire so easily? 2. Are my morning headaches caused by "allergies" or is the fracture somewhat responsible? 3. Why do I still have anxiety dreams? 4. What causes the buzzing in my left ear? 5. Will it be necessary to consider the fracture in my future activities, i.e., can I skate, dance, run, swim, and drink occasionally? 6. Is anything apt to develop later, i.e., brain tumor or loss of vision?

[Dreams.] While in the hospital I had very few dreams. At one time I dreamed that the doctors were persecuting me. I was on my way home from the hospital (traveling up and down the streets in a bed), but couldn't make any progress because a doctor in white seemed to step out from every doorway and elicit my reflexes. I was bruised and exhausted and called for Dr. S. Finally, I jumped out of the bed and ran for a telephone, the doctors chasing me. When I got to the phone I hadn't any change and began banging my head against the wall. It all sounded like metal banging. I awoke to find the girl in the next room kicking around in her fracture bed. On another night I dreamed that I tried to get up and found I was too dizzy to walk. It wasn't until I left the hospital that I had really disturbing dreams. Very often I would become engaged in some kind of street brawl, and people would chase me with clubs. I tried to tell them I had a fracture, but couldn't stop for a split second or they would overtake me. I awoke completely exhausted from these dreams. On several occasions I found that my pillow was wet with saliva. One dream was somewhat alarming. I dreamed that I was insane. Men, women, and children gathered round my bed to poke fun at me. They seemed highly amused at my antics. I "swung" at them but they only laughed. I knew I was hallucinating, but couldn't stop myself from seeing things that didn't exist; there was someone in blue velvet sitting at the foot of my bed. I couldn't determine if it were a man or a woman because the back was faced toward me. I tried to look away, but wherever I looked there were funny-looking people seated. I could not decide whether they were men, women, or children. All during this time my tormentors continued to plague me. Again I awoke lying in moisture.

> [After six weeks the patient returned to her work.]
>
> I had only one bad dream since I returned to work. I dreamed that the subway doors couldn't close because my head was caught between them.

She was entitled to compensation by the taxicab company, but didn't show any interest in it at all. She has continued to work and has made complete adaptation. Only slight anxieties occasionally arose.

This observation has been reported in detail because it shows: (1) A specific attitude toward head injuries. (2) Terrors, with the attempt to overcompensate them with displacement (syphilis). (3) Dreams reflecting the terror, chiefly in the form of persecution. (4) Hypochondriacal fears. (5) A hysterical episode. In this case acute terror prevails. This is a neurosis following head injury in which there is no reason to assume that the neurosis is facilitated by organic lesions of the brain. The psychological attitude concerning the head is a fundamental factor. The patient was given psychotherapeutic aid and made a full recovery. It is easy to understand that such a neurosis might persist under less favorable circumstances. Furthermore, it should be pointed out that there is good reason to believe that a very great number of cases of head injury go through similar experiences, which for various reasons are less clearly expressed. Strauss and Savitzky (1934b) report similar cases in which a like picture became the basis for a more lasting neurotic elaboration. Kardiner (1932, pp. 385-386) reports an observation of a patient with a fractured skull:

> He sleeps fitfully; he is at first awakened from his sleep by terrors, the content of which is that he is being annihilated. Then there is a series of dreams in which he is no longer in danger, but in which he witnesses race riots with Jews fighting Chinese, etc. Following this comes a series of dreams in which he is witnessing combative sports, such as football games; then a series in which he is at work, but subject to repeated frustrations. In one dream, finally, occurring about two weeks after the traumatic event, he is at work and is interrupted by a fire in a school, but the dream terminates with the remark, "Oh H—, I don't go to school any more!"—he wakes

up, and goes back to a dreamless sleep. This is the last dream of the series.

Pictures of this type can also be observed in children.[1]

Arthur, twelve years old, was admitted to a hospital March 7, 1938, with a history of having been struck by an automobile and thrown on his head. On admission he was conscious, drowsy, but answered questions clearly. He told a fantastic story in relation to the accident, complained about pain in his head, right shoulder, and right chest, and vomited shortly after the admission. There was a large hematoma over the left parietal and right frontal brain regions. There were bilateral Babinski toe signs and ankle clonus. The spinal fluid was bloody. Throughout the patient's stay in this hospital he was difficult to control on the ward, tried to get out of bed, pleaded to go home, and stated that his father or mother would die if he did not go home. He threatened to cause the doctors and nurses to disappear by magic. He was transferred to Bellevue Hospital (Psychiatric Division) on March 16, 1938. At that time he was oriented and gave a rational account of his accident. However, he was dominated by anxiety and restlessness. He showed quick changes of mood, called continually for his mother and father, and did not stay in bed. He reported dreams in which he was an aviator who crashes and gets killed; also, that he put a bear trap in the chimney to catch Santa Claus. The X-ray examination revealed a vertical fracture of the squamous portion of the temporal bone on the left side. The spinal fluid was negative. There were bilateral Babinski toe signs and a dropping of the left arm. On March 18, he was tense and overalert, very anxious to hold his contact with persons around him, and continually seeking assurance. He now described the accident in the following way:

He was playing in the park with other boys and told them: "Well, I will go home." He thought about it and hoped it wasn't late because to warm up dinner again would make trouble for his

[1] The children reported upon here were observed on the Children's Ward of Bellevue Hospital (Psychiatric Division) in charge of Dr. L. Bender.

mother. He remembered that he crossed the street half-heartedly and did not look at the lights or notice that a car was coming. The next thing he remembered was that he awoke in the hospital. He said that it is very bad to be hit, and if he ever finds that he is hit by an automobile again he hopes we will "sock him in the eye." He certainly will be careful in the future. He had thought about other boys who were "hit by automobiles, and were run over their stomachs, and crushed their heads, and they are dead." When telling this he started to cry and wanted to go home to his mother. (The day before, he had called the nurse "mother.") "I wanted to get to my mother and had a feeling that whoever was taking care of me was my mother." The boy asked constantly to go home and to get to his mother. It seemed as if he would be sure he was not dead, and nothing could happen to him once he could reach his mother or father. He said that in the first hospital he had been told that his mother and father were dead. He said: "I awoke in the hospital and I saw my father and he told me what happened. My father said there was no blood. If I bled out of my nose and ears, I would have had a hemorrhage, and it would have been bad." His death fears and anxieties expressed themselves in restlessness, talkativeness, and the continuous wish to go home. At the same time he reassured himself continually. At the time of discharge on April 18, 1938, the restlessness had completely subsided and there were no obvious fears and anxieties. He proved to be very dependent on his parents, especially his mother. He had an average intelligence.

Immediately after the accident the boy showed the psychotic picture described by Blau (1936). As the illness developed, the psychotic picture retreated into the background and a neurotic picture filled with fright and anxiety appeared. It is interesting to note that in this fear and fright he had a particularly strong longing for his parents and parent substitutes. Furthermore, he reassured himself continuously. There is no question that a brain injury was present and that organic factors may have played a part in the initial psychosis and in the neurosis. However, the picture is essentially a picture of fright and subsequent restlessness and an attempt to escape the fright and fear of death. The picture is essentially the same as in the case previously reported.

According to Huddleson (1932), traumatic neuroses are rare in children. He quotes several observations by Oppenheim (1889), Fetterman (1928), Gabrio (1920) and others. Most of these observations were not concerned with head injuries. In a discussion of Wechsler's paper (1935), Hall and Mackay (1934) even deny the existence of neuroses in children following head injuries. I think that acute fright reactions in children following head injuries have been overlooked. I believe they are not uncommon, and have convinced myself in my analysis of adults of the long-lasting effects of injuries in children, and especially of head injuries. Acute fright reactions bear a close relation to the psychotic cases described by Blau. It is an open question whether such experiences might not later on lead to behavior difficulties. It might be very difficult to differentiate such situations from the behavior difficulties found in children following head injuries dependent on an organic basis (Kasanin, 1929).

Neurasthenic and Hypochondriacal Reactions

We now turn to a second group of neuroses following head injuries, namely, the neurasthenic hypochondriacal group. Our first case complained of fatigue and had a series of hypochondriacal ideas.

M.S., a 43-year-old married woman who had three children, did not show neurotic trends, according to the reports of her family and the physician, before an accident which occurred one year prior to her admission to Bellevue Hospital, March 20, 1936. The patient fell, and a dress-dummy figure fell on top of her head. She then complained of headaches, dizziness, and fear of falling, and was fatigued and unable to work. According to the report of an indemnity company, she was unconscious for a short time and stayed in the hospital for six days. At an examination three months later, there was an increase in the deep reflexes, bilateral Babinski toe, and Rossolimo signs. The encephalogram was negative. The patient received compensation of eight dollars a week, which stopped one month before she came to the hospital. She complained chiefly about headaches, dizziness, and nausea, which came on whenever she tried to work. Her eyes bothered her; she could not sleep; she had dreams that she had gone crazy and that a horse and wagon would kill her. She was continually under tension, agitated, and on the verge of tears. There occasionally was trembling of psychogenic character; her hands sweated; her pulse rate ranged between 120 and 144; her basal metabolism was normal. There were no organic signs referable to the nervous system. An intelligence test showed that she was not defective. Her memory was poor, but the memory disturbance was not of an organic type.

It is an open question whether cases like this should be called neurasthenic, in view of the headaches, fatigue, and dizziness, or whether one should speak of a hysterical picture. Unquestionably, the patient had a head injury with a brain lesion. Whether one wants to consider the tachycardia as a part of the concussion syndrome or as psychogenic is immaterial. Friedmann (1892) observed the vasomotor syndrome after head injuries. It consists of headaches, dizziness, nausea, and vasomotor and vegetative phenomena of all kinds. There is no question that this is an organic syndrome. However, it may lead to neurasthenic attitudes and may be fixed by psychogenic mechanisms. It might be emphasized that, in our case, the condition was exacerbated when compensation stopped.

Hypochondriacal pictures often are based on an alteration in outward appearance, which is then regarded as an impairment of one's body image.

A.W., 22 years old, was run over by a car. He was operated upon for a compound fracture of the skull. Upon admission six years later, a trephine opening over the right frontal bone 4 cm. in diameter was seen in the X-ray. There were no organic neurological signs. His I.Q. was 108. There were no disturbances in memory functions. He complained about restlessness, and one year before admission he had run away from home for no particular reason. He also complained of loss of memory and whirling sensations in the head. Sometimes he felt blank and talked automatically. He fatigued very easily. When he became dizzy, things seemed to turn around: for instance, the faucet in the bathroom. He gave an enormous amount of attention to the opening in the skull. He experimented with it, blowing it out, and was particularly afraid that he might get hurt in that area. In general, he was greatly concerned about his health. He thought that his sex urge was too great, although careful questioning showed that his sex adaptation and attitudes were about average. He had had sex relations with prostitutes.

Protracted observation did not prove that his blank states were epileptic. The whole picture must be considered a neurotic consequence of the severe head injury. A plastic operation covering the trephine hole in the skull gave him a greater feeling of security, and his difficulties diminished considerably.

The complaint of memory disturbance is common after head injuries. A psychiatric examination almost always makes it possible to differentiate organic from psychogenic memory disturbances following head injuries. The same complaint was present in the previous case. This type of psychogenic memory disturbance is of neurasthenic character and must be differentiated from the amnestic gaps on a hysterical basis. The patient reported that he once ran away because of restlessness. There is no reason to believe that this was due to an epileptic fugue. Differential diagnosis may sometimes be difficult. I have previously observed an individual who showed character changes after severe head injury; without any reason he occasionally decided to leave home for a long time. I was inclined to believe in an organic character change due to a brain lesion. In this instance, irritability (missing in the case just described) was present, and organic memory disturbances had preceded the character change.

A case similar in many respects, but psychologically more accessible, was seen on the children's ward:

Frederick, eleven years old, was of low average intelligence.

His I.Q. was 92. Educational tests showed that he was able to do fifth grade work. He was a normal boy until October, 1935, when, at the age of nine, he was playing on a freight train and fell on his head. He was temporarily dazed, but got up and walked home; then he lost consciousness, but regained it before an ambulance arrived. In the hospital, he became unconscious for the third time. The diagnosis was made of a depressed fracture of the skull in the right posterior parietal region, with additional fissure fracture in the temporal bone around the mastoid involving the base of the skull. He was operated on the second day and the depressed pieces of bone were removed. A later X-ray showed evidence of a resection of an area above the right mastoid two and one half inches in diameter. Since the accident, the boy has been emotional, unstable, and liable to outbursts of irritability, during which he attacks other children; he even choked a boy with a rope. He was also subject to headaches which developed in the region of the injury when there was a change in the weather. He described these headaches as maddening at times. There were vestibular phenomena in which he felt dizzy, things whirled about him, he became nauseated, and vomited, and felt hot and as if the bed were moving in wavelike motions. There were also petit mal episodes in which he felt that his mind left him for a minute. The boy was extremely sensitive and terrified by his condition, and felt that he could not fight because of the opening in the skull. He was admitted February 18, 1938, to the children's ward. He was acutely distressed by the sequelae of the accident:

"Yes, I used to say I wanted to die. I don't know why . . . . Yes, I wished it before the accident. Sometimes I would not feel it when stuck with pins. I used to feel hot and cold. Things looked different before my eyes. The bed would move up and down. . . . Yes, I would lose my memory for hours. . . . Yes, I had my appendix out a few months ago. I was more afraid to have that scar touched afterward than to have my head hit."

The psychotherapeutic approach revealed a deep underlying fear concerning the defect in the skull. On the 16th of March, a plastic operation was done to cover the skull depression, with good results. He was seen on the 17th of May and said that he felt much better. His irritability had diminished, and he adapted well to school.

Although this case undoubtedly showed an organic concussion syndrome, there was deep concern of a hypochondriacal type in relation to the cranial defect, and his behavior disturbances were not on a purely organic basis.

Hysterical Reactions

The largest group of neurotic pictures following head injuries is made up of hysterias. Most of the cases reported in the literature, for instance, by Strauss and Savitzky, are hysterias as far as they are neurotic. It seems that hysteria following head injuries can occur without any organic residuals due to the head injury as such.

Wechsler (1935) saw 56 hysterical reactions among his 100 cases of head injury. However, his material consisted of the chronic sequelae of head injuries in which severe organic consequences were not predominant. Among 360 cases with manifest injury of the brain, Pfeifer (1924) found 28 with hysterical admixtures. Pfeifer's material came from an institute of war veterans who had suffered brain lesions. In similar material, Poppelreuter (1917) found between twelve and fifteen percent of hysterical cases.

R.F., 43 years old, was admitted to Bellevue Hospital July 30, 1937. The patient complained of headaches: "It feels like someone painted varnish on it. I have had it, off and on, for nineteen years. I wish I were dead. I can't sleep or do anything." He also complained about weakness on the right side, falling to the right, and there were convulsions on the right side.

In 1922, he was struck on the head by a rivet and then fell twenty feet from a scaffold. He was unconscious, but later went back to work. Two years afterward, he went to the hospital where a right Babinski toe sign was found and a slight right horizontal nystagmus. A right temporal decompression was performed. An encephalogram in March, 1937, was negative. An encephalogram repeated in our hospital on August 30, 1937, was again negative. An ophthalmologic examination showed a dystopia of the right iris and lens, with impairment of vision. Both visual fields were contracted, especially the right one. There also seemed to be a pallor of the right disc. Hearing was only slightly impaired on both sides. There was a right-sided paresis and hemianesthesia of typical hysterical character. The patient would fall to the right. The outstretched arms deviated to the right.

The patient reported that he had headaches for the first time in 1919 when he was afraid of being attacked by a jealous lover. At that time it felt like a band around his head. However, the real headaches started after the accident. The patient was oriented, clear, of average intelligence; he had a slight memory impairment. He was rather definite concerning his report that an accident had happened; but the details varied. His complaint about headaches was likewise not very consistent.

However, on the basis of the report of the hospital in which he was operated on two years after the accident, we may suppose that an organic injury of the brain was present. The picture at the present time is chiefly of psychogenic character, although the falling to the right side might indicate organic components. One might also suspect that the headaches of which the patient complained were organic. A sympathetic nerve block was tried, but was without effect. The patient never got compensation. A superficial psychiatric examination did not reveal sufficient reasons for such lasting signs.

The outstanding symptomatology so far described consists of hemiparesis, convulsions, and monocular polyopia. However, the entire gamut of hysterical symptoms can be seen in such cases.

In another case, a severe accident for which a small amount of compensation was paid led to attacks of sleepiness during the day, insomnia during the night, and vasomotor attacks in the left arm, which ended with a sort of unconsciousness. The patient also had some kind of attacks in which he fell down. Careful examination failed to reveal any organic signs. The patient, a plumber, had had many accidents before, mostly involving the hands. In the few dreams which occurred during the lengthy observation, he was often bitten on the hands by animals. The patient maintained a carefree attitude, although the accident and the neurosis had deprived him of his livelihood, and he was on welfare. He had a particular attitude toward death. He felt that he could predict the death of others, and that he had prophetic dreams. Extended psychotherapy did not bring any definite relief. A considerable amount of time was spent in clearing up the early history. Throughout his whole life he had felt that he had been put at a disadvantage. His older brothers were continually preferred to him, and his mother did not give him much attention. He always felt that he had been pushed into an inferior position. After careful analysis, the accident could not be considered in any way connected with his personal attitudes. It was merely an incident. The compensation question was very soon settled. However, the patient was later shuffled between jobs in the Works Progress Administration and Home Relief and felt that both of these agencies did not give him as much help as they should have.

This case illustrates a variety of psychogenic symptoms and gives a deeper insight into some of the psychological conditions that are operative in traumatic neurosis in which the feeling of social injustice plays some part. Although the roots of this patient's attitudes go back into his childhood, his difficulties started in immediate relation to the accident. It could not be decided whether the vasomotor phenomena, undoubtedly present, are psychogenic or a part of the postconcussion syndrome.

Another group of hysterical neuroses following head injuries is represented by amnestic states.

B.W., 30 years old, was admitted to Bellevue Hospital as an unknown white male who had come out of a restaurant looking for a job, and could not remember if he was married or had a child. On January 29, 1928, the following notes were made: (What is your name?) "I don't know, sir. I am trying to remember it. I can't." (How long haven't you known your name?).... (Do you know where you are now?) "A hospital; the nurse told me. I don't know what the name of it is. Who am I?" ... (How long are you here?) "Since yesterday." (Are you sick?) "I get pains right along here" (patient indicated his forehead). "I didn't know I was brought here. I don't know who brought me." (Where do you live?) "I don't know." (Are you dizzy?) "Right now I just have little pains in my head." (Where did you live before you came in here?) "My mother." (What does she look like?) "A woman around fifty; short-built woman." (Do you like her?) "Yes." (Where does she live?) ... (When did you see her last?) "Yesterday morning." (Did she make breakfast for you?) "My mother is in business." (Who makes the breakfast?) "It is right on the stove." (Who puts it on the stove?) "I got dressed afterward, and I went to look for a job." (What kind of a job?) "Driving a truck. I went into a restaurant on Broadway, and that's the last thing I remember. When I came out everything went blank." (What did you do then?) ... (Did you go to a policeman?) "A policeman stopped me because he saw that I was crying...."

The patient was very bewildered. Neurological examination showed tremor of the fingers, ankle clonus of organic type, and exaggerated reflexes. The amnesia was considered psychogenic; however, an old organic brain lesion was supposed to have given the pattern to the psychogenic picture. In the meantime, information was received from his physician that he had sustained a head injury in May, 1935, in which he was unconscious for fifteen minutes. Following that, there were post-traumatic headaches and dizziness. It was a compensation case, since the accident happened while he was at work. There had been no previous periods of amnesia. During the last year he had become irritable and had an exaggerated opinion of his own importance, and had spent too much money, which he took from his mother. He cried very easily. The X-rays were negative after the accident and also at the time of the examination. The patient refused an encephalogram.

Cases of this type are not uncommon. Abeles and I (1935) often found that a head injury may provide a pattern used later on in a psychogenic amnesia. I have seen cases in which there was at least the probability that a head injury at the age of five gave the pattern to amnestic attacks in later situations. It seems that in such cases the head injury was connected with an attitude of acquiescence and passivity. One may raise this question in such cases: What was the relationship between the organic and the psychogenic picture? It seems that the accident with its partially organic consequences threw the patient out of his orbit, and psychogenic difficulties followed, of which the amnesia was one expression. In this case, it seems probable that there were psychogenically conditioned changes in character. It is worth while emphasizing that neurotic pictures may occur years after an accident and still may be consequences of the accident.

We may hope to get a deeper psychological insight in studying the case of a child in which a hysterical picture followed a head injury:

Oliver was a ten-year-old black boy. He was on the children's ward from January 20, 1938 to February 17, 1938. He was seen in the Mental Hygiene Clinic on December 22, 1937. The case was referred to the hospital by his school, with the statement that he was subject to violent outbursts of temper when he would "shoot spitballs"; once he attacked a child with a pocket knife. The teacher stated that, "although he is considered bright in school, he constantly beats and threatens other children, and he can close his mind like a door, and will not learn the things he doesn't like. He even closes his eyes and stuffs his ears with his fingers. He rarely plays with other children, preferring to work on little projects of his own." The father stated that there was nothing wrong with the boy until he suffered a skull fracture in September, 1935. "When the moon is full, Oliver always acts up," he said.

The history was as follows: The father and mother have

been separated for three years. The father is 57. At one time he appeared to be a fairly capable person, but he is gradually deteriorating in his social standing and working ability. At the present time he drinks to excess. The mother is much younger and works as a domestic in a suburb. There are two children by this marriage, Oliver and his sister who is eight years old. The mother is responsible for the girl and either keeps her herself or boards her out in a pleasant home. Oliver has lived with his father practically since the time of his parents' separation and, as indicated above, they have lived in squalid surroundings. There seems to have been too close an attachment between Oliver and his father. Frequently during the boy's stay in the hospital the father visited him, usually under the influence of alcohol, at which times he would become lachrymose, assuring us that he was more than a father to Oliver; in fact, the two of them were more like brothers. He also said that he could not live if Oliver were taken away from him. In addition to the squalid surroundings and inadequate care, Oliver also had to share the bed with his father's paramour on occasion. It was noted by his school teacher that he was always in a dazed and more irritable condition on Monday morning than on other days during the week.

His birth and early development were normal; there had been no severe illness until September, 1935, when he was struck by a taxicab and suffered a severe cerebral concussion, serious injury to the right leg, and fracture of the right clavicle. Skull X-rays showed no fracture. Head X-rays taken in Bellevue, December, 1937, were normal. He seemed to have been unconscious for a few hours following the accident. When he awoke he thought he had saved a girl from a fire, but did not know anything about the accident. He was drowsy and semiconscious for several days. He was discharged after ten days in the hospital. Both the school authorities and the father date his behavior disorders from this accident.

Our examination (December 22, 1937) disclosed a mental age of eleven and a half with an I.Q. of 115 on the Stanford-Binet, 4A School placement when he was only doing third-grade reading, arithmetic, and spelling. It was felt that he had a moderate reading disability. During the psychiatric examination the child was friendly and talked freely, giving the following information: First, feelings of inferiority because he was black. (It should be added that the father attributed a great many of the difficulties in school to the fact that he was black.) He described "spells" over which he had no control, during which he felt dizzy and was nauseated. He would look at an object and it would suddenly become very large and close to him. At other times the object would become very small and far away. Sometimes he had feelings of heat in his head or of being suffocated. Sometimes he felt his brain "separated in the middle and went back and forth"; sometimes it lifted off the skull or "went to the top." He also saw colored spots before his eyes. He wished he were a girl because he likes girls' dresses, bright colors, and partly because his sister received much better care and had more things than were given him. Spontaneously, he complained of not being able to defend himself among other children, being afraid of aggression in other boys. (It has since been reported to us that during his summer in the country, he was said to have been constantly afraid that other boys would do him bodily harm, and he ran to the counselor for protection. He still is entirely dependent upon other people, particularly his father.) He also had a masturbation complex and feelings that he was sexually weaker than other boys of his age.

On the ward he made a very good adjustment. There were a few periods of instability, but taking him away from the group and giving him assurance was sufficient to ward off one of his attacks. He had no hysterical features at this time.

There is reason to believe that there were organic changes present in this case since there had been a severe head injury, with unconsciousness. We may suppose that his spells of dizziness and nausea were of organic origin. The vasomotor phenomena described may belong to Friedmann's vasomotor symptom complex, or, in other words, to the organic concussion syndrome (1892). However, whether we believe in such an organic nucleus or not, the picture gets its final meaning through an interpretation of the psychological problems related to the boy's attachment to his father, toward whom he felt completely passive. There was a hysterical symptomatology consisting of micropsia and macropsia. Furthermore, there were behavior difficulties which were the expression of the fright to which he had been exposed, which had accentuated the feelings of passivity and helplessness.

The problem in the next case is very similar; however, it was subjected to less psychologic investigation, and the organic nucleus of the symptoms was more obvious.

F.L., 21 years old, had a fractured skull when he was six years old. He was run over by a car and was unconscious for a short time. He said: "For eleven years I have had dizzy spells; when they happen I say, 'Hold me, hold me,' and I groan. I want to hold on to the ground because I have a feeling that my body is getting lighter. I get spells as often as I want to, just by going into open spaces. When I look at an object, all other objects seem to fade away, and I see only one at a time. I see different colored spots. Faces become blurred; everything becomes very large and I become very small. Things don't become distorted; they come closer and become larger. They don't incline to one side or another. I don't go on bridges because I would have a spell. I never fall down; anything which goes off the ground makes me dizzy. I haven't had relations with girls. Sometimes I dream about sex, though. Other times I dream I am drowning in the middle of the ocean. I haven't any ambitions; I just don't want to do anything which is not easy to do and makes demands on me." His I.Q. was 82.

There was a calcified area in the left parietal lobe. The patient had a weak bilateral Hoffmann sign and a slight tremor of the hands; no other palpable signs. When the patient was standing with outstretched arms during an examination, with his eyes closed, he had a dizzy spell, reached for a chair, and cried loudly.

The dizziness in this case had a partly organic origin but also facilitated neurotic attitudes of hysteriform type which led to changes in character. The interaction between organic changes due to lesions of the brain and psychogenic elaboration can be very complicated, as Pötzl (1917) has shown.

On the whole, it is astonishing to note that, once hysterical symptoms are developed, anxieties and terrors with corresponding dreams sink into the background. However, there are rare cases in which anxieties are transformed into hysteriform pictures.

E.O., 35 years old, was struck on the head with a telephone when he was attacked by six political enemies. He was unconscious, but physical examination did not show any organic signs. He complained of dizziness and headaches. One year later, he was still afraid that someone was after him and imagined he saw strange people in his room at night. The structure of these illusions proved to be of hysterical type (Schilder, 1934b).

In summing up the data concerning hysterical cases after head injuries, one comes to the following conclusions: Psychogenic pictures develop more often in cases in which there is no severe organic impairment. However, they also occur (as Strauss and Savitzky, 1934b, have emphasized) in cases presenting marked organic defects. It seems that more or less persistent dizziness is in itself a factor which encourages neurotic attitudes.

Very often, the postconcussion syndrome is the basis for psychological elaborations of hysterical type, which can also occur when the head injury is not severe enough to lead to impairment of cerebral functions.

In the majority of cases reported here, the neurosis developed in individuals who previously had shown no neurotic symptoms. In some cases a superficial investigation did not even show a personality one would have suspected as easily falling victim to neurotic tendencies. I do not doubt that personality characteristics have an important influence on the later formation of the neurosis and its symptomatology. However, one must not overlook the etiological importance of the fact that a head injury has taken place, that unconsciousness has occurred, and that the individual suffers from organic consequences of the head injury which, even in themselves, may facilitate neurotic attitudes.

Psychological factors which facilitate a hysterical attitude might be found in a wish for deep dependence on either parent, with a tendency to masochistic subjection. At the same time this may be a factor which leads the victim to expose himself to the chance of accident. The hysterical symptom may, furthermore, substantiate the feeling that injustice is done to the individual, and, finally, the individual may claim love and support through the hysterical symptom.

From this point of view one understands the frequency of hysterical manifestations after injuries and especially after head injuries.

The symptomatology of hysteria after head injuries is as varied as the symptomatology of hysteria in general. However, it seems that hysterical hemiparesis, sensory disturbances, and amnesia play a particularly important role in the material which we have at our disposal.

Hysterical blindness and deafness have often been observed after head injuries. They did not play an important part in our material. Monocular polyopia was often present. After head injuries one may find all the symptoms otherwise found in hysteria. These symptoms are determined by the total psychological situation of the individual and express deep-seated emotional problems. The symptoms are, of course, also dependent upon the social setting in which the individual lives. Imitation and suggestion may have a share in their production. However, the individual does not imitate consciously or unconsciously unless such imitation helps to express his own emotional needs. Human beings in general, and patients with head injuries in particular, are only amenable to suggestion insofar as the suggestion is accepted by unconscious strivings.

It should be emphasized that compensation questions play a comparatively small and unimportant part in our series of cases. This is obviously due to the fact that the material has been collected from psychiatric wards and not from institutions taking care of compensation cases. It is also important to stress the fact that the clinical pictures of patients with such syndromes who demand compensation and of those who do not demand it are basically identical.

It is well known that severe character changes occur on an organic basis following head injuries, in children as well as in adults. Some character changes may lie in the field of hyperkinesis or epileptoid manifestations. Memory disturbances of an organic type may be present. However, a long-lasting neurosis obviously also changes the character of an individual, and it sometimes may be difficult to differentiate the psychogenic alterations in character from the organic; this is equally true of adults and children. The character changes and the disturbances in memory and intellect observed in prizefighters are obviously due to organic conditions (Martland, 1928; Winterstein, 1937). However, in cases I have observed of prizefighters who had to quit the ring after several defeats, psychogenic depression complicated whatever may have been present of organic nature.

Social and Compensation Factors

The hysterical patient addresses himself to society and makes it clear that he suffers and demands help. Among cases of head injury, those with hysteria demand help more urgently than others; moreover, this syndrome is often combined with the demand for compensation. The feeling of social injustice may come more and more into the foreground, and the demand for help and compensation will become more and more outspoken.

Even in cases of so-called malingering, this social factor and the wish for help play a very important part. It is obvious that prolonged litigation will increase the feeling of injustice and make adaptation more and more difficult. However, even when the litigation is settled by a lump-sum payment, the processes underlying the neurosis do not come to an end. Although definite financial settlement is of incontestable value, it in no way ends the neurosis. Schnyder (1936) has emphasized this point of view in its relation to head injuries. Eliasberg (1927) and Riese (1929) stress the fact that traumatic neurosis is not merely a medical problem, but also a cultural and sociological one. Furthermore, it is not correct to emphasize only the question of whether or not the individual is capable of doing work again. The important question is whether the individual suffers by reason of the psychological consequences or does not suffer.

Schnyder (1936) has also emphasized the difficulties in potency in traumatic neurosis following head injuries.

Psychology of Neuroses Following Head Injuries

It is perhaps worth while to summarize the psychological problems encountered in neuroses following head injuries. We have first to consider the psychology of the trauma as such. During the trauma, the individual experiences a threat to the integrity of his body—a threat of death or deformity. At the same time, he acknowledges the superior force of the traumatic agent, which might become a symbol of the power of the parent. The individual may experience masochistic gratification in the trauma and may even have sought the trauma for a similar reason. When a head injury has occurred, unconsciousness may be followed by a period of organic disorientation with a severe disturbance in brain function.

Here we are interested in those cases in which the organic consequences are not in the foreground. There may be a more or less outspoken difficulty on a psychogenic basis in the reorientation of the body and the outside world (Kardiner, 1932). The terror of annihilation may be revived again; it may recur at the specific hour of the accident or as a mere terror or as a revival of the traumatic scene of the accident, in imagination, hallucination, or as a dream. The dreams may be an unchanged revival of the traumatic scene or they may constitute a more or less symbolic interpretation of annihilation: e.g., drowning and catastrophes of other types; and finally, there are often dreams of persecution. It seems as if the individual cannot get over the dangerous situation, and again and again tries to become acquainted with it. This is the meaning of the so-called repetition compulsion, which, according to Freud (1920a), is proven particularly by repetitive dreams in traumatic neurosis. He is of the opinion that the repetition compulsion is connected chiefly with the ego instincts and less with the libidinal instincts.

There cannot be any doubt that the individual does not get over the entire situation which he has once experienced. Furthermore, he may derive some masochistic gratification from his suffering. All his previous doubts and fears may express themselves in death fears. It is rather interesting that the fear of syphilis was a temporary substitute in one of our patients for the fear of disease through head injury. The terror may finally be replaced by the fear of a lasting defect in the intellectual and, in some cases, even in the sexual sphere. One may speak of this as fear of impairment of the body image. Sadger (1920) has described castration fear.

When the organic signs of headaches, vomiting, dizziness, and vasomotor phenomena are present, they add to the insecurity and terror. Hypochondriacal and neurasthenic signs will be more outspoken when the body image is changed, e.g., after a trephine. It depends upon the previous structure of the personality whether the individual will overcome the continuous threat of annihilation or whether a more chronic neurotic picture will occur. Difficulties in memory may lead to a deep fear of having lost the integrity of one's brain and personality. Hysterical pictures may express the wish that the suffering should be compensated for by the love and appreciation of others around one. The hysterical symptom emphasizes the suffering in its social aspects, and its demands arise frequently in connection with previous deprivations of love; these symptoms are often related to the need for emotional and financial compensation. Hysterical syndromes are frequently built upon somatic compliance, i.e., a somatically impaired function. All these reactions are based not only upon the present situation, but also on the individual's past. However, in the case of traumatic neuroses following head injuries, the head injury with its psychological consequences is an indispensable factor in the total development. In cases in which the question of compensation comes to the fore, the feeling of social injustice is of paramount importance.

Diagnosis

It is necessary to have a clear picture of the accident as such. Careful somatic examination immediately after the accident, especially X-ray and spinal fluid examinations, will often help toward a later understanding of the picture. A careful physical examination with all the aid modern neurology can offer is indispensable, as emphasized by Strauss and Savitzky. One should keep in mind that organic signs do not exclude the possibility of neurotic ones. Correct appraisal of the situation is necessary for the understanding of neurotic signs. The vasomotor phenomena and dizziness are often organic. One should also keep in mind that retrograde amnesia, memory disturbances of the Korsakoff type, and specific types of irritability are psychological signs which are not neurotic. These organic psychological signs might be interwoven with psychogenic ones, or they even might be the nucleus around which psychogenic pictures are grouped. Furthermore, it is probable that dizziness and disturbances in consciousness facilitate neurotic attitudes. Particular attention should be given to the hysterical sensory and motor hemiparesis, especially with involvement of the special senses on the same side. Monocular polyopia can be organically determined, but is most often a sign of hysteria. The various psychological types of gait disturbance should be considered.

Traumatic neuroses may be acute or chronic; they may immediately follow the accident or may occur after the acute organic signs have passed. Moreover, it seems that we may encounter a traumatic neurosis first appearing at a long interval following the trauma. This time period may depend partly on the fact that organic traumatic signs also may come to the fore after a long interval.

One should refrain from all statements which are too schematic. One should not speak about traumatic neurosis when a trauma has been merely an insignificant episode in a neurotic's life history. A traumatic neurosis may be diagnosed only when a decided change has taken place in the individual following an injury. Neurosis and malingering can best be differentiated from each other when one considers the total situation and the entire development. Sometimes the proof for malingering can only be adduced from external data concerning the behavior and the remarks of the patient when he does not know he is being observed by the physician.

Oberholzer (1931) has used the Rorschach test in the differential diagnosis between organic and psychogenic mechanisms. Further investigation on this point is necessary.

Treatment

It should be kept in mind that many individuals with traumatic neuroses in general, and especially those following head injury, suffer not only from their neuroses but also from typical organic consequences of the trauma. One should keep in mind that many persons can, and often do, force themselves to work, even if they suffer and work under great difficulties (Riese, 1929). There is no reason why one should expect any worker to put forth a great amount of self-sacrifice and work under conditions of distress which surpass the average difficulties encountered in working. It is perhaps necessary to remark that organic symptoms often can be overcompensated by a specific effort, but the necessary effort may be very great. The diagnosis of neurosis is unjustified merely because an individual gives in to symptoms instead of making extraordinary efforts. One should also remember that ability to work as such is not a sign that an individual has no symptoms. Furthermore, the organic consequences of head injury are almost always increased by work; this may have a bad influence on a concomitant neurosis. If one deals with neurotic manifestations, one has to keep in mind the symbolic significance of work. It frequently symbolizes sadistic aggression which the individual does not want to exercise in order not to be exposed to counterattacks. Tools and machinery may present additional fears. Phobic reactions may be connected with scenes reminding him of the accident. Work means also that the individual is independent and strong and has no further claim for consideration by others. Finally, it may mean that the individual is no longer entitled to compensation. Under such conditions, it can readily be seen that the advice or order to go back to work is of very great psychological significance and should not be lightly given. In the majority of cases there will be no special reason to rush the patient back to work as long as he has complaints, irrespective of whether or not there are organic residuals. When there are no organic residuals and the patient continues to complain, the advice to go to work has to be considered only as a part of general psychotherapy, subject to the rules which are valid for active therapy.

It is preposterous to believe that any neurosis of severe degree can be "cured" by changing the external situation alone. It is true that among the traumatic neuroses the compensation question may play a more or less important part. This will depend partly on the type of the neurosis. In general, we may expect that the compensation question will be less outspoken in the acute terror reactions, will gain a greater importance in the neurasthenic hypochondriac reactions, and will find its greatest role in hysterical reactions which demand attention and love. It is generally conceded that the medicolegal complications arising in connection with compensation might increase the neurotic symptoms. However, in most cases the roots of the neurosis lie deeper, and a neurosis which consists merely in the claim for compensation is obviously either malingering or at least very near to it. It is usually acknowledged that a speedy ending of the compensation question, by settlement or otherwise, is preferable. Riese (1928) and Schnyder (1936) emphasize that even after lump-sum settlement, difficulties of neurotic character often remain. On the whole, it is advisable for the physician who treats a patient with traumatic neurosis to be aware of the compensation element, but he should not approach the traumatic patient with the idea that the main question is whether or not the patient is entitled to compensation. Even the individual with a traumatic neurosis who demands compensation suffers and has the right to be treated as a patient. It is therefore advisable to approach the case as one would any other neurotic patient. Psychotherapeutic procedure should consist of the steps usually followed in such cases: (1) winning of the transference; (2) working through the transference; (3) breaking of the transference. The physician should listen to the complaints of the patient and let him express himself as freely as possible.

Psychoanalysis has taught us that we are more certain of building up the transference of a patient correctly if we are not too active. According to the character of the case it may be advisable to use forms of short psychotherapy or the classical technique of psychoanalysis. It is more important that the patient understands the situation than it is for him to get advice. I think it is essential that the patient should also have a clear understanding of the physical findings in his case. There is no reason why the whole problem should not be discussed with the patient freely and in intelligible terms as soon as he shows any interest in it. The patient is entitled to a discussion of X-ray findings, serology, and so on. Our own observations show how easily patients misinterpret what they have been told, and one should make as certain as possible that the patient has a clear understanding of the extent of his difficulties. In many cases it may even be advisable to see that the relatives and individuals around him should have a similar understanding. It will depend upon the skill of the psychotherapist to decide at which part of the treatment the situation should be discussed with the patient. According to the general rules of psychotherapy, active therapy can only be started when a positive transference has been gained.

As already mentioned, the advice to go to work is very active therapy. Moralizing, scolding, and threatening have no place in the therapist's scheme. In some cases it might become advisable for the physician to take an active part in shaping the total reaction of the patient. In the majority of cases it will be advisable to try to drive the psychotherapy sufficiently deep so that the patient is enabled to do that himself. In many cases, it will not be necessary to help the patient gain an insight into his own psychosexual development and to go systematically into early childhood experiences. In some cases this will be unavoidable, as in other forms of neuroses. Group discussion and group psychotherapy have never been tried systematically in cases of this type. This seems to be a method for the future. For the present, there should be a planned psychological approach to the patient. At any rate, the physician should recognize his own attitude toward the social problems involved and should especially guard himself against the negative countertransference so often shown by those who have written on compensation neuroses. It might be well for the physician to be aware that he is not a referee to decide on compensation questions, but that his chief task is to help the patient to understand himself so that he can find a way out of the neurosis.

CHAPTER ELEVEN

Problems in the Technique of Psychoanalysis

An eighteen-year-old patient whom I analyzed in the Phipps Clinic of Johns Hopkins Hospital recounted the following as his first dream: He saw a water tank which he and a friend blew up. A big strong man caught them and whipped them so severely that streaks of blood ran down their legs. This dream was brought out in the first analytical hour. Now, we know that these first dreams outline the patient's whole life situation and point to important materials in early childhood.[1] This I want to demonstrate in this case.

Appeared originally in *The Psychoanalytic Review*, 17:1-19, 1930. Reprinted through the courtesy of the Editors and the Publisher, National Psychological Association for Psychoanalysis, New York, N.Y.

[1] [This idea has gained such wide acceptance that it might be wise to set the record straight. Dr. Francis Baudry, in an unpublished report to the Treatment Center of the New York Psychoanalytic Institute in 1967, noticed that "the special significance of the first dream seemed to be taken for granted by most authors who made any mention of it." Baudry traced the origin of the idea to Stekel (1943, p. 551) who sometime between 1931 and 1935 cited Missreigler (1932) as having been "able to prove that the very first dream may bring to light the dreamer's whole life history. . . ." Missreigler, however, credited Stekel with the idea.

In any case, the nearest Freud came to dealing with the subject was in connection with the dreams of severe neurotics, not with initial dreams. In "The Handling of Dream-Interpretation in Psycho-analysis," he wrote: ". . . in cases of severe neurosis any elaborate dream-productions must from the nature of things be regarded as incapable of complete solution. A dream of this kind is often based on the entire pathogenic material of the case, as yet unknown to both doctor and patient (so-called 'programme-dreams' and biographical dreams), and is sometimes equivalent to a translation into dream-language of the whole content of the neu-

The most striking feature in this patient's neurosis is found to be his fighting with his father and his family. It is very likely that his father really was severe with him and often beat him. As the associations showed, the father did this in the same manner as the big strong man in the dream. These experiences have created in the patient a feeling of hatred against the father and a desire to kill him; they have also created a great dependence on the father. Throughout his life the patient needed somebody to treat him badly. In other words, this type of discipline created in him a masochistic, passive attitude. Passivity played an important role in his life and made him feel, whenever he was with someone older than himself, that the other person was influencing him. He experienced no will of his own. At the same time, he felt that he could not remain in this masochistic, homosexual position, that he should be more active, independent, and efficient. From time to time, therefore, he had wild outbursts by which he proved to himself that he was active and independent. The blowing up of the water tank in the dream represents such an act of rebellion and self-assertion against the father. The question then arises, why this particular kind of aggressive activity?

When the patient first told me the dream, I had the feeling that birth fantasies might be present behind it and some special relation with water, but the patient's associations did not fit in with this supposition, and I was compelled to drop the idea. His associations showed that he has always had a peculiar attitude toward urination. First of all, he had been eneuritic for a long time and had been punished and laughed at for this. This bedwetting also had a sexual meaning. He often dreamed about swimming, and these dreams always ended with either sexual

roses. . . . The full interpretation of such a dream will coincide with the completion of the whole analysis; if a note is made of it at the beginning, it may be possible to understand it at the end, many months later. It is the same as with the elucidation of a single symptom (the main symptom, perhaps). The whole analysis is needed to explain it;. . . Similarly, no more can be expected of a dream occurring in the early stages of the analysis; one must be content if the attempt at interpretation brings a single pathogenic wishful impulse to light" (1911, p. 93).—Ed.]

intercourse or an emission. We thus see that the rebellion against the father which appeared in the dream was partly connected with the patient's sexual attitudes and the punishment he received for something closely related to sex.

His attitude toward this big strong man, however, was also rather closely related to the psychoanalytic situation. This leads us to a very important consideration, namely, that such an initial dream not only brings forth a situation from the early life of the patient, but also points to something about the analytic relationship. Such a dream enables us to gauge what the patient's attitude toward the analyst will be (cf. Rank, 1924). The present technique of psychoanalysis not only lays stress on the interpretation of the patient's past, but asks at the same time for the meaning of a dream, an association, a symptom as regards the psychoanalytic situation and the transference. In other words, we never give an interpretation which concerns only the past; every interpretation must also be related to the interaction of the psychoanalyst and the patient. The psychoanalyst must assess in the beginning of the analysis what the trend of the transference is going to be when the patient brings forth a dream such as this one. We must ask ourselves just exactly what is best to tell the patient about the psychoanalytic situation at the very beginning of the analysis. Should we be very active in the interpretation of the psychoanalytic situation or should we proceed in the more classical analytical manner and wait with our interpretation?

After having explained the basic psychoanalytic rule about free association, we should induce the patient in the beginning of an analysis to tell us something about his previous life, and perhaps we should give special consideration to all that he can remember of the events between his third and fifth year. In doing this, however, we must immediately begin by preventing the patient from giving us an artificially logical tale. His opportunity to produce free associations must be encouraged right from the start; we must not hinder him from going off into side paths. Neither should we interrupt the patient too frequently. It is better to remain passive.

But how should we proceed when a dream such as this one, which seems to give the key to the whole neurosis, appears right off? Should we or should we not tell him what we know, and further, what should we tell him about the transference situation? I am of the opinion that we should not begin too early with elaborate interpretations. I would not begin by telling the patient what I think about such a dream, and I would especially refrain from telling him what I think about the psychoanalytic situation. It is necessary that the relationship should develop to some extent, and that the patient should gain some insight by himself. Only after the patient has gained some degree of insight would I begin very carefully with the interpretation, and even then I would not speak too much about the transference. During the first two or three weeks of the analysis, I generally prefer not to disturb the spontaneous development of the transference. Only when I get a rather obvious expression of transference do I begin to speak about it with the patient. We must ask: What is the nature of the transference in the beginning of analysis? It is to be expected that the patient will show a positive transference in the beginning, as every patient does who goes to a physician. It is precisely that which brings him to the physician. The positive transference toward the physician is, however, already mixed with some distrust and some negative feelings, and it is a question whether we should begin by trying to bring out the patient's negative transference. Should we show him with what distrust he has come to us, that in some way he hates to be frank and open with a stranger, that he has the very worst ideas about the analyst? Usually the patient is indeed suspicious, feels that the analyst is concerned only with the interesting case, with the money, etc.

Reich (1933) is of the opinion that it is best to begin the analysis with a dissection of the negative transference. If we were to follow this rule we would have to speak with the patient who brings the above dream in the following way: "You hate your father. It is not very probable that you hate only your father. If you dream such a dream and bring it to me, the whole analytic situation which you experience with me must remind you of all the things you have suffered at the hands of your father. You are reacting to me in a similar manner as to your father. You must have negative feelings toward me. Please tell me what these negative feelings are. What do you have against me or the analysis?" This procedure would constitute a rather active method. We would immediately provoke rather strong reactions in the patient, and the whole relationship would become tense. While it is possible to analyze in such a way, it is very likely that in psychopathic individuals such an active technique which stresses the negative transference, would evoke the masochistic and hostile attitudes toward the father and toward the psychoanalyst. The danger of such a procedure is that it would be difficult to handle such a strong degree of negative transference. We might provoke such a violent outburst of hatred in the patient that we could not direct it into the proper channels and the analysis would have to stop. I personally, therefore, prefer not to be active in the beginning and to initiate the analysis along classical lines.

Being Active

Reich formulates his technical procedure so that he sometimes recommends that the resistance be analyzed first. I would like to make some general remarks about this. Resistance means the force which prevents repressed material from coming to the surface, that is, into consciousness. The resistances are practically the same as the repressing forces. But repressions always have motives, and we deal not only with the question of what is being repressed but of why the repression took place. The motives of the repressions are to be understood only when we analyze the superego. The analysis of the ideal ego[2] is certainly as important as the analysis of the id. But it is possible to analyze the ideal ego only when we have analyzed the id; it should only

[2] [Schilder used this phrase as the term "ego ideal" is used today.—Ed.]

be carried out parallel with the analysis of the id. An analysis of resistance pure and simple, therefore, is impossible. We may ask the patient why he does not wish to produce his material, and we may show him that his resistance is really not connected with his transference or with his distrust of the psychoanalyst. But we must not forget that the negative transference is in no way identical with resistance. On the contrary, repressed material comes to the fore in the negative transference. The analysis of resistance consists largely in showing the patient from the very beginning the shortcomings of his character from too intellectual a point of view and forgetting the libidinal foundation of the superego. I am certainly not in favor of the so-called analysis of resistance.

There is, however, still another form of activity in the beginning of analysis, and that is the method advocated by Rank (1924). Rank would begin by telling the patient that this blowing up of the tank must have something to do with the feeling that he is too closely bound to the family, that he has too strong a fixation to his mother and that he wants to be rid of the family. As I have already mentioned, I did not get any association from the patient which made it probable at that time that the water tank had anything to do with birth and birth fantasies. In the later course of the analysis, however, as was to be expected, the water tank appeared to refer not only to urinary desires but also to birth fantasies. He proved to be especially fond of being in a tub. There, he felt complete satisfaction, and often said that he wanted physical treatment such as baths and the like. Only then did he feel relaxed; otherwise, sex desires harassed him terribly. It was at this time, too, that he had dreams about sexual intercourse after swimming. A tub was very likely the symbol of the mother's womb for him and an expression of the tendency to return to the mother's womb as well as to get rid of her.

I am nevertheless of the opinion that it is not useful to give the patient too much interpretation in the beginning of analysis. I prefer not to tell the patient more than he can understand in the beginning. If I should speak with the patient about birth trauma and the birth situation, he could not readily experience it, and if he did not feel it, it could not be more than purely intellectual comprehension. Such purely intellectual understanding is not only useless, but is often a weapon of resistance.

I believe with Rank, of course, that birth fantasies are present in every person and that there is also a tendency to develop ideas of both returning to and leaving the mother's womb. This is undoubtedly an important part of every analysis. These special fantasies, on the other hand, are not the only important ones to be found, so it is not advisable to direct the analysis only toward the birth fantasies or the birth trauma. To me, this seems wrong not only from the practical point of view but also from the point of view of theory. It has not yet been proven that birth fantasies are actually based on real memories. Nor is it probable that the birth situation, as such, can ever be revived. We are therefore speaking about theoretical conclusions when discussing the birth trauma from a psychological point of view. We know nothing about individual differences in birth trauma. To believe that the birth trauma is responsible for a neurosis seems, therefore, an assumed construction. As regards our patient's dream, we can see that the masochistic and passive attitude toward his father plays at least as important a part as his attitude toward the mother's womb. We are nevertheless able to determine a specific Oedipus situation and an individual infantile conflict in the patient.

Transference

The first few hours of an analysis usually reveal the general trend of the transference. The positive transference generally overshadows the negative. But I remember one patient who was in love with a previous psychoanalyst and who had been disappointed by him. Her hatred for him remained largely unconscious until she came into analysis with me. She identified me to a great extent with the other analyst and developed a strong transference toward me, which, of course, contained a great deal of hatred. In such a case, where negative transference crops up immediately, we naturally must speak with the patient about it.

We should also proceed along the lines of the patient's material. In general, we should restrain ourselves concerning interpretations and be especially careful with interpretations of the transference in the beginning unless the material is such that we are forced to do so. There is a generally accepted technical rule which states that it is usually not damaging to refrain from speaking about the positive transference, but that it is dangerous not to speak about the negative transference if it protrudes rather sharply into the analysis.

The patient I am discussing was a man who from time to time really blew up, and the blowing up of the water tank could also be considered a symbolization of the emotional tendencies of the dreamer. Shortly after this dream he went into a state of great excitement wherein he was rather threatening and in an aggressive mood. He thumped his head against the wall, cried, shouted, etc. The behavior lasted for several days. This, and other similar attacks, were always a protest against his father and his family. On the other hand, the attacks showed him that he was not as passive as he seemed to be. Indeed, this first dream reflected the whole psychic situation of the patient, his vacillation between activity and passivity. During the periods in which he behaved in such a manner, he expected to receive special attention from the physicians. They were compelled to take care that he did not commit suicide. At the same time he complained that the physicians could not help him. We see, again, that such a blowing up, such an outburst, is to be understood not only in terms of the family conflict but also in terms of the relationship between the patient and the physician. We see here that in his relations with his physicians he manifested a considerable degree of distrust. The physicians, he said, could not help him nor did they care enough about him.

When we hear such a complaint, we know that it can only be a reflection of a childhood situation. As a boy he greatly desired that his parents should take special care of him and should give him special love. His wish was never gratified, however, and he succeeded in gaining his objective only when he was obstinate. Then the parents granted him attention by punishing him. It is to be expected that the same situation would return in the guise of transference. He could never acknowledge real love for his parents, although he desired very much to do so. He was always in fear lest the parents reject him, and this attitude came out in the transference. He was always undecided about whether he should really transfer his love to the physician; he was always ready to withdraw the transference at any moment.

In actual psychoanalysis, we must at all times stress the present situation, must show the patient that it is closely connected with memories of early life situations. In psychoanalysis, early memories and experiences come to the surface rather quickly. One of the earliest memories of this patient, for example, was that when he was about four or five years old his mother and father were absent and he felt very lonely. He experienced a very great longing for them, and this longing was one of the motives of his life. It was certainly very closely connected with his active sex wishes, for which he feared punishment.

The patient's father had often warned him against masturbation, so he felt that sex was something very dangerous, that he could perish as a result of sexual abuses. His fears about sexual matters went back to a very early age. His one line of thought was that he was sexually impotent, that he had masturbated too often. It all goes back to a very early state when he had already begun to feel that he was weaker than both his older brother and his father, and that he was too passive. At the same time he got the idea that he was too girlish, too feminine, and he began to think about bisexuality. More than that, he had always felt that he had the body of a boy but the soul of a girl. These ideas were manifestly very closely related to his masochistic attitude in his conduct. This masochistic attitude toward the father was also linked with the punishment he had received from his father.

We know that a passive attitude in such a case is closely

connected with the idea of castration. The castration then gives him the characteristics of a girl. We must say here that we find similar ideas and fantasies in many neuroses. In this complex, masturbation had an important place and was a part of his masochistic attitude when he tried to get the attention of the physician by being sick, by being physically ill. These were his reproaches against his parents. He accused them of being the cause of his condition. He said that he got his neurosis and all his troubles from them. He built up interesting masochistic fantasies concerning his mother, saying that he had a deformity of the skull, which in reality did not exist, and that this resulted from his having been thrown down by his mother when he was a child. On other occasions, he complained that his illness was due to heredity and that for this reason his parents were guilty for his suffering. These ideas concerning his abnormal skull and his inherited nervous system were closely related to his complaint that he was too passive and that he was not a male person but had some feminine characteristics.

When, under the influence of the psychoanalysis, he began to get rid of these ideas, he built up the notion that the hair on his face and on his body was growing faster than usual. All of these ideas of bodily inferiority came to the fore in the course of time and were found to be similar to the usual ones observed in many young men and women. They build up an elaborate system by which they prove to themselves that there is something wrong with their body. I have observed two other patients of a very similar type who also had the feeling of physical inferiority. The inferiority feeling concerning their body is related to their sexual concerns—for example, that the growth of the hair involves something related to the development of the sexual organs.

How shall one handle such an elaborate system in terms of psychoanalytic technique? It is well known that we generally do not discuss our psychoanalytical interpretations with the patient. We know that the final decision will be revealed in the patient's subsequent associations. We do not even answer the patient's questions directly, but respond with counterquestions. In the beginning it will be necessary to get all of the ideas connected with such problems, but when they are out and we can see that there is a whole system, then it is necessary to discuss this with the patient. We find that the system is built up in a logical way and that the patient defends it by prejudices that he has acquired by reading literature or the newspapers. To believe that one can destroy such a totally erroneous system of ideas by always asking the patient for associations would be false.

It is at this point that we have to be somewhat active in our discussions with the patient. Passivity in such a situation would be a mistake. We must, of course, be able to show the patient how he came to such a construction and for what purpose he has developed it. But we also have to show him that all the things he has gathered in such a way, in such a system, are wrong in themselves. But one must not rely on the interpretation alone; the interpretation must be combined with discussion. At this point in the psychoanalysis—which is generally not reached in the first or second month but in the third or fourth month and even later—the patient can also be shown that he uses the neurosis for a special purpose in daily life.

These are the mechanisms Adler (1907) has described. That they exist is without doubt. But they are only one part of the neurosis. The infantile sexual conflicts form the deeper basis. What Adler says is not wrong in itself. Feelings of inferiority as well as feelings of overcompensation certainly exist and play an important part in neurosis. But in the case we are discussing here, the primary basis of the neurosis is the patient's passive attitude toward his father and mother. Along with this passive masochistic attitude, he developed the idea that there was something wrong with his genitals and his masculinity. He tried to overcompensate for his passive attitudes by his outbursts. He desired in this way to be freed from his brother and his father. Instead, he became dependent upon necessary medical care. In addition, he made use of his suffering for a secondary gain. The parents now had to take care of him. He tried to be superior by "blowing up" and frightening them, and now they had to pay the hospital and physicians. These secondary mechanisms, as we pointed out, were based on a sexual complex.

The male protest of Adler, the inferiority feeling and the subsequent overcompensations are, in other words, closely connected with what we call the castration complex (cf. Freud, 1918). The castration complex and the Oedipus situation are indeed the important primary situations. The secondary reactions are nevertheless of very great interest. In the course of almost every analysis we have to show the patient what use he makes of his neurotic symptoms. They usually aid him in commanding attention and ridding himself of every responsibility and independent action. Our particular patient diminishes his responsibility by his idea that he is suffering from some pathology of the skull because of his mother's negligence and by his idea that he is inferior by heredity. Through his outbursts, he gets greater care from the physician and more considerate solicitude from his parents. It is therefore essential to discuss this situation with the patient. In doing so we have to be active in some way because mere passivity would be a technical fault in such a situation.

We might, of course, say that in this case there is a special problem, that another neurosis might not have such a logical superstructure and that it would therefore not be necessary to hold a discussion with the patient. In such an instance an analysis along the lines of free association might be all that is necessary. Nevertheless, in most cases such a logical superstructure does exist. A discussion with the patient would, of course, be based on the material which has been produced by free association, and should take place only when the transference situation is sufficiently clear. We have to remember that the transference will sooner or later begin to reflect all of the important events of the patient's life. We know, for instance, that in transference the psychoanalyst will play the part of the father in the same way as the father appears in the patient's consciousness.

I once had a patient who always quarrelled with his father. The father wanted a place of superiority in the family and did not allow anyone to contradict him. In fact, the patient secretly always harbored mutinous ideas against his father. In the analysis it soon became evident that the patient was treating the analyst in the same manner as he had his father. He did not want to believe anything that the analyst said and always expressed doubts about the analyst's statements. He showed considerable rebellion, but this attitude toward his father was actually superimposed upon a great love for his father of which he was not aware. As the analysis progressed, the patient's great love for his father began to show in the form of his transference to the analyst. In the early part of his analysis it was only his relation to his father which came out. In the second part of the analysis his relation with his mother, which had been almost wholly unconscious, began to crop up; at that point the analyst began to take on the role of the mother.

These cycles where the analyst plays the part of the father or the mother in different ways repeat themselves very often in the course of a psychoanalysis. As the analysis proceeds, the analyst may play the part of the father at the level of the Oedipus complex, and that may be the first part of the analysis. In the second cycle he might play the part of the father on a lower level, perhaps on the level of sadistic/masochistic attitudes. We can say, in other words, that in a complete psychoanalysis the analyst will not only play one facet of the father image, but the role at every level where the father actually played an important part.

It is understandable that such a complete analysis will naturally take a long time. We not only have to analyze the positive and negative transference toward the father, we also have to analyze the negative transference toward the father in the Oedipus complex and the negative transference toward the father in the pre-Oedipus situation. In each of these phases we may meet prejudice on the part of the patient. One or another logical structure has to be destroyed, and in destroying them we must enter into a discussion with the patient at special points. We must first try, of course, to enable the patient to see his errors by means of his free associations, but if we do not succeed we have the right and even are duty bound to enter into a discussion with the patient.

The actual conflict of the patient naturally reflects his infantile situation and will also influence the transference. We should not neglect such conflicts. Analysis is never only the analysis of the past but also the analysis of the present, and this present is the actual life situation as well as the psychoanalytical situation. The analysis of the present is the most important factor because the conflict can never be understood on the basis of the past, due to the persistence of a few irreducible elements.

Now we come to a very important point in the development of the psychoanalysis. The first phase consisted chiefly in the analysis of unconscious desires, of the id, an analysis which had not very much to do with the ego. It was a psychoanalysis of repressions, of the repressed self. We know that every psychoanalysis is incomplete which is not also a superego analysis (Freud, 1923). In other words, we must analyze not only what is repressed, but, what is more important, we must analyze the forces that repress. These repressing forces are very closely related to the ideal ego. Speaking in a psychoanalytical sense, the superego advises the ego what to repress. We shall now turn to an analysis of the ideal ego.[3]

In analyzing the repressions, we will find much material which will help us in understanding why the patient has built up this or that moral ideal, and we have then to interpret to the patient his special moral attitude. In the present case, it should be made clear to the patient just why he possesses a masculine ideal, why he is of the opinion that it is very bad to be feminine, and why he feels masturbation is so bad for him. This patient lived in fear that he might masturbate. He became very much excited whenever his libido was on the increase. The outbursts, which I have described, would appear especially at times when he had a feeling that he could no longer restrain his sex desires. At such times he would want to get into a tub. We will never cure the

[3] [See footnote, p. 225.—Ed.]

patient if we interpret to him only that he has desires and wishes relative to the Oedipus complex and do not explain to him that he has built up an ego according to what his father told him—i.e., that he should not be excessively sexual, that strength is possible only to those who are not too sexual—if we do not destroy his ideal of being excessively strong and masculine. In other words, a complete psychoanalysis is not only an analysis of what has been repressed, but it is also particularly an analysis of the repressing forces. By changing the patient's attitude toward his father and mother we shall also be able to change his ideal ego. We must in some way change the patient's ethical attitude; if that is not done, the psychoanalysis will usually not succeed.

I once analyzed a very interesting case of perversion in a man of about 30. His perversion consisted in his deriving sexual pleasure only when he had the opportunity of observing other men urinating. This perversion went back to a very early stage in his development. He experienced his first excitement when he was about five and was in a public toilet. It is very likely that his urinary homosexual tendencies were closely related to early experiences related to his father. The patient's family preserved an interesting story from his history, namely, that, when he was born, the first thing he did was urinate on his father who was bending over him. It is certainly of interest that what is reported about his first action in life is so closely related to his later perversion.

This patient loved his father very much and respected him very highly. His father was a remarkable personality, but did not know much about sex matters. He often asked the boy to tickle the soles of his feet, and he also played with the children, telling them jestingly and in funny words that he was going to castrate them. It is doubtless a fact that these playful habits of the father increased the patient's passive homosexual attitude toward him. The father was a man of very high moral standards, and no one in the family dared speak about sex matters. Even in his business life the father's morals were rather strict. The boy tried very hard to emulate his father as much as possible, and consequently, over the years, built up a superego which looked upon all things sexual—and especially all perversions—as absolutely immoral. He felt that they were to be repressed, and that it was absolutely necessary for him not to have feelings of that kind. To insure his repressions, he built up the idea that whenever he succumbed to such ideas and got sexual pleasure out of going to a public toilet, some failure in his business would result. Although he was a very intelligent man, he frequently reported that following some sexual experience in a public toilet he suffered some business reversal.

Now, this ideal ego, directed against sexuality with the help of superstition, was a great hindrance to the psychoanalysis. I did not discuss it sufficiently, nor did I destroy it carefully enough; as a result, the patient never dared bring out his sex fantasies in a clear way. Because I failed to bring the ideal ego into the transference, the analysis of the patient was unsuccessful. The mistake that I made was that I did not pay sufficient attention to the patient's very strong superego, and that I did not sufficiently analyze, and thus destroy, the ideal ego. I did not show the patient that his attitude toward his father was wrong, that his ego ideal was ultimately related to homosexual tendencies toward the father. Nor did I analyze sufficiently his positive transference toward me. I did not show him that his positive transference was based on the same homosexual tendencies he so much feared. My conclusion on this case is that in every successful psychoanalysis we have to ask ourselves what constitutes the patient's ideal ego. How can we effectively transform the patient's superego and, along with it, his system of repressions?

One of the cardinal marks of every neurosis is that it contains a faulty construction of the ideal ego and of the system of repressions. But the fault is comparatively minor in the neuroses as compared with the psychoses. Nevertheless, if we do not give this our attention, the analysis will invariably be a partial failure. We can say that a psychoanalysis must not only bring out the repressed material, but that it must also show the patient how he has built up his ego ideal. Every analysis also consists, therefore, of an analysis of the superego as Freud (1923), Reich (1933), and Alexander (1927) have pointed out. The superego is partly built up along the lines of identification with the parents, but it is also an overcompensation against this.

Not infrequently, one sees persons who have become what they are because they have tried to avoid everything their parents or their brothers and sisters have done. It is evident that such an ideal ego, based as it is on hatred, needs some correction. From the technical point of view, therefore, every psychoanalysis must be directed toward a transformation of the identifications which build up the superego. Thus, every psychoanalysis is an analysis of the patient's character. Character is built up on the basis of sublimations and overcompensations of the id. It has the same psychological structure as a neurotic symptom. Our character is nothing but those of our neurotic symptoms with which our personality agrees. It is, to a great extent, identical with the consciousness of the ideal ego. If we want to change a character we must first show the individual that what he considers good sublimation is not, in fact, good sublimation at all but a neurotic symptom. In other words, every psychoanalysis must change the patient's identifications. While this change will come partly through free associations, it will also be essential to discuss with the patient the manner in which he has built up his ideals, his character, and his attitude toward the world. In short, some activity will be necessary in the course of the analysis.

But what is going to happen after we have destroyed the character of the individual? It is, after all, impossible for such a condition to last. Something else will have to replace what was formerly the patient's character. The patient will usually form a new character on the basis of identifications with the analyst, but the analyst must still remain in the background. The psychoanalyst becomes, as it were, the outline of a personality which has adapted itself to reality. But in so doing, the personality of the analyst must not interject itself into the analysis. The identification effected with the psychoanayst, which occurs at the end of every psychoanalysis, must not be identification with one particular personality; rather, it must be identification with someone who is looked upon as a useful member of society, one who is able to cope, to be happy. It is an imperfect psychoanalysis if the analyst creates persons too much like himself. But that is precisely what will happen if he is too active and instills too many of his own ideas into the patient. It should be the psychoanalyst's objective only to destroy the patient's imperfect adaptations and to afford the individual the opportunity for acquiring new adaptations, adjustments which fit a whole new situation, an entire life, the total character of the patient. At the end of a truly successful psychoanalysis this identification with such an abstract image of the analyst takes place and, of course, this image of the analyst now becomes a real father or mother image for the patient. We could say that the end of the analysis is marked by an identification with the father and with the mother, not the father and mother who are weak personalities in reality, but a father image and mother image who are adapted to reality.

It is at this point that the psychoanalyst becomes unnecessary to the patient. Sometimes we have to be very active in order to make it clear to the patient that he need no longer be dependent upon us, and sometimes our activities are directed toward showing him that he has a tendency to cling to his father and mother and to the psychoanalyst who is substituted for them. The patient has to become an adult personality. We are confident that the neurotic person liberated from the unfortunate influences of early experiences will be able to build his new personality by himself. The reconstruction, therefore, is effected, not for the sake of the analyst, but for the sake of the patient. By just giving advice we return the patient to the infantile level and fixate him there. Advising the patient is permissible only when special circumstances are present which make us doubt the patient's ability to reorganize his superego in the right way.

Terminating the Psychoanalysis

Rank (1924) recommends declaring the termination of the psychoanalysis when the patient has identified with parent images that are adapted to reality. But this method of ending the psychoanalysis often gives us real problems should we be forced to continue the analysis although we have told the patient we are going to stop. Even though we may feel that the analysis has progressed far enough, it is usually not good practice to set a special date for its termination. Rather, we should insist, during these last phases of the analysis, on showing the patient that he still clings to us, that he is clinging to his father and mother, that he must get rid of us, get rid of his dependence by identification.

As Rank (1924) has excellently observed, toward the end of the analysis the psychoanalyst takes on to an ever greater degree the role of the mother. The analyst increasingly becomes the symbol of the general principle of protection where one is at home and safe. The psychoanalyzed person has to feel that he is able to lose this protection and that he is able to leave his mother. Then, if the psychoanalysis has been successful, the rebirth fantasies set in. At this phase of the analysis, they play a very important part. It is now that we observe the presence of two tendencies: one is identification with the analyst and the other is the fantasizing connected with rebirth. The latter tendency, however, indicates real independence from the mother and from the analyst. It is in these last phases of the psychoanalysis that we have the right to be active, to show the patient that he must become independent, that he can not always cling to the mother, father, or psychoanalyst. It is also necessary to show him that he must construct an ideal ego in which dependence on the mother, father, the psychoanalyst, or other substitutes plays no important part. The end of the psychoanalysis very frequently brings forth very primitive material of early stages, along with the rebirth fantasies. The end of the analysis is the only time the rebirth fantasies may be taken for more than a metaphor. It may be that the great emotion engendered by separation from the mother substitute provokes a revival of primitive catastrophes in life as far back as birth itself.

We have described the common type of psychoanalysis. It is not possible to lay down any rigid scheme, but in the course of a special analysis we will naturally be more or less active; actually, we can never be completely passive, asking only for associations and giving only interpretations. We shall never make a mistake if we stress the idea that psychoanalysis is to a great extent the analysis of the superego. There are, of course, always some situations in the psychoanalysis which need a greater amount of active treatment as, for example, when the patient has a tendency to make peace with his symptoms.

We know that patients who are impotent sooner or later compromise with a neurosis and build up a secondary personality in which they are more or less at peace with their impotence. The impotence, paradoxically enough, becomes a part of their superego. Such an individual will say that it is not moral to be always looking for intercourse, and he will consider such attempts both useless and immoral. Whenever we see that the patient is trying to make peace between himself and his symptoms we must step in and try to prevent it. In other words, we have to try to prevent the patient from letting his neurotic symptoms become a part of his adjustment.

Anxiety neuroses offer us a similar situation. In such cases the patient sooner or later comes to the point where he says to himself that it is no use struggling against his anxiety, that it is better to accept the symptoms and live at peace with them. Whenever the patient shows passivity toward his symptoms, whenever he tries to sacrifice a part of reality in order to achieve peace with his neurotic symptoms, whenever the ego ideal tries to effect a compromise with them, then we have to be very active (Ferenczi, 1925). It is then that we have to force the patient to act against his tendencies, to go through his problems over and over again. It is necessary, of course, that we have the benefit of some positive transference before we can force the patient in such a way. We must rest upon some authority. But we must nevertheless increase our activity at any point that our patient becomes too content with his neurosis. This is the one type of patient for whom great activity is absolutely necessary.

Ferenczi (1925) even goes so far in his active technique as to advise certain of his patients to retain their feces and urine as long as possible in order that this may produce repressed material related to these partial tendencies. In other cases he asks the patient to invent and act out scenes bearing upon any direction in which he supposes the hidden material may lie. I am not in favor of this type of activity, which is so dependent upon the personal initiative of the analyst. After all, we try as much as possible to search for a technique which will permit natural growth without the influence of the analyst's personal initiative.

We must not forget, however, that the tendency to be reconciled with the neurosis lies in the neurosis itself. The neurosis always offers the patient the symbolic gratification of the perverse states of childhood. It also satisfies the feeling of guilt. Alexander (1927) has pointed out that the suffering in a neurosis is the price the neurotic pays for his infantile satisfactions. The gratification of the tendency to self-punishment (Reik, 1925) is one more motive for the development of the neurosis in the first place. The analysis of the superego will, of course, recall these feelings of guilt, which play such an important part in the illness. The activities in the analysis of the ideal ego will generally be sufficient to destroy this course of the neurosis. We must see to it that the transference situation never gives the patient complete satisfaction, since we also know that establishing the transference is another means by which the neurotic tries to make peace with his neurosis. As Freud (1919) put it, every analysis should take place with the patient suffering "abstinence." The patient should never feel too comfortable in the psychoanalytical situation. The term "abstinence" in this respect has a double meaning: The patient should not enjoy too much either the transference situation or the neurotic symptoms.

Countertransference

It is at this point that I wish to make some remarks on a subject which has not yet been sufficiently treated in the psychoanalytic literature, namely, "countertransference." There is a general law in psychology which states that whenever one person possesses a feeling or an attitude there must be a complementary feeling in the other person toward whom this feeling is directed. When one person feels a strong love, there must be an answer to it in the other person. When one person exhibits a narcissistic attitude, there must be a masochistic answer in the other person. I am of the opinion that this law is one of the most important psychological laws regulating human relations. I once expressed the view (Kauders and Schilder, 1923) that the masochistic infantile attitude of the hypnotized person must call forth a corresponding active sadistic attitude in the hypnotizer. But the hypnotizer must be aware of this and has to keep these impulses in the background and under the control of his superego. In the psychoanalytical situation, the analyst's feelings are necessarily complements of the patient's feelings. But the analyst must know himself to the extent that he will not permit himself countertransference impulses consciously or unconsciously. This is the real reason why we insist that the analyst must know his own unconscious. Only then will the analyst not run the risk of forcing a positive or negative transference according to his own wishes. We should enjoy neither the positive nor the negative transference of our patients too much. If we experience impulses corresponding to the impulses of the patient, we must be aware of them and try to express them only in so far as is permitted by the ego ideal and the psychoanalytical situation.

One of the real difficulties in a psychoanalysis lies in the fact that we ask our patient to tell us everything that he thinks about us, and we, on the other hand, are never allowed to answer him. We have to take on the mask of an impersonal observer and physician. If we leave this straight and narrow path, we are no longer analysts.

We have confidence in the ability of most neurotic persons to be able to reorganize their own superego in the melting pot of the analysis according to the deep layers of their personality. We generally prefer not to disturb this process of self-rehabilitation. We believe that the psychoanalyst and the psychotherapist should not consider themselves omniscient gods. They are in real danger of such an attitude when under the influence of the transference. Advice and education in the commonsense manner will generally be unnecessary in a neurosis where there are forces enough to hold up the sublimations in their adjustments to reality. It is this strength in the rebuilding forces of the superego of the neurotic which permits us also to be ruthless in telling the patient the truth about his repressing tendencies. If, however, we are dealing with a psychopathic individual who possesses a genuinely weak superego or with a psychotic who has undergone great changes in the ideal ego, then we must be more active in the sense of education and reconstruction. In such cases we cannot rely on free association. We must always discuss with the patient the present actual situation. We must discuss with him his general attitudes and his attitudes toward life. In a psychosis we must consider carefully whether a patient's superego is strong enough to resist his wild and primitive instincts. Sometimes it is necessary to help this ideal ego, as for example, by resorting to such adjunct treatment as occupational therapy. If we tell a schizophrenic patient that he is sadistic, he will agree with us and then act in a sadistic way. What should we do? Either we should not speak to the patient about his sadism until we are convinced that his superego is strong enough, or we should indicate his sadism and aid his ego ideal by showing him how he can compensate for his sadistic tendencies.

According to the general ideas that I have developed here, psychoanalysis is, to a great extent, an analysis of the ideal ego. We have to pay attention to the ideal ego of every one of our psychotic patients, and we have to be constructive in reorganizing their superegos. The analysis of a psychosis will therefore be much more closely related to educational measures in the general acceptance of the term than will the analysis of a neurosis. The analysis of a psychosis is therefore akin to the analysis of children (Anna Freud, 1927). We can say that the primary difference between the neurotic and psychotic patient is that the neurotic patient has forces within himself with which to build up a superego adapted to reality, whereas the psychotic individual, especially the schizophrenic, lacks this ability. In schizophrenia, free association will very often be unnecessary as a technical method. Here, the repressing forces are impaired, and talking will often substitute for free association. In the neurosis, however, the task is often a disintegration of the ideal ego which has become deformed by the struggle of the ego against the id. In the psychosis, the task is rather the reintegration of dissolved systems of repression.

I will finish by emphasizing that we are generally passive in psychoanalysis, but we must not remain passive when we have before us the job of changing character formation. If the character does not change in the course of a passive psychoanalysis, we must become active in destroying any wrong developmental tendencies. If the patient does not himself see that he has built up an erroneous character, we must show him that he has done so, and we must help to make him feel that what he has believed to be his character has been a neurotic symptom. In character analysis we have to be active, and character analysis is one of the most important features of any psychoanalysis.[4]

[4] [See also Schilder (1938a), especially Chapter 7, The Relation Between the Physician and Patient, pp. 158-170.—Ed.]

CHAPTER TWELVE

Results and Problems of Group Psychotherapy in Severe Neuroses

The problem of adequate psychotherapeutic care for neurotic patients who frequent the outpatient departments of public hospitals is an urgent one. Psychoanalysis is undoubtedly an efficient therapeutic weapon, but it makes great demands on the time of both the physician and patient. It has thus become in our economic structure a method employed only for the wealthy. In addition, the general trend in psychoanalytic technique is to prolong the treatment; indeed, daily treatments for two or three years are not considered unusual. If psychoanalysis is the best treatment available at the present time, the community should utilize it; but if this is impracticable, experiments should be conducted in an attempt to find an alternative. In public hospitals, surgical cases receive care that is in no way inferior to that given the private case. It is our social duty to set up the same standards for the care of the neurotic patient.

Psychoanalysis is based upon a definite and well-studied relationship between two human beings—the analyst and the patient. Other human beings appear in a way suggestive of

Appeared originally in *Mental Hygiene*, 33:87-99, 1939.

ghosts during the analysis. The patient confides in an analyst whom he trusts not to divulge his secrets. To be sure, the analyzed person, re-experiencing his past life with the analyst, finally finds his way back to the social situation in which he lives. There is no doubt but that the transference situation, carefully as it has been studied, is still full of pitfalls. When one considers that isolation and secrecy are basic factors in the psychology of the neurotic, one is tempted to discard both of them in the therapeutic situation. In group psychotherapy, a number of patients are seen simultaneously by the physician, and each patient is aware of the problems of the others. A second physician may join the group and add his interpretations.

In 1934 I began an experiment in group psychotherapy in the Outpatient Department of the Psychiatric Division of Bellevue Hospital. Up to the present time (1939) about 50 cases of severe neuroses and mild psychoses have been treated. Only severe cases have been taken into this group. Most of the neuroses were of long standing and had been treated previously by other methods. A definite therapeutic plan was followed.

Human beings live not only in a group—they live also as comparatively independent entities. A therapy dealing only with the group would be as one-sided as a purely individual treatment. Every patient was seen individually before he joined the group, and these personal interviews were continued throughout the treatment. The groups met once or twice a week, from two to seven patients participating. This type of therapy emphasizes the leadership of the physician through the mere fact that he directs the group. Patients should have insight into this relationship. They should not be blind believers. The physician should not be an authority, but a leader; and it should be clear that his leadership is based, not upon any intrinsic superiority, but upon the particular task to be solved by the group. Basically, he is a fellow human being confronted with the same problems as any other member of the group.

The various forms of psychotherapy emphasize specific aspects of interpersonal relations. If a physician gives orders to patients without giving them any insight into the nature of these orders, his therapy is based upon the necessity for authority in human life. In hypnosis, therapy is based upon the human relationship of erotic submission. In cathartic hypnosis, the patient is forced into insight. Again, one may treat a patient as a sensible fellow human being with whom problems can be discussed. An attitude of friendly helpfulness may be added.

In psychoanalysis the semblance of an impersonal relationship may be insisted upon, but the patient is in reality in a state of submission which is more or less one of complete surrender. In the further course of analysis, insight accrues, with the revival of significant childhood attitudes. The therapeutic situation, if in any way valuable, is based upon a human relationship of fundamental importance. Hypnosis, for instance, which stresses submission and surrender to a magic power of love, reveals at least one important side of human relations. The technique immediately reaches a higher level if the patient has insight into this. The part truth of the hypnotic attitude and of any psychotherapeutic attitude should be seen at its real value. The final aim of psychotherapy can only be insight. Psychoanalysis comes nearest to this goal. Insight means more than verbalization. It means the ability to see the structures of the real world and to act accordingly.

Psychoanalytic insight was utilized in this group treatment. In every case the life history of the patient was discussed and elucidated in detail, and early infantile material, especially, was studied. A written report was asked of the patient after he had gained partial insight. Not only had he to write his life history, but he also had to discuss his relations with father, mother, siblings, and any parent substitutes. In addition, a report of his sexual development was required. Further reports were called for according to the needs of the therapeutic situation. Dream interpretation and so-called free associations were used both in the individual treatments and in the group treatments. Sexual development was studied as completely as possible. Besides a historical approach to the personality, the ideologies of the patients and their general orientation to life were investigated. No individual can be understood unless his objective is known—his goal and his life plan. One must know his expectations for the future. The individual must also gain deeper insight into his own needs and wishes. He must learn to understand the social setting and his social and sexual ambitions.

The basic problems may be formulated briefly as follows: (1) body and beauty; (2) health, strength, efficiency, superiority and inferiority in a physical sense; (3) aggressiveness and submission; (4) masculinity and femininity; (5) the relationship between sex and love; (6) the expectation for the future; and (7) the meaning of death. Particular attention must be given to the language in which the patient expresses his attitudes toward these basic problems. The patient often uses certain phrases in order to enable him to hide his real attitudes from himself. Phrases not fully understood in their true meaning are often found at the turning point of an individual's life. It is necessary that the individual's conscious and unconscious goals come into full light with insight. Modern psychology has all too often forgotten the social nature of human experiences. I have been able to show that even the experience of one's own body, the body image, acquires its final expression only in a continuous interplay with the body images of other human beings.

Hartshorne (1934) has emphasized the social character of every sensation. Any problem of money, occupation, and sex that may be met has its true meaning only in a social setting of which it is a part, and cannot even be thought of apart from this social setting. Obviously, then, the significance of any detail of an individual life history will be clearer if it is brought forward in a group and appraised by a group. In one discussion, for example, a patient remembered an attempted sexual assault against his sister. It was astonishing how many members of the group recalled similar experiences in their own lives, so that a correct appreciation of such an event became possible. On Mother's Day one of the patients brought forth bitter complaints against his mother, who had curtailed his freedom, had not given him enough love, and had had a sex life of her own. This outcry provoked a whole series of similar associations from the other patients. The deeper social meaning of the Oedipus situation revealed itself, and the patients experienced their specific attitudes merely as variations of a general attitude. The relief patients experience when they no longer feel excluded from the community because of urges and desires that society does not openly tolerate is remarkable. To be sure, in the strictly analytic situation, the analyst offers a like relief, but there he is merely the representative of a group, whereas in the group treatment the patient actually experiences the breaking through of similar or identical impulses in others. Group treatment is in this respect a step nearer to reality.

Feelings of guilt result from sexual drives and actions, and from aggressiveness. Both seem to excommunicate the individual from a society that sets up for him a system of ideals that cannot be fulfilled. Mothers are supposed always to love their children, and children are expected always to love their parents. There should be no destructive impulses against any one; good deeds from the individual are not enough—the demand is also that he think only good thoughts. Morally, we live in a state that punishes, not only actions, but thoughts as well. In a general way we feel that the authorities of a country should permit liberty of thought. But the unwritten ideologies and prejudices, the demands of misunderstood morality are much more tyrannical than written laws, since the former punish for thoughts. Thoughts must come out into the open the same way as do ideologies if individuals are to be liberated from their feelings of guilt.

In a group, the patients realize with astonishment that the thoughts which have seemed to isolate them are common to all of them. This enables them clearly to see their aggressive instincts and helps them to understand that aggressive instincts and social conduct are compatible.

The thoughts and ideologies of one patient become the common medium for the group in their continuous emotional interplay. Most of the threads are united in the person of the analyst, who enters into the discussions, the language analysis, and even into the free associations of the patients. The definite interpretation of a patient's symptom or action is the work not merely of the analyst but of the whole group.

The phenomena of positive and negative transference to the analyst are not less outspoken in the group than in the usual psychoanalytic treatment. They express themselves in generally known terms. The reaction of one patient to the transference situation of another patient is very often remarkable. The patient in a state of positive transference feels a need to defend the analyst against the negative transference of another patient. In the negative transference, the group particularly stresses that the physician is not sufficiently interested in their fate, that as a public employee he must spend his hours with them regardless, and that he is less interested in the fate of the patients than in the scientific problems they offer. Discussions of problems of this type frequently have a very important effect upon the fate of a group. They can be shown that nobody has the right to expect the complete emotional surrender of another person—that the other person has to live his own life even if he does happen to be one's father or one's relative or one's physician.

The patients brought together in one group are not particularly selected, but men and women have been treated separately. It has been my general plan to bring every patient who is at a given time under treatment into contact with the other patients of the same sex. I hope it will be possible to have persons of both sexes in the same group when we have gained a deeper understanding of this method.

The method I have described (Schilder, 1938a) will not escape the reproach of being too intellectual and of putting too much emphasis upon the factor of insight.

Skepticism may be increased when I confess that I do not refrain from using an elaborate system of questionnaires. These contain such questions as what the patient remembers about his father, what he thinks about him, and what fantasies he has had about him. These questions are concerned not only with the sexual problems relating to the father, but with every phase of the father's life—whether he was considered strong, healthy, gifted, clever, successful, and so on. Similar questions are elaborated about the mother, siblings, nurses, and teachers. A further series relates to ideas about one's own body. Others probe the castration complex, masturbation, intercourse, breasts, urination, defecation, the attitude of the family and of the patient toward disease, food habits, and so forth. A different set sought to discuss aggressiveness and attitudes toward death, the opinions the individual has about himself, his goals in life, and, finally, the general attitude of human beings toward one another. At least one should try to discover the basic attitude of an individual in the following spheres of experience: (1) the need to love and be loved (according to Watson, 1924, love means stroking); (2) the need to maintain one's own support (in childhood, against gravitation); (3) the need to maintain the integrity of the body (sudden noise, sudden impressions are a threat in this respect); (4) the need to eat and drink and to get as much property as possible, to acquire and to retain; (5) the need to expel what the organism can no longer use and to push away what is threatening; (6) the need to handle and to destroy objects and human beings and to get an insight into their structure; (7) the need to help others in the pursuit of the same aims.

This is a reformulation of the problems that are considered most important in an individual's life.

One of the discussions arising out of the individual problems of the patients is here reproduced in a slightly altered form. I have prefaced it with brief remarks about each of the patients. Every one in the group knew the histories of the others.

B., 21 years old, had a severe social neurosis which caused him to withdraw from contact with others and to suffer from severe feelings of inadequacy; his speech was actually hesitant. He stammered when he checked impulses of rage directed against those he believed were ridiculing him. Excessive ambitions had developed to overcompensate for his sense of being threatened.

In school games he did not want to be on the losing team. He was interested in auto races and in all speed races involving motor-driven vehicles, seeming to feel that their force was added to his. He did not like sports in which he was dependent only upon his own ability.

E., 21 years old, with a low basal metabolism (minus 23) had felt that he had no energy and no drive. Accordingly, he would exert himself too much, feel bewildered, and then give up almost completely until he really had become inefficient. His sexual energy seemed to have little vitality. There were no sex fantasies or sex impulses when he came for treatment. In spite of a rise in the basal metabolic rate to minus 8 under the influence of thyroid medication, he did not change until psychotherapy had given him insight into his problems. Sexuality then awakened. The question is, where did he get the energy with which to drive himself forward?

F., 21 years old, an anxiety neurotic with the fear of sudden death, had no problems of this kind. He lived in an emotional attachment to his mother and brother and expected protection from them against the dangers connected with his own lack of strength. It did not matter whether this attachment to the mother was sexual or not, but it was important that he have no inferiority feelings in the ordinary sense.

C., 24 years old, suffered from inferiority and guilt feelings because of obsessional sex drives against children and men, and obsessional aggressions such as kicking and pushing. He had been forced into this situation by his mother, who overpowered him. If there were feelings of inferiority, they were the result of a complicated sexual development. He was very much frightened by his impulses, whose strength he overestimated.

In the case of W., nineteen years old, the fight against the father and the protection of the mother against the father (also sexually) were prominent. In W.'s attempt to substitute for the father, he cultivated intellectuality. He denied himself sexuality because he condemned it in his father and mother. Since he wanted to convince himself and others that he was superior to his father, he was concerned only in having others acknowledge his superiority. He was shy and self-conscious with people who he believed gave him exaggerated attention.

Modern men suffer from the idea that they should be perfect. They expect perfect health and are unduly perturbed and excited by minor symptoms. W., for example, had palpitations when in bed. One should have patience with one's own body, and not be afraid of being weak and tired. People want to be highly efficient, to show speed and energy, when they should have the courage to be slow and adynamic. It is easier to be tolerant toward oneself if no comparison is made with others. Humanity should be considered as consisting of varied types; those who are not highly gifted are still an important part of society as a whole. The imperfect human being is needed as well as the one approaching perfection, and one should be tolerant of one's own stupidities. The stupid person is more than a mere background for the intelligent.

Perhaps too much is expected of us in a moral way, and it should be acknowledged that there are impulses which go against the standards of society. One should be lenient about one's own morality, especially if it harms no one. It is probable that tolerance of one's own impulses does not strengthen them, but reveals them as inefficient and weak—that is, if they do not fit into the structure of the personality and into society. One may draw the conclusion that human beings should willingly acknowledge their shortcomings. They should be taught neither to overcompensate for them nor to brush them out of consciousness. Everyone should be aware of the necessity of having shortcomings. The ideal of general efficiency and of striving to be blameless is a wrong one. If one is a minus variant as a personality, one should accept the fact. Minus qualities in ourselves and in others make us human, and the attempt to be perfect only makes us into caricatures.

If humans ask of themselves speed of movement and of speech and strength, why should they not ask to be beautiful in all parts of their bodies? The perfection sought for oneself is demanded of others, and intolerance ensues. This intolerance is greater toward the members of one's own family, who are expected to be ideal figures without blemish. Of course, they can't live up to these images. Parents have to pay dearly for every perfectionistic ideal they put into their children's minds. The child will soon measure his parents against the ideals implanted in him and find them wanting. When parents teach children suppression of sex, children retaliate by fighting against the sexuality of their parents. Asexuality belongs to the perfectionistic ideal. Sometimes it is expected that sexuality will awaken only at the conventional signal. Perfectionistic ideals exist for one's strivings as well as for physical functions, and can be positive as well as negative. They demand, for instance, from oneself and from others (1) absence of hate, (2) a continual flow of love toward one's love object, (3) continuous sexual impulses toward a socially acknowledged love object, and (4) absence of promiscuous sexual impulses.

There is no reason to believe that only one fundamental problem lies at the base of neuroses. One should evaluate life situations as human problems in their varieties of expression.

The foregoing paragraphs summarize the essence of one group treatment. The objection of intellectuality may again be raised. The account given here does not indicate how closely these general remarks were related to definite experiences of the patients. It should not be forgotten, either, that this is only one of the phases in the treatment. The truth of the formulation is considered only as partial truth, which must be completed by the other aspects of the situation. In connection with this specific record, for instance, a discussion would be necessary to show how the individual fits his impulses into society.

In modern psychopathology, the difference between intellectual and emotional processes is too greatly emphasized. Though it has never been formulated, there is an underlying assumption that intellectual processes are pale and without strength, and this at a time when everybody speaks of the "personality as a whole." Attitudes express themselves in thinking as well as in emotions, and emotions also have goals and aims. A separation of intellect and emotion is artificial and is justified only if one considers them as two sides of the unified attitude of an individual, one or the other facet scintillating more strongly according to circumstances.

One might further object to the procedure as recorded because it showed the physician taking a more or less definite stand, whereas psychoanalysis has professed an attitude of neutrality on questions of morals and values. But as I have stated, Freud (1920a) deceived himself in holding that he was purely scientific and had no *Weltanschauung.* Psychoanalysis has, in fact, a definite attitude toward certain moral problems. A body of definite knowledge contains in itself a definitely moral point of view and invites definite actions. One should know this.

As one would suppose, group psychotherapy is especially effective in cases of what I should characterize as social neuroses. These are patients who do not feel comfortable in the presence of others. They feel that they cannot concentrate, they cannot think, or they are merely embarrassed and uncomfortable. Physical symptoms such as palpitations or discomfort in the gastrointestinal tract may be present. Sweating, blushing, awkwardness in movement may become obvious signals of this discomfort. The individual feels that he is the center of attention, that not only is something wrong with him, but that others realize it. Every object becomes, in this respect, an important object on a sadomasochistic level. To be seen and to be observed means to be hurt and to be pushed into an inferior position.

Twelve cases of social neurosis have been treated by this group method. Three can be considered as cured. In the case of E., mentioned above, sexuality, which had been dormant, appeared in spite of the organic background. Only two cases showed no improvement. The remaining seven were decidedly improved, and some of them are still under treatment.

In one case of stammering, the stammering was not overcome, but there was an improvement in social attitude.

Nine cases of obsessional neurosis have been treated. There

has been no complete failure in this series. Two severe cases were cured. In a third, an involuntary bromide intoxication led to a complete disappearance of the symptoms. Two cases with slight encephalitic signs showed a very decided improvement. Two other cases, both severe and of long standing, were mildly improved; both were still under treatment at the time this paper was written. The two remaining cases improved to the point where they are adapting well to society and enjoying themselves.

Of three cases of anxiety neurosis, two were cured and one was improved.

Of four hysterias, two were cured, one was unchanged, and one ceased treatment too early.

Three cases of hypochondriasis were not influenced by the treatment. Two cases with organic vegetative symptoms adapted better, but the organic symptoms did not disappear.

Of three cases of character problems, one was discharged and was well adjusted at the time of writing; the other two were considerably improved and are still under treatment.

Of six depersonalization cases, one was cured and one decidedly improved; one who did not come back for treatment was slightly improved at the time the treatment was broken off. Three were unimproved. One of these three was a schizophrenic and another a depressive.

Two cases of depression (in addition to the depersonalization case) were unimproved. One of them committed suicide. The family had been warned.

Among four cases of schizophrenia in which treatment was attempted (besides the depersonalization case) two cases were not influenced. One case, in which the diagnosis was dementia simplex, adjusted much better. The fourth case completely recovered, and was socially and sexually adapted at the time of writing. Fear of homosexuality and homosexual ideas of reference had been in the foreground. I was in no doubt about the diagnosis of schizophrenia when I started the treatment, which lasted several months. The possibility of an atypical depression might have been considered, but I adhered to my original diagnosis.

Many of the cases treated in this group could not have been treated individually even with the classical analysis. They reacted only in the group. This is especially true of social neuroses.

This is only a very brief report of the experiment. It is difficult to judge therapeutic results after so comparatively short a time, and perhaps I have been too optimistic. If this should be so, it lies in the nature of the psychotherapeutic approach. It is probable that not all of the results are permanent, and there may be relapses sooner or later. But I believed, as did the patients, that they were helped in getting a better orientation to life. I have had an opportunity to compare the results of this method with those of others. In some cases the approach is preferable to the strictly analytic technique, and, again, there are cases in which the psychoanalytic approach is doubtlessly superior. However, one will have to learn. A definite technique has been utilized. I hope that this technique can be taught and can be learned.

A method of group psychotherapy has been developed which attempts to give the patient a deeper insight into his individual life history, his ideologies, his problems and his expectations for the future. The basis of this treatment is a written report of the patient concerning the various phases and aspects of his life and of his relationships to the persons in his world. Sexual development is elucidated. Dream interpretation and free association are utilized. The patient must understand how much he has been under the influence of merely verbal formulations in his life plan. In individual interviews and in group discussions various aspects of the personality come into the foreground. The analyst as a member of the group is compelled to greater activity. The patients gain a new direction and new orientation in life.

The therapeutic results so far are promising, especially in the social neuroses and obsessional neuroses. This truly social method, though it too requires much time, enables the physician to treat a relatively large number of cases and to help them in the development of their personalities.

CHAPTER THIRTEEN

The Treatment of Depersonalization

Depersonalization is a state of the personality in which the individual feels changed in comparison to his former state. This change extends to the awareness of both the self and the outer world, and the individual does not acknowledge himself as a personality. His actions seem automatic to him; he observes his own actions as if he were a spectator. The outer world seems strange to him and has lost its character of reality. We find, therefore, in this picture changes of the self, or depersonalization in the narrower sense, and changes in the environment, or feelings of unreality, alienation of the outer world, *Entfremdung der Wahrnehmungswelt.* For this latter phenomenon, Mayer-Gross (1935), Guttmann and Maclay (1936) have suggested the term, derealization. Pictures of this type occur, according to my own studies (1914), Haug (1936), and Mayer-Gross, in a great variety of clinical conditions. The picture has been observed as a passing phenomenon combined with *déjà vu* in the normal. It may appear in connection with organic diseases of the brain, especially before and after epileptic attacks. It has been observed in depressive psychoses and schizophrenia. In the beginning and in

Appeared originally in the *Bulletin of the New York Academy of Medicine,* 15:258-272, 1939.

the phase of disappearance of severe neuroses, it is not uncommon.

However, this picture occurs also as the dominant symptomatology of a very severe and chronic type of a specific neurosis. Patients of this type complain year after year about their changed experience concerning the self and the world. Cases are on record with a duration of twenty or 30 years. This study deals merely with this nuclear group, the neurosis depersonalization.

The philosophical and psychological interest which these cases offer is considerable. Taine (1870) was the first to use the picture as proof for his philosophical theories of perception. Besides the complaints of changes in perception and emotions, there are complaints concerning the experience of one's own body and about changes in the perception of time and space. Accordingly, the philosophers have used every one of these complaints as proof that this particular function is the most important one in our relation to self, body, and world.

The picture of depersonalization has also attracted the attention of psychoanalysts, among whom I may mention Sadger (1928), Nunberg (1924), Reik (1927), Federn (1926, 1928), Oberndorf (1934), and Bergler and Eidelberg (1935).

The various authors have stressed different aspects of the psychological problems. Reik stresses the constant self-observation, which, according to his opinion, is based on sadomasochistic attitudes. Oberndorf puts the main emphasis on the erotization of thought and especially upon the wish to adopt the way of thinking of the opposite sex. Other authors stress the exhibitionistic and voyeuristic components in the picture. Bergler and Eidelberg are of the opinion that there is a strong tendency to anal exhibition. This exhibition is transformed into an increased tendency to self-observation. I am inclined to stress the fact that the patient with depersonalization has been admired very much by the parents for his intellectual and physical gifts. A great amount of admiration and erotic interest had been spent upon the child. He expects that this erotic inflow should be continuous. The final outcome of such an attitude by the parents will not be different from the outcome of an attitude of neglect. Dissatisfaction has to ensue even if the parents live in a state of continual admiration of the child, since every such relation does not consider the child as a total human being but merely as a show piece. The child's dissatisfaction and deprivation has to express itself in an increase of aggressive and submissive tendencies. These combine with sexual tendencies to sadomasochism. Finally, by identification with the parents, self-observation will take the place of the observation by others and it will be blended with sadomasochistic tendencies. The individual will at first be able to admire his body as well as his thinking. Since such a detachment from the love object cannot remain satisfactory, the self-adulation will be followed by hypochondriacal signs. To the denial of vision in the sphere of perception is now added the loss of admiration of oneself. The individual, however, does not completely give up and will at least enjoy the self-observation, which represents the sadistic components as well as the voyeuristic and narcissistic (self-admiring) ones. The patients, furthermore, preserve their intellectuality in this way and are able to continue their activities in the social and physical world. These activities may appear outwardly successful, although empty of emotional satisfaction for the individual. Depersonalization is the neurosis of the good-looking and intelligent who want too much admiration.

It is understandable that a neurosis of such depth will need psychotherapy of long duration. The best observers in this field agree on this point. Oberndorf, for instance, has treated his cases for a long time and Bergler and Eidelberg write as follows: "We think that this absolute pessimism (concerning the treatment) is not justified; however, it is a prerequisite for the therapy that one knows the mechanisms and starts on the right point. Furthermore, a very long time is necessary. While the analysis of a more severe case of obsession neurosis takes at least two to two-and-one-half years, double the amount of time is the requirement for the treatment of depersonalization. It does not seem to be very hopeful if one demands half a decennium for a treatment.

However, *'amicus Plato, magis amica veritas'* " [Schilder's translation]. The experiences of Oberndorf and myself are, however, better. Some of my cases were treated with individual psychoanalysis, some of them were treated in group psychotherapy. Two cases may be mentioned, one briefly, the other in more detail.

R.H. came for treatment at the age of 25 with depersonalization symptoms which had existed for two years. She was good-looking and of superior intelligence. As so often occurs, the symptoms had suddenly started during an episode of petting in which she had felt that she had lost herself and her emotions. Her sexual feelings also vanished suddenly. This episode had followed an incomplete and disappointing love affair with her employer. The final rejection by him had revived the humiliations she had experienced in early childhood from her father. The psychological treatment led to a recovery after two years. The symptoms disappeared completely; however, one year after the treatment, the patient had not yet made a sexual adaptation.

G.W. came for treatment at the age of 21. Depersonalization symptoms had persisted for several years. She complained that things were moving up and down before her eyes. She felt that her head was empty. "There is only black inside. My head has no top. The inside is withering. If you took it out it would be very small. I must have a tumor. I don't think at all. It is as if I were asleep all the time. I don't know how time passes. My whole intelligence and personality have disappeared completely. I have no desires anymore. I might as well be dead. The emotions are not in my head any more. My voice has changed completely. My sensations do not reach my head. I do not recall things properly. There is no soul, no real 'me' in my head. I feel myself like a puppet."

On physical examination she had a suggestive male distribution of pubic hair with a growth of hair on the chin. There was a slight rectocele. The gynecological examination, which had to be incomplete because of the small introitus, made a hypoplasia of the uterus probable. The family history was without interest. The patient considered her mother and especially her younger brother neurotic.

The patient had a fractured clavicle at three, a fractured elbow at seven, a partially fractured right ankle at sixteen. The present illness began with constipation, gas, and belching. When constipated, she put her finger up her rectum. A rectal prolapse followed. She thought that her other organs were also falling. She first blamed this on putting her finger into her rectum; later she blamed her masturbation. This was around Christmas time when she was fifteen. Perception of moving objects before her eyes followed three weeks later. The depersonalization symptoms described above developed gradually. She graduated from high school and became a copywriter, but during the subsequent five years had about eighteen different jobs. Sometimes she left a job because she felt tired, but apparently she had never been discharged because of incompetence.

In her earliest remembrance she saw herself as a baby riding in a baby carriage with her mother pushing from the back, putting her foot on the brake to stop the carriage and then making it go. She also recalled staring up from the carriage at the elevated trains as they grew from tiny black specks in the distance until they passed overhead and continued away. Her psychosexual development can be traced back to her fifth year. At that time a very large family lived in the next farm house. The children had a rather rough stepfather. The children presented themselves in her mind when she masturbated. "I would picture them being stood in line according to size and then each one would get up in a hammock, would turn upside down while holding on and would be whipped with a stick across the back and behind until they fell out." Later on during the frequent masturbations, she thought of the old colonial methods of punishment where the offender was sitting in a stock in front of a board wall with openings just big enough to hold his hands or feet or head. Sailors were lashed across their backs with cat-o'-nine-tails, their hands stretched above their heads. Around age thirteen with the onset of menstruation, she almost stopped these fantasies, which were only vivid during masturbation. She felt that she had overtaxed her imagination through these masturbation fantasies. The fantasies were very elaborate. Later on, pictures of various torture chambers in which the victims were chained in hideous positions, quartered, and guillotined, were fantasied. None of the victims ever thought of protesting. In another fantasy, a woman had to go around the streets naked and feeling humiliated. Sometimes the patient would be nailed to a cross. She also pictured horses being cruelly whipped by the driver. She imagined Negro slaves sold at auction, or Christ nailed on his cross with a double amount of nails, with one nail also sent through his abdomen. There was also a boy drowning. Nobody cared for his distress and struggling. She fantasied Joan of Arc sitting in her carriage while being driven to her execution. Caesar was murdered, and the bier was carried through the streets very fast. Very often the patient had the feeling that she was the person tortured in this way.

With the increase in the depersonalization symptoms, masturbation stopped and, with it, the fantasies. The patient herself had the feeling when entering treatment that she had abused her thinking and that her brain had been injured by so much masturbation. She also believed that she had injured her genitals and her rectum in the same way.

She was very intelligent. She had skipped several grades in school and had the feeling that it had damaged her when she was with older girls on a social basis. She reported proudly that a nurse had said about her when she was one year old that she was such an intelligent, lively, and restless child that she would have mental troubles in her later life. It could not be ascertained when the patient had been told of this episode. She was very proud of her intellectual faculties and observed herself very carefully. She thought that women had to be more clever than men. She identified herself in a dream with her physician's wife, who she supposed was the brain behind his work. In early childhood she admired her own father for his ability to play pinochle. Otherwise, she considered her father efficient but in no way intellectually outstanding. She had no particular admiration for the intellectual capacities of her mother whom she otherwise considered efficient in womanly arts. The patient was inexhaustible in self-observation and took a great interest in her own case. She wrote voluminous notes about herself and wrote her dreams out regularly.

She described her father as stubborn, severe, and aloof. She was frightened by him, although he had never beaten her. She considered her mother overprotective. Neither of her parents were demonstrative. The patient reported repeatedly how much her parents were disturbed by her illness. She considered her brother similarly affected as she was. Her brother had particularly resented the emotional coolness of their father. She had no deeper relation with any of her relatives or with her girl chums. She always felt isolated in advanced grades at school because she was so much younger than her classmates. She also felt isolated as a Jewess since her family had lived in a non-Jewish neighborhood since she was ten years of age.

One of her first dreams dealt with a diary which she had given to her physician. She wanted it back and was suspicious that the woman in his office to whom she had handed the diary had not, in fact, actually given it to him. In her second dream she was threatened by a voice over the telephone. She wondered if it were her father. "I fell down on the floor; I wanted to die; he had killed me through the telephone." In the same session she reported a dream about a man making physical love to her. There was a continual tendency to project her difficulties onto her love objects. She dreamed that the boy in whom she was first interested was in a hospital, crippled in the hip—he was a hunchback. After her physician had told her that he was Jewish, she wondered how he could walk in the hall. "Your physical self seemed to waver and go into your spine. And your head seemed nothing, as if you had no feeling there."

Another dream: "As I was sitting down on the toilet, a rather big and wild cat appeared either out of the air or out of the toilet bowl with mouth open as though it wanted to bite at my anus." In the associations it came out that her uncle had mentioned to the patient how brave her grandmother had been when she had piles. This brought to mind her prolapse. As a child she was not clear about the difference between anus and vagina.

This case has not been presented from a psychoanalytic point of view. Its outstanding features are: (1) the extreme narcissism of the patient, especially in the intellectual sphere, partially due to her superior intelligence and probably fostered by the disappointment concerning the affection of her parents; (2) the subsequent gratification by sadomasochistic fantasies where the victim comes into intimate relation with the cruel father substitute with whom she has the tendency to identify herself; (3) the emotional coolness of her parents leading not only to sadomasochistic attitudes but also to the reinforcement of the anal component; (4) the overemphasis on the visual fantasies in connection with masturbation; (5) the repression of pregenital satisfaction with the onset of puberty and heterosexual drives, with the subsequent symptomatology involving all organs which were previously libidinal centers. Her neurosis started with symptoms centering around the genital-anal region and passed from there to overerotized vision and thinking.

She was treated in group psychotherapy, during which the past was elucidated by psychoanalytic technique. This was modified since the physician talked more freely with the patient than is customary and encouraged her to write out more biographic notes and dreams. Sessions were shorter and more irregular. Strong transference developed very soon and was especially outspoken in dreams, with a marked jealousy of the analyst's wife whom she mostly depicted as sensual and not intellectual.

She lost almost all her symptoms. However, in this case, too, no sexual adaptation was reached.

Three other depersonalization cases were treated by L. Bender with good results. However, several years later all three cases relapsed under difficult external situations. In one of my cases no therapeutic result was achieved in three months, and the patient discontinued the treatment. In two cases psychotherapy resulted in minor gains. These cases will be mentioned later in another connection.

Psychotherapy in depersonalization cases takes a great amount of time, is technically difficult, does not always remove all problems, and does not protect the patient from relapses. There is no question that every case of depersonalization needs a great amount of psychological help, and there is no reason to be pessimistic concerning psychotherapy in these cases. The treatment has to be psychoanalytic or has to utilize psychoanalytic insight.

Considering the difficulties of the psychotherapeutic approach, one might ask what could be done for these patients by medication. I have occasionally tried benzedrine in depersonalization cases; however, the results were temporary, and the psychotherapeutic approach was in no way helped by medication as in other types of neuroses (Schilder, 1935a).

Guttmann and Maclay (1936) have studied the influence of mescaline on depersonalization symptoms insofar as they consist of changes of the surroundings (derealization) but not of the self. However, the improvement was of short duration, not lasting longer than one day. The authors came to the conclusion that it may be used as an adjuvant for psychotherapeutic activity. A drug which brings a relief of short duration is obviously not of great therapeutic value with such chronic problems. It is usually not very helpful in psychotherapy when one proves to the patient by the temporary relief with drugs that he can feel better. Drugs which allow the patient to come to a deeper insight by increasing the transference situation and changing the state of consciousness help the psychotherapeutic approach much more than drugs which merely relieve symptoms.

Other biological methods of treatment for schizophrenia have been tried occasionally in severe neuroses. Glueck (1936) mentions a case of severe obsessional neurosis which improved by insulin treatment. In the series of cases treated in Bellevue, one case of severe obsessional neurosis reacted only temporarily to the treatment. At Bellevue we generally found the application of metrazol therapy simpler from a technical point of view and decided, therefore, to make an attempt to treat this particular type of neurosis with metrazol. The depersonalization cases constitute a comparatively well-defined group of neuroses. The psychotherapeutic approach to these cases is difficult. Results obtained in such a group with metrazol might be of use in evaluating the treatment for neurosis in general. We have followed the technique of Meduna (1937) and used a ten percent aqueous metrazol solution. Injections were given intravenously in doses varying from four-and-a-half to fifteen grains. We tried to produce three convulsions in a week. One case has been reported in a short abstract, as an example.

J.L., 31 years old, came from a family in which the father and one aunt had severe psychotic states, probably of manic-depressive character. She was always considered an outgoing personality. Her brothers and sisters were also energetic and successful. She was the oldest of five children, three girls and two boys. She had two children, one of whom was only a few months old when she got sick. The family was at that time in straitened financial circumstances. The illness started five months before admission to Bellevue Hospital. She complained that she always felt too tired and was disinclined to sexual intercourse. She ate very little and claimed that she had lost her sense of taste. She thought this was as a result of a cold. She became untidy in appearance and was preoccupied with the care of her children. She complained that she had lost interest in things; that she didn't belong to this world, and that she couldn't cry. She was sent to a sanitarium. There she stated that she was not alive, but had turned to stone and had no feelings and no emotions. In the sanitarium she swallowed several needles with suicidal intent, and was therefore sent to Bellevue Hospital, on September 10. She said: "I don't feel at all; I just got fear of life; everything became complicated; the whole world just looks flat. Nobody can help me. It feels as if I had no place on earth; nothing in the world belongs to me; I seem to be inside out. Time neither passes nor stands still. It doesn't seem like another day; there is no penetration of enjoyment. My mind goes round and round all the time in circles, the whole world looks flat to me. I know what torture you and everyone else is going through but no torture is greater than my misery." On the ward she was seclusive and did not talk spontaneously. However, she was very productive when one talked with her. On one occasion, she tried to grab iodine in order to drink it.

On October 4th, metrazol treatment was instituted. She received four-and-one-half grains intravenously and had no convulsion. From then on, until November 7, fifteen convulsions were produced: the first four with injections of six grains, the subsequent three with seven-and-one-half grains, and the last eight with nine grains. There were no particular incidents during the treatment. The improvement started after the third convulsion and progressed steadily. The clinical symptoms had practically disappeared after the tenth injection. The patient was discharged fully recovered and with full insight, but she still received psychotherapeutic help.

We have treated nine cases so far. Table 2 shows the most important features of these cases. The patients were treated in the hospital, with the exception of two who were treated in the outpatient department. These two patients could not be induced to have more than three convulsions. They felt improved, but experienced a sensation before the convulsion so terrifying that they did not want to continue voluntarily. We have had the same experience in other patients whom we have tried to treat in the outpatient department. We have discussed all the details of the treatment, not only with the patients, but also with the relatives, and treated only those patients who could themselves be convinced that the treatment might be effective. There were no untoward incidents in the treatment, except that one patient dislocated his shoulder, but the effects of this disappeared in a few days.

Not much has to be added to this table. Everyone who

TABLE 2
NINE CASES OF DEPERSONALIZATION TREATED WITH METRAZOL

Name	Age	Additional Symptoms	Duration before Treatment	Previous Psycho-therapy	Number of Con-vulsions	Maximal Dose in Grs.	Result
J. L.	31	Suicidal attempts Severely depressed	5 months	Incomplete	15	9	Cured
R. O.	29	Slight residual signs of previous encephalitis	Several weeks	None	9	9	Cured
L. R.	31	Severe psychological conflicts for years	4 months	Incomplete	10	15	Much Improved
S. H.	30	Neurotic conflicts preceding suicidal attempts	1 year	Incomplete	7	7½	Improved

B. A.	19	Catatonic pupils	3 months	None	8	13½	Cured
S. S.	32		4 years	Moderate improvement	3	10½	Further but still incomplete improvement
S. R.	18	Hears his own voice continually as an obsession	15 months	None	25	12	Improved
W. T.	23	Flatness of emotions	4 years	Incomplete	22	10½	Slightly improved
A. S.	26		4 years	Partly successful	3	10½	Further but still incomplete improvement

has worked with depersonalization cases will agree that the results surpass the results reached by other methods. One may doubt the diagnosis in one or another case, as for instance, where emotional flatness is noted. This case was diagnosed by others as one of schizophrenia. The borderline between endogenous depression and depersonalization may sometimes be difficult to draw. However, these diagnostic difficulties lie in the nature of the subject.

It is obvious that insulin and metrazol treatment have a justifiable application outside the field of schizophrenia. They have been tried in manic-depressive psychoses. My own experience with the metrazol treatment of manic-depressives is too small; however, there have been startling results in two cases of confused mania. I have also observed improvements in depressions. Bennett (1938) reported that ten consecutive severe depressive psychotic patients were all relieved by shock therapy. The improvement started two weeks after the treatment began. He also quoted literature which asserted that hysteria and anxiety cases derived benefit from metrazol treatment insofar as the patients established a better rapport for psychotherapy after its use.

In most of our cases the first signs of improvement appeared after the first three or four injections, and in the majority of cases the symptoms had cleared up. The symptoms may disappear without further psychotherapy, but of course the individuals still have unsolved psychological problems. I am therefore of the opinion that every depersonalization case which is treated with metrazol needs extensive psychotherapy even after the patient is free from manifest symptoms. We have acted accordingly in all cases in which the outward circumstances made the application of psychotherapy possible. This is the same point of view which Orenstein and myself (1938) have taken in respect to insulin and metrazol treatment of schizophrenia.

One may, of course, raise the question whether the results of this treatment of depersonalization are due merely to psychological factors connected with the treatment. The patient indeed experiences terror and fright and even a threat of death. The transference is increased when he regains consciousness. However, it seems to me that such psychological phenomena are obviously the reflection of deep-lying changes in the organic functions. Furthermore, experience shows that deep-lying neurotic pictures cannot be influenced by mere fright. I am therefore of the opinion that organic changes in brain function connected with metrazol treatment have a therapeutic effect on the depersonalization neurosis. It is not possible to say at the present time whether one can generalize this statement for other neurotic conditions. It is even too early to state that the cure in depersonalization cases and in manic-depressive psychosis and schizophrenia will be a lasting one. One of my recovered depersonalization cases is free from symptoms and has worked steadily for more than ten months.

Summary

The picture of depersonalization is a rather well-circumscribed chronic neurotic picture which offers great difficulties for psychotherapy. Psychoanalysis or methods akin to psychoanalysis give good results if the treatment is continued for several years. Treatment with mescaline and benzedrine is ineffective. Nine cases are reported in which the intravenous treatment with metrazol in doses sufficient to give convulsions gave good results. However, some of the cases were not completely cured. This treatment should be combined with psychotherapy. The effects of treatment are probably due to organic changes. The psychological effects of the drug treatment are not sufficient to explain the results. Metrazol treatment is not only effective in schizophrenia but also in manic-depressive psychoses and in specific types of chronic neuroses. The question arises whether other types of so-called psychogenic disturbance (neurosis) will be responsive to this treatment.

CHAPTER FOURTEEN

Psychogenic Loss of Personal Identity: Amnesia

In psychopathology every state of forgetting is called amnesia. We are interested here merely in states of amnesia in which the subjects forget their own identity. To one's own identity belongs the connection with a specific structure. One has relatives, friends, a place where one works, and another where one lives. But the names and addresses are symbols of one's identity. In everyday life one identifies people by these criteria, and they identify themselves in the same way. A person's knowledge, insight, and faculties are much less important in this respect. We speak about amnesia in this paper only when consciousness is not deeply clouded, orientation is retained, and the possibility of forming impressions is not completely lost. However, when knowledge and general information have been impaired, in addition to the loss of identity and address, the case is still classified as amnesia.

Although this condition is well known, special studies have rarely been devoted to it. At the Ninth Annual Meeting of the American Psychiatric Association, Leavitt (1935) discussed the

---

Appeared originally in *Archives of Neurology and Psychiatry*, 34:587-604, 1935. Milton Abeles, co-author.

problem. Newspapers often report such cases. During World War I amnesia as a defense reaction was often observed. Price and Terhune (1919) and Henderson (1918) reported such cases and were particularly concerned with the differentiation from malingering. Amnesia in relation to crime has also been carefully studied by Hopwood and Snell (1933). In not many cases has a thorough study been made and the cases psychoanalyzed. Hamill (1925) reported a case of pathological stealing associated with amnesia, and Gordon (1926) described a case of dual personality with amnesia. In both of these, psychoanalysis was carried out. In both cases there was intense parental repression followed by rebellion in the form of amnesia. Ribot (1881, 1882) was more interested in the spectacular case of double personality. In the book of Pierre Janet (1889), one also finds a few remarks about this specific type. Though psychoanalysis has drawn new attention to the subject, the compilations of Fenichel (1931) do not touch upon it. Braun (1928) in the German *Handbuch* gave merely a short description of the picture. Wechsler (1929) gave two interesting cases of amnesia, one of which lasted a year and a half. Brown (1934) also briefly mentioned amnesia in one case.

Amnesia is a well-recognized pattern with social implications. We have therefore undertaken to study the problem based on the rich material from the Psychiatric Division of Bellevue Hospital. It is well to begin by presenting a typical case.

N.C., a woman aged 38, approached a policeman in the street and said she could not remember her name. She was admitted to the hospital. She said, "I don't know anything about myself." The time of admission was about 2 A.M. She was depressed and agitated. After sleeping through the night, she was interviewed by a physician about eight hours after admission to the hospital, by which time she had spontaneously recovered. She gave the history that she had been twice married. The first marriage was unsuccessful because of the husband's sterility (due to mumps). She had married again ten years before coming to the hospital, but had not had sex relations in five years. She had been faithful to her husband, nevertheless, until eight months prior to her amnesia when she had fallen deeply in love with another man on a vacation trip to Florida. She would have liked to remain in Florida. She would also have liked to get a divorce, but did not want to disrupt her social life. She enjoyed sexual relations and missed them. She had arrived back in New York two weeks before the episode of amnesia. The night of the episode she felt hungry and cold and went out to get something to eat. In the street she accidentally collided with a man and was shaken up. From then on she remembered nothing until she recalled her memory in the hospital.

The psychogenesis in the case is very clear. From the warm climate of Florida where she found love, she came to a colder climate. She felt "hungry and cold" before the episode. She wanted to be warm and with the man she loved in Florida.

The onset of amnesia usually occurs when a change in some long-standing disagreeable situation becomes imminent. There is a preceding period of depression. The patient most often finds himself wandering in the street or in some public place such as in a hotel or a railroad station. Sometimes the patient wanders around for days before seeking help. It is of interest that none of our patients has had sexual relations during the amnesia. Frequently the actual behavior during this period remains rather vague. Then, with dismay, the patient realizes that he has forgotten his identity and becomes alarmed. The most frequent course of action is to go to the first policeman with the problem. On admission to the hospital, the most common mood is one of depression and perplexity. The patient is agitated and apprehensive and often cries. Occasionally he is terrified, mute, and unresponsive. Most patients make an apparent effort to recollect the past. Only rarely are they calm.

The depressive features in our cases generally continued during the period of absence of memory, although they frequently became less severe; when the amnesia disappeared, the mood became normal. In one case, however, the recollection of the unpleasant incident which led to the amnesia made the patient irritable and depressed for several days following recovery. As has been stated, in rare cases the mood was calm, cheerful, or even hypomanic. In most of these cases, simulation had to be considered.

Background Histories

During the past three or four years, 63 cases of psychogenic amnesia have been collected and studied at the Psychiatric Division of Bellevue Hospital. Twenty-two patients were admitted between January and June, 1934, when the total number of patients admitted was 8,298, or 0.26 percent of all new patients.

Thirty-one amnesia patients were male and 32 were female. The oldest patient was 56 and the youngest fourteen, although another patient had a history of a previous episode at the age of twelve. By decade age, there were none in the first, thirteen in the second, 21 in the third, seventeen in the fourth, eighteen in the fifth, four in the sixth. There was a definite preponderance in the earlier decades, eighty percent of all patients being in the second, third, and fourth decade.

In our series, fifteen patients had had one or more previous episodes of amnesia. In addition, six had histories of dizzy spells and fainting attacks. Three had made suicidal attempts at some time in the past. One had a history of somnambulism. Another patient had a history of antecedent manic-depressive psychosis.

The next two cases are reported in some detail because of the significant earlier history.

I.P., a man of 37, was admitted on December 10, 1933, saying: "I don't know my name. I don't know where I live or whether I am married." He recovered spontaneously after two days. He recalled that he had been attacked by several men immediately preceding the loss of memory. Interesting and probably significant was the history of being attacked by several men at the age of three when he was extremely frightened.

N.Q., a woman of 54 who was admitted on December 5, 1932, had approached a policeman because she could not remember anything about herself. Her memory was restored in less than a day with the aid of hypnosis. The history was that five years before she had been in an automobile accident in which she was injured, with resulting right hemiplegia and aphasia. She recovered from this except for slight residual effects. On the day of loss of memory, she looked out of the window and saw her daughter get into an automobile. She said, "I was so nervous. I was afraid she was lost."

In both these cases, a previous distressing and unpleasant memory was recalled just before the onset of the amnesia. Even more interesting were the circumstances in the next case.

I.C., a woman aged 29, was admitted on July 27, 1933, very depressed and in a state of amnesia. Although her mind was deeply clouded and she did not recognize her mother or father, she was fairly well oriented about impersonal things.

She was found in the subway and had apparently fallen down stairs. The amnesia continued for six days before she recovered with the aid of hypnosis. She then gave the history that, eight years earlier, the father of her illegitimate child died. Since then she had had periodic amnestic episodes. These had usually followed a period of depression, once following the death of a sister. Six years before the present admission, she had fainted in the subway and had fallen off the platform in front of a train, her right arm being cut off. It is of interest that this present attack also accompanied a fall in the subway. At the time she was on the way to visit her brother (possibly a substitute for her father). Here, again, an unpleasant memory was recalled.

Etiology

In a number of instances there were either psychic or physical trauma immediately preceding the amnestic episode and precipitating it. For instance, in the first case (N.C.) the last thing the patient remembered was unexpectedly colliding with someone in the street. Episodes in some of the other patients were initiated by quarrels. In the second case (I.P.) the fright of the assault by several men was followed by the loss of memory. In two instances the patients were startled by approaching automobiles. In still another case, a woman was alarmed by a black man who accosted her. The next case is a good example of fright as a precipitating factor.

N.M., a girl aged fourteen, was brought to the hospital by her father because, several days before, she had lost her memory and the next day was found on a park bench unable to tell where she had been. Although she had already recovered, he brought her in for observation. The patient told of a quarrel with her aunt the night before, in consequence of which her mother had slapped her. She had had a similar amnestic episode ten months previously which lasted for two days and was accompanied by mutism. This attack followed an encounter with two rats, one of which she had accidentally stepped on. She said, "One of them jumped for my throat."

All of these events, however, were mere stimuli for more significant conditions and conflicts which were usually uncovered on going deeper into the backgrounds of these patients. By far the majority had some familial difficulty or an imminent economic problem. An interesting example of the first is furnished by the next case.

G.B., a woman aged 30, was admitted on March 22, 1934, while depressed and unable to identify herself. The next day, with some persuasion, memory partially returned, and from then on she gradually recalled more and more information about herself, although she still retained some blank periods even on discharge. The story was that, several years before, she had run away from home because of a domineering father. She said that since then, every time she made plans and prepared to go home for a visit, some partial or complete loss of memory would develop. For instance, while packing her clothes preparatory to the trip she would forget what she was doing. She was afraid to go home for fear she would have one of these attacks.

The desire to flee from some unpleasant marital situation also frequently led to loss of memory. For example, one of our patients, who was the wife of a man with chronic alcoholism with whom she had many difficulties, lost her memory and found herself wandering on Broadway. Another woman, whose husband expected perverted sexual relations, fled into amnesia. There were four unusual cases in which there was latent or conscious homosexuality, the amnesia being the result of some conflict arising from the sexual psychopathology. The next case is an excellent example of this situation.

M.K., a woman age 24, was found in the street unable to remember her name or where she lived. She was depressed and anxious, and showed some twitchings of the muscles, especially of the left leg. Three days later, under superficial hypnosis, she revealed her name and address. She lived in a suburb of New York with a woman much older than herself for whom she apparently had a very deep unconscious homosexual attachment. She said she never cared very much about men. Earlier in life she had been very much devoted to an aunt, who, she said, "got along in the world without being married." She said she had not wanted to live after this aunt died five years before. She dreamed about her frequently. On the day of the amnesia, she quarreled with the woman with whom she lived because she gave a gift to another friend. Feeling very unhappy, she came to New York, and the amnesia developed.

As a variation, a male homosexual of the overt type, in a fit of jealousy over a boy friend, experienced a short period of amnesia.

In another important case, because of feelings of guilt arising from a conscious hate of the mother, the patient had an episode of excitement in which she called for her father. This was a black girl, age fifteen, who was transferred to Bellevue Hospital from another hospital where she had been hospitalized for pulmonary tuberculosis. While there she had acted peculiarly. At first she was restless and noisy, then she became mute and uncooperative. On admission to Bellevue she continued to be uncooperative and refused to answer questions. She frequently called out, "Daddy." After a week of this behavior, she recovered and became cooperative. She denied any recollection of the entire episode. In the antecedent history, it was found that she had a very strong attachment for her father from whom she had been separated by her mother. In consequence, she did not feel a proper regard for her mother. The idea of guilt arose out of the realization of the unnatural feeling for her mother. This patient was on the borderline of amnesia (in the wider sense) and of the loss of personal identity in which we are interested.

Generally, amnesia patients are apprehensive about economic difficulties, including financial reverses, unemployment, and impending poverty. The condition in the next case was unusual in this respect.

S.R., a man age 36, entered the hospital in a dazed, bewildered state, very depressed. He had been found overcome by gas, apparently in a suicide attempt. He continued in this perplexed state, unable to grasp the situation or to remember what had happened. He frequently gave contradictory answers, sometimes remembering things which he had just said he had forgotten. However, he gradually improved. Significant in his history was that the day before the suicide attempt he had been promised a more responsible position with more salary.

This was an interesting reaction to a sudden increase in responsibility, probably owing to a feeling of inadequacy. Of note in this case also was the patient's intense subjective feeling of impairment of judgment and memory and his concern over it.

The next case is described because a partial analysis was possible and revealed important facts in the early history.

O.A., a 36-year-old woman, was found in the subway unable to identify herself. On admission, she was extremely agitated and depressed. She continued to be so, and all she could remember was "Johnny" and "Rue Galilée." Several hours after admission she was identified by a man; she did not recognize him at first, but then recalled everything. This man was "Johnny." She was married to a man twenty years older than she was. She was dissatisfied, and felt superior to her husband. For the past three months she had been participating in a clandestine affair with Johnny. A week before the illness she had had an argument with her husband and had left him to stay with Johnny. On the day of the amnesia they had agreed that she should go back to her family. That idea was extremely disagreeable to her, and as she went down to the subway suicidal ideas entered her mind. Instead, amnesia developed. She recovered eight hours later in the hospital.

A short analysis revealed that her mother had always been very strict. Her father died when she was three, and her only memory of him was that he had a beard. "All men with beards are disgusting," she said. She had definite desires for self-expression; she wanted to be an actress and to write. Because of these ideas, she came in conflict with her mother. She envied her older sisters who were artists and lived on the Rue Galilée in Paris and never married. She said she was the "ugly duckling" of the family. She entered a convent school at an early age where restrictions continued. Her mother wanted her to teach, and, in order to escape, she had married at seventeen. She did not love the man she married. He was much older than she, and he probably became a substitute for her father. She even exaggerated the actual differences between their ages. He was also strict, did not care much for social activities, and did not approve of any excessive activities on her part. During the early part of married life the patient often walked in her sleep. She would leave her sleeping husband and go on somnambulistic jaunts, occasionally walking out of the house. During the twenty years of married life she made abortive attempts at self-expression, but for the most part she led a life of intense repression. Her early resentment toward her parents was transferred to her husband, who was the father substitute. The amnesia was a rebellion and a protest against authority.

Duration of Amnesia

The duration of amnesia in our cases was anywhere from a few hours (three hours was the shortest time that could be estimated) to about a month, as in the next case.

F.H., a man of 34, was found on the street complaining of a sudden inability to see, and was admitted to the ophthalmologic service of Bellevue Hospital on April 17, 1934. Complete examination of the eyes revealed no pathologic change. The patient refused to eat or to give any information, and was transferred to the Psychiatric Division. The blindness disappeared on the second day. He professed complete amnesia for his whole previous life and could not identify himself. His attitude was rather silly and indifferent. He continued to be amnestic in spite of hypnosis with and without the aid of hypnotic drugs. His amnesia was anterograde; he forgot things that happened in the hospital. For instance, he declared that he had never seen the examiner the day after he had seen him. The amnesia reached a ridiculous point at one phase, so that a Ganser syndrome was seriously considered. He even denied recognizing his own face in the mirror, and professed other impossible losses of memory. In spite of this, a psychometric examination showed that the patient was of at least average intelligence. His manner continued unconcerned and silly, and he made little effort to recall his memory. On May 11, 25 days after the onset, without being asked, he volunteered the information that this was the day on which he had landed in this country thirteen years before, saying that the date in the newspaper reminded him. He gave his true name and details of his past life. He stated that he had had financial difficulties in the past year.

In this case it was remarkable that practically nothing of importance was discovered about the psychological etiology. It may be mentioned here that, the longer the duration, the more one has the impression that a secondary mechanism exerts a part. In many of the spectacular cases of dual personality, the actual cooperation of the physician plays an important part in prolonging the amnesia. Notably among these cases are those mentioned by Azam (1887), Sidis and Goodhart (1905), and Prince (1916).

In another case the patient had fugues lasting one, two, or three months, during which he was amnestic. However, he had an organic background, so that this case cannot be included among those of purely psychogenic amnesia. These cases will be reported later. In several other instances, the patients wandered about for several days or a week before asking for help. Sometimes, during these extended attacks the patient roamed far from home. The next case is a good illustration of this type.

J.Q., a man age 34, was referred to the Mental Hygiene Clinic of Bellevue Hospital for help. The story was that on August 30, 1933, he received his pay check in New York, bought a glass of beer, and was on his way home from work. The next thing he remembered was when he was in Indiana on the bank of a river, feeling weak and with a chalky taste in his mouth. After wandering around for a while, he returned home. He could not recall how he got there or account for himself. Memory for four days was totally gone. No obvious reason for the fugue was elicited. He went away with his pay check. When memory returned, he had spent it, which is a common occurrence in amnesia.

Statistically, in 27 cases, the amnesia lasted less than 24 hours; in 21 cases, the amnesia lasted one to five days; in seven, it lasted a week; in two, about two weeks; and in two others, three weeks or more. In two cases, the duration was not definite because the patient had recovered by the time of admission, but the attack probably endured less than a week.

Intellectual Functions

Many patients recover quickly before the depth of amnesia during the attack can be estimated; in these cases, it can at best only be surmised. The main symptom is the loss of identity. The patient does not know his name or address. He approaches someone in the street, most often a policeman, and complains that he cannot remember his name. One of our patients was unusual because she knew her name but not her address. Frequently, the patient can give some approximate information or isolated data about himself, which is of little or no use in identifying him or in locating relatives. Not infrequently, he hints at the cause of the absence of memory; he may mention money or some conflict of opinion. One case was unique in that the problem was not so much the loss of past memory as the inability to remember the present circumstances of his life, i.e., whether he was married and details about his business. Sometimes, the memory loss is spotty, so that one is reminded of Ganzer's syndrome. In most cases, the condition is not amnesia in the sense of loss of memory of the past. The next case is interesting because the patient denied recognizing his face in the mirror during the amnesia.

J.F., a married Jew age 50, was admitted February 9, 1934, complaining of complete loss of memory and identity. He was supposed to have left a town in Pennsylvania and to have arrived in New York a week before, but he did not remember anything that happened previously. His memory for the events that had happened in New York the week before were hazy. He had some recollection of going to see a lot of shows. His knowledge of general current information was almost nil. He declared that his mind was a complete blank. When his sister and a niece visited him the next day, he did not recognize them. He even said that he could not talk Hebrew, which he evidently knew. He denied understanding the most basic conceptions of everyday life. When asked if he recognized his face in the mirror, he said, "My face looks strange; it does not look natural." On the fourth day in the hospital the patient partially recovered with the aid of hypnosis. The history was that he believed himself a "mental healer." He would hypnotize people and believed that he helped them. Several months before his illness, a girl he was treating in order to make her quit a bad life accused him of having sexual relations with her. He was arrested, and it cost him $500. On the day of the onset of the amnesia he had been near the railroad station, saw an advertisement for an excursion to New York, and took it.

General information about current events and about everyday familiar knowledge and experience was frequently poor, as demonstrated by the routine informal memory test in the psychiatric examination. Some of the patients professed no knowledge at all; their minds were a complete blank. Some could not even do ordinary calculations. Others retained an adequate fund of general information. The next case is paradoxical.

A.G., a man of 40, was admitted on Nov. 13, 1932. He had gone to the home of a minister and had asked for help. He could not remember his name. He was brought to Bellevue Hospital. He remained amnestic until November 26, when the sounds of piano-playing on the ward helped to restore his memory. He had been completely amnestic. However, during the period of amnesia, a memory test revealed a memory span well above normal. Thus, though his past was a blank, actual formal testing of the efficiency of memory indicated good function.

In some cases in which the name of the person was known and presented to him, he did not recognize it. Similarly, patients would occasionally not recognize close relatives. The relatives often treated the patient as a malingerer and doubted the genuineness of the amnesia. Nevertheless, the inability to recall was usually retrograde and did not include events that transpired following the onset of the amnesia.

Quantitative memory-retention tests were not given to many of the patients during their amnesia, but from their general behavior and replies to routine questions it appeared that their ability to retain new material was not impaired. In five cases, standard intelligence tests were given during the amnestic period, and in some instances the patients made at least an average score in spite of the loss of memory recall. In three instances, because of mutism and unresponsiveness, the extent of the patient's knowledge could not be determined.

Complications and Atypical Cases

In a large percentage of the cases, the condition was uncomplicated, being straightforward amnesia. Alcoholism was a factor in only a few cases, and then it was incidental to the general depression and had no appreciable effect on the clinical picture.

There was one case, however, in which alcohol played an important part.

J.K., a man of 28, was admitted to the hospital on June 14, 1934. He had acute alcoholism and was mute and very depressed. Several hours later he began to talk, but was unable to tell his name or address. He said that his father had died a month before and that he had been drinking since. He soon recovered completely from the amnesia, but professed amnesia for the mute episode.

In two cases the condition was complicated by hysterical blindness. One of these (F.H.) has already been cited. In the next case, the blindness dominated the picture.

L.M., a black woman of 24, was found in the hallway of her mother's home saying she was blind and going to die. She was brought to Bellevue Hospital and continued to be depressed, complaining of blindness, though she made movements that indicated she was not totally blind. Twelve hours later, after sleeping through the night, she awoke and said she could see. The story was that she had been to a party and had a drink of whiskey. Someone there said something about her brother being killed (he had been killed about a year before). Following this, she remembered nothing until she found herself in her mother's home and was "blind."

As already mentioned, hysterical fainting, headaches, noises in the ears, and other somatic complaints may be involved in the clinical picture. The following case is an interesting variation in what is otherwise a classic case of amnesia.

L.B., a twenty-year-old girl, left a difficult home situation in Florida and went to a neighboring city. There, she lost the memory of her identity for about a day. After recovering, she hitchhiked to a point near New York. She took a train into New York and, on arriving at Grand Central Station, again became amnestic. She was brought to Bellevue Hospital where, with the help of hypnosis, she remembered everything.

This condition was similar to a fugue except that the amnesia punctuated rather than involved the entire flight.

Recovery

Of the total number of 67 cases, 47 recovered spontaneously. A number of them recovered automatically on the appearance of a relative, although some gave no indications or made no effort to recognize relatives. One patient reacted by becoming extremely agitated and running away from the relative. On the other hand, many recalled their identity spontaneously. Often, in the middle of the night or on awakening in the morning, the patient would announce his identity to a nurse.

In 25 cases hypnosis was attempted. In some it was attempted after the memory was recovered, but with a residual blank space for the events during the time of the amnesia. In three this period was recalled with the aid of hypnosis. Of the 25 cases in which hypnosis was attempted, eight cases were wholly successful and six partly so. The patients recovered during or immediately after the procedure. Sometimes the hypnosis was merely an aid in completing the recovery from amnesia which had already partially disappeared spontaneously. One of the most remarkable cases in which hypnosis was used successfully was the following.

B.H., a man age 26, was admitted on January 6, 1933, totally amnestic for his whole previous life, although his general information for current events was intact. He continued to be amnestic until January 10, when he was hypnotized with the aid of paraldehyde. During hypnosis he revealed many identifying details and, in disconnected fashion, the events preceding his amnesia. He told of a fight with a friend over a watch. Hypnosis was then discontinued, and memory was completely restored except for the events during the amnesia and the period of hypnosis. He asked where he was and who the examiner was. His story was that on the night of January 4 he had a fight with a friend whom he was choking when two other men knocked him down. Following this he got up and had a few drinks. The next thing he remembered he was sitting on the hospital bed with two doctors questioning him after the hypnosis.

In another case, suggestion with pressure on the eyeballs was used effectively to produce recovery. In still another patient, who was involved in a law suit, the threat to expose the patient to the police produced a speedy recovery. Here, the question of malingering was considered. In a number of cases the patient was given a pencil and told to allow his hand to write automatically. In three cases, significant information was obtained in this manner. In some cases the name was recalled piecemeal, letter by letter, with the persuasion of the physician. In two cases, association with dream material was contributory in the recovery of the patient.

A.W., a man of 28, entered the hospital in an amnestic state which continued for five days. The past history, which was obtained later, was that he was the son of an English sea captain who had been stationed with the fleet at Hong Kong. The patient had been trained in the English navy. Ten years before, he had had an accident, falling 65 feet, which incapacitated him for further service. On admission to the hospital he said that he had been frightened by a taxicab. Hypnosis was attempted on the fourth day, and he re-enacted the traumatic scene. He said, "I am falling, I am falling." The next day he was hypnotized again and had two dreams. In the first he was sailing on the Japanese sea and saw two sharks swallowing meat. From this he remembered Shakespeare, which he kept repeating, and became very excited. In the second hypnosis he said: "We are going over the river Avon to the funeral of Caesar, and that is how I got to Mark Antony." Then he associated sharks, Shakespeare, Brutus, Antony. He said, "what General von Lochinvar—Clive—Clive—That's my father's name. My name is Anthony Wallace."

It is of interest that the memory of two patients was restored by hearing piano-playing on the ward. Another patient regained his memory when he hallucinated his mother's voice calling his name. In the majority of cases, when memory returned, it did so completely and at once, although some patients did take several days, recovering gradually. Some were even discharged from the hospital with fragments of the past still missing. Frequently, there was a blank period which was apparently permanent and never recalled after recovery. This was the period from the onset of the amnesia until the patient decided to confide his difficulties to someone else. This blank sequence was occasionally recalled with the help of hypnosis, but more often it was not.

Differential Diagnosis

Differential diagnosis is not always simple; often, the diagnosis is only certain after the patient has recovered. Practically the entire range of psychiatric classification has to be considered in differential diagnosis. Schizophrenia, manic-depressive psychosis, organic disease of the brain, including trauma to the head, cerebral arteriosclerosis, presenile dementia, aphasia, carbon-monoxide encephalopathy, alcoholism, Korsakoff's syndrome, and simulation are some of the possibilities to be considered. It is best to demonstrate these contingencies with cases.

J.G., a man of 40, walked into the police station on October 23, 1932, and stated that he did not know his name or anything about himself. He was very untidy, with a beard and swollen feet. He appeared to be somewhat depressed, although he said he was happy. Under hypnosis four days later he was not able to tell his name, although he was able to tell a few facts of his life. He thought his troubles had started seven weeks before, and told a number of other things. On November 14, three weeks later, he remembered everything. He said, "I couldn't get my name out of me. I was frightened. I had the idea I wouldn't use my name any more. I got too frightened to tell it." He told of organized persecutory trends that he had. He thought that the Masons were after him at one time. According to his relatives, he was very seclusive. He had been put in a sanitarium about seven years before, but had disappeared and had not been heard from since.

In this case the diagnosis was schizophrenia. In the next case the diagnosis of manic-depressive psychosis was made.

C.H., a man age 59 when admitted to the hospital on January 16, 1934, was extremely depressed, apprehensive, and bewildered. He complained of pain in the back and said he did not know who he was or where he came from. He stayed in the hospital for more than two weeks, during which time he continued to be profoundly depressed and made numerous hypochondriac complaints. After a few days, with persuasion and suggestion, he spelled out his name and gradually recalled many of the facts of his previous life. However, his depression continued to be so severe that he was transferred to a state hospital. No cause for the depression or amnesia was determined.

It is interesting that in our psychogenic cases, injuries of the head and carbon-monoxide poisoning producing amnesia were not rare. This shows how difficult it is even in cases of organic involvement to evaluate psychogenic factors. In the next case, in which amnesia followed injury of the head, the etiology was subsequently discovered to be on a merely psychogenic basis.

C.P., a man of 35, was admitted on May 14, 1934, with a marked discoloration and swelling of the right eye and the history that he had been hit over the head and robbed. He said, "I cannot remember my name or anything." He did not remember being hit and could not tell anything about his past life. He did not know whether he was married. Two days later he recalled his name, and the amnesia completely disappeared except for the traumatic incident. The spinal fluid and X-ray examination of the skull were negative. The Wells Memory Test on May 21 showed a quotient of 82. He was discharged with a diagnosis of organic amnesia caused by trauma to the head. About three weeks later he was readmitted to the hospital, again amnestic, without any evidence of trauma. He presented a clear-cut case of hysterical amnesia and had sufficient family and financial difficulties to account for it.

The usual picture associated with trauma of the head is loss of memory for the traumatic event, especially if it is accompanied by unconsciousness and subsequent confusion.

The next case had definite organic disease of the brain, but the patient had fugues which were at least partly psychogenic.

A.R., a man age 50, was brought to Bellevue Hospital for

observation in February, 1934. Three or four weeks before, he had had financial reverses and had lost most of his money. After this there was a change in personality. Whereas formerly he had had many friends and was a good mixer, he now lost most of his friends and became morose and irritable. Family disagreements began, and he disappeared from home for two or three days at a time. He would explain that he had been away on business, but never told where. Then he began to have longer fugues. First he disappeared in February, 1933 with a few dollars in his pocket. In May he was found in the neighborhood, dirty and neglected. He was very depressed and cried; he could not tell where he had been or how long he had been away. He came home and was happy for a while, but in August he disappeared again and was found in October in circumstances similar to those of the previous attack. This was again repeated from November, 1933 to February, 1934, when he was admitted to Bellevue Hospital for examination. At the beginning of his stay in the hospital he was depressed and somewhat dull. However, he gradually became more amiable and cheerful. He told little about what had happened during the fugues. Psychometric examination revealed intellectual disturbances of a general sort, especially in memory retention and perceptual tests. The Wells Memory Test Score was 55 percent. Physically, except for some slight sclerosis of the peripheral vessels, he showed nothing abnormal. Encephalography showed a small amount of air in the lateral ventricles and a considerable amount of air in the subarachnoid space, probably indicative of cortical atrophy. He was discharged from the hospital with the diagnosis of cerebral arteriosclerosis, with fugues probably of psychogenic origin.

Amnesia for the events occurring during and following a convulsive seizure are well known. The next case is an unusual example.

J.A., a man age 36, was committed for observation to the Psychiatric Division of Bellevue Hospital from the magistrates court. He had been found suspiciously wandering around a cellar and was booked for unlawful entry. When he was found, he said he was looking for his brother who, he said, lived only two blocks away. The address he gave for his brother, however, was in another city. When he was brought to court, he claimed that he did not know how he got in the cellar or what he was doing there. On transfer to the hospital he maintained this story. He had no recollection of the events which transpired in the cellar. A Ganzer's syndrome and even schizophrenia were considered, but the diagnosis remained in doubt for over two weeks, when the patient had a major convulsive seizure in the hospital.

The usual picture in such cases is for the patient to be found in a dazed condition after a convulsive seizure. When admitted to the hospital without any previous history, and at the same time unable to identify himself because of postepileptic confusion, a diagnosis of psychogenic amnesia is on occasion incorrectly made. The correct diagnosis is established only after the patient recovers from the confusion and gives a history of previous epileptic seizures.

The next case shows unusual features in which both hysteria and simulation played parts.

A.O., a girl of nineteen, approached a policeman on the street and said she could not remember anything. She was brought to Bellevue Hospital on November 30, 1930, and remained amnestic for more than two months. She was given every freedom about the hospital. Hypnosis was attempted. At first she was a poor subject. She would go into a deep sleep and would not make any contact. Initially she gave a fictitious name. And she was also very unstable emotionally in the beginning. About two and a half months after her admission, another amnestic patient was admitted. Our first patient watched the second one respond quickly to hypnosis. After that, she gave significant information during hypnosis. She could not talk during hypnosis so that she made all her answers with hand gestures. In this way she gave her father's and her sister's names. After hypnosis, her father's name was presented to her, and she became wildly excited and even hallucinated her father. Finally, her relatives were located and identified her. Before she left, the patient admitted that she had no amnesia at all and that she knew all about herself from the beginning. She said she went to the policeman because she "wanted to get away from it all." She thought she would be sent to a state hospital where she would starve herself to death. She had refused to eat at times in our hospital. She had refused to be hypnotized when she first came because she was afraid she would give herself away. During her stay she often wondered why her people did not come to the hospital to look for her. As a matter of fact, they had been there and asked for her, but she had given a fictitious name. She finally submitted to hypnosis because she was afraid we would think she was "fooling," but she had always asked for sleeping medicine in order to go to sleep and not talk.

The next two cases are examples of obvious simulation.

F.R., a twenty-year-old girl, was admitted to the hospital on February 28, 1933. She had approached a police officer and told him she could not remember her name or address. The day after admission she was recognized by one of the hospital employees as a former patient. At first she denied the identity, but she soon admitted that she had simulated the amnesia to get away from her husband. Investigation revealed that although she was only twenty, she had a long history of asocial behavior, including many sexual misdemeanors and superficial suicidal attempts, and had been in various reform institutions from which she had run away. Wherever she had been, she was found to be unreliable in her statements and even fantastic in some of her confabulations.

E.H., a woman of 24, was admitted to the hospital June 6, 1934, complaining of inability to remember her name and address. She stated that the last thing she remembered was being startled by a loud noise. She was calm and not depressed. In the hospital she was agreeable and happy, even singing and entertaining the other patients. She continued amnestic until the next day, when her sister identified her and she was discharged. On being released she stated that she knew her name all the time, and had used simulation as a means of escape from her family who had oppressed her.

This study does not deal with amnesia in criminal cases, but one can see in the preceding examples how fluctuating the borderline between true amnesia and simulated amnesia can be. However, we hope that our description of cases of patients without criminal background will help in the differentiation of simulated and nonsimulated cases.

Psychological Meaning of Amnesia

Although none of our patients was observed long enough to allow deep psychoanalysis, the material allows some conclusions concerning the psychologic structure involved. In one case where the amnesia occurred after the death of a lover, the amnesia led to an accident in which the patient lost an arm (run over by a subway train). In another case the patient contemplated suicide by throwing herself in front of a subway train, but she did not do it, and amnesia developed. In these and other cases one has the impression that the amnesia is self-punishment arising from a feeling of guilt; it is a partial suicide. The psychogenic blindness in two cases preceding the amnesia probably had a similar meaning.

In many cases one finds a deep disappointment in a love object. Then one wishes to be dead for the love object and removes oneself by suicide. But one removes the disappointing love object at the same time. The tendency to punish is often obvious.

Financial problems are often given as the reason for amnesia. We should be skeptical about such a possibility. There are usually deeper motives. A man forced to sell a valuable picture became amnestic; he needed the money for the defense of his mother, who was accused of murder.

Amnesia is often a "giving in" to a stronger force. One of our patients became amnestic after being robbed of money he needed for the family. Amnesia was seemingly a simple way out. In another case the patient became amnestic when pushed by a car, but in this case a deep love conflict was in the background. It is remarkable that, as far as our information goes, no sexual relations took place during the amnestic period.

In amnesias one deals with a well-known pattern which can be easily used. Comparatively superficial conflicts are sufficient. Because the pattern is generally well known, it is comparatively often used for direct simulation.

In some cases there is an organic nucleus. Amnesia of the organic type, after an attempt at suicide with gas or by accident, may serve as an easy pattern for getting attention.

On the whole, amnesia is a weak attempt of a weak personality to escape problems which are chiefly conflicts of actual life. These conflicts have relation to more infantile levels, especially to the Oedipus complex. It is the fear of being punished by the family, by the father or mother or their representatives, that leads to an effort at escape which does not harm the person too much.

Therapy

In the interest of the patient and the family, the amnesia should be removed as quickly as possible. When urgent questioning does not help, automatic writing or hypnosis should be used. The psychotherapeutic task is not finished when the amnesia has disappeared. One should try to secure insight into the problems of the patient and to find the deeper motives which have led him to attempt to escape from reality and from his identity.

Summary

Sixty-three cases of psychogenic amnesia have been reported here. Thirty-one were male and 32 were female, of which 80 percent were in their second, third, and fourth decade of life. Fainting attacks and suicidal attempts were important in the patient's previous history.

Some unpleasant social conflicts, either financial or familial, were significant as the immediate cause of the amnesia. There were four cases in which homosexuality played a part.

The duration of amnesia varied from a few hours to several months. Twenty-seven cases, or almost half, recovered in 24 hours, 21 in one to five days, seven in about a week, two in about two weeks, and two in more than three weeks.

Cases of so-called amnesia are characterized by loss in memory of personal identity. In addition, general knowledge, information, and memory for past events are usually poor. The ability for retaining new information is often preserved, but not adequately. The patients are usually puzzled and perplexed.

Forty-seven patients recovered spontaneously. In 25 cases, hypnosis was attempted, and in fourteen of these it was partly or wholly successful. Other methods, such as persuasion, automatic writing, and association with dream material, aided in recovery.

In differential diagnosis, schizophrenia, manic-depressive psychosis, organic disease of the brain, trauma of the head, cerebral arteriosclerosis, presenile dementia, aphasia, carbon-monoxide encephalopathy, alcoholism, Korsakoff's psychosis, epilepsy, and simulation have to be considered.

Psychologically, behind the superficial conflict which precipitated the amnesia, deeper motives are found. The conflicts of actual life are related to more infantile conflicts, especially the Oedipus complex. It is an attempt to escape from punishment and at the same time receive self-punishment by effacing one's own personality (psychologic suicide).

The amnesia as such should be removed by persuasion, suggestion, and hypnosis. When the patient has recovered from the amnesia, one should try to help him obtain a deeper understanding of his emotional conflicts.

CHAPTER FIFTEEN

Remarks on the Psychophysiology of the Skin

Human beings know very little about the insides of their bodies, but they seem to know about the surface, their skin, and they seem to have a clear perception of it. They do not feel it as a living part of themselves, but they are aware of sensations streaming from the skin continually, and the eye observes the skin in a rather objective way. Indeed, according to the investigations of D. Wechsler and myself (Schilder and Wechsler, 1935), children between the ages of four and five can name the skin and have a clear perception of it at an age when they conceive of the inside of their body as merely the food which they have just eaten. Still, two of the children answered the question, "What is under your skin?" with "Me." The skin evidently appeared to them as merely a protection and shroud of the real body.

Investigations of Hartmann and myself (1927) offer further insight. When adult persons close their eyes, they can tell very little about the surface of their bodies. They can describe only a distinct feeling of those parts of the skin which are tense over boney areas. The surface of the skin in other places is experienced

Appeared originally in *The Psychoanalytic Review*, 23:274-285, 1936. Reprinted through the courtesy of the Editors and the Publisher, National Psychological Association for Psychoanalysis, New York, N.Y.

as vague and indistinct with unclear borderlines, together with vague sensations of temperature. Even when we touch an object we experience the object and its surface, and next to this is an empty space, and underneath only the mass of the body; the skin is not in the immediate field of perception. It is as if the body lies underneath the skin. Only if we touch the skin very lightly is there a real sensation on the skin, but this, again, seems to be on the outside of ourselves.

In pathological cases, patients may demonstrate the same principle in an exaggerated way. A sixteen-year-old girl with a severe chorea minor complained about the sensation of a thin rubber membrane which covered her body. She complained that this was not her real skin and that she would not get well until this skin was removed.

Even optic perception does not give us a definite experience concerning our skin. We are unable to judge its appearance correctly. Even if we look at the naked bodies of others we marvel about the color and the structure of their skins. The partially naked bodies of bathers on the beach astonish us again and again by their varying colors. Painters have tried to catch these evasive hues. It seems as if the uncertainty concerning our own appearance prevents us from having a clear perception of the bodies of others. We have no stable experience concerning our skin. We acquire the knowledge concerning it by a continuous dynamic process by which we gain a definite borderline between ourselves and the outer world.

Language preserves these various attitudes concerning the skin. One is "fond of one's own skin." One "comes off with a whole skin." One "protects one's own skin." But one also "jumps out of the skin." In German, too, one says: *"Ich wehre mich meiner Haut"* (I don't value my skin) and *"Das ist zum aus der Haut fahren"* (My skin is my armor). It would not be worthwhile to go into such a discussion if the psychological plasticity concerning the experience of the surface of the body did not indicate that active dynamic processes are building and constructing our knowledge of our body surface. How we experience the outside of our body is determined by the total personality as well as by the configuration of the outside of our body.

The total experience consists of perception and sensations. But there are also imaginations and self-representations, and the objective side is profoundly modified by and interwoven with the emotional attitudes and problems of the individual. Psychic processes are not a mere addition to the clear experiences of the senses; the attitudes of an individual are an inseparable part of the sensual experience. It is not correct when we say that our emotions change the experiences of the senses. Every emotional attitude is a sensual experience at the same time and every experience of the senses includes an emotional attitude.

Twenty-four-year-old J.D. came into the hospital in an extreme state of excitement, continually complaining that he felt an itch all over his body, especially in the hairy parts. He repeatedly said: "Now it is itching in my nose, now in my eyebrow." A few months before, he had acquired pubic lice in the rooming house where he lived. He was cured by one treatment. But then his excitement started. He was convinced that the lice were coming from the feathers of his pillow. He saw the lice flying around in fantastic shapes. He saw them settling and crawling on him. He saw about 30 at a time. They had shapes like feathers, some like curved lines, and others like straight lines. Still others had the shape of small discs. He felt that he should report the house to the police. Others would be affected too. In the course of about ten days his agitation subsided. He was a rather excitable boy who felt unhappy in the city. He was trained in farming and wanted to go back to it. He told about his experiences in farming, especially chicken farming. Two years before, after cleaning a chicken coop, he felt itchy. He thought it came from chicken lice. The itching disappeared after he had washed himself. The patient was rather interested in his appearance, proud of it, and especially of his complexion; he had always been a health apostle.

This simple case leads to a basic problem. There was at first a sensory experience. It came from the outer world. It came from the periphery and modified the person. His itching was, from the beginning, the specific itching of a specific person. In the second phase, the experience did not go from the periphery to the center of the personality, but from the center of the personality to the periphery. It was the same process but in reverse order. One might say that the experience of the senses had an aftereffect. And this aftereffect made the flow from the center to the periphery possible. We have sufficient proof that this aftereffect in the periphery was not necessary. When the patient began to talk vividly about his itching, the persons around him also started to feel itchy. It is true that the itching of these other persons was not only in the central nervous system but it went into the skin. Of course, it was imagination, but this imagination was connected with material changes in the periphery. I have said that this itching was the patient's personal and individual itching. His disgust concerning the uncleanliness of the rooming house revived memories of chicken farming. The lice flying in the air like chicken feathers with the same shape also recalled chicken farming. He wanted to go back to farming. His previous experience was the pattern according to which the sensual material was shaped and molded. But what about the itching of the bystanders? They, too, must have had actual experiences before. Their centrifugal process led back to a reality they had previously experienced. Imagination always leads back to realities. The imagined world and the real world are fundamentally the same world. There is nothing new in this observation. Psychogenic itching has been observed, among others, by Klauder (1924) and Sack (1926, 1933). If we look at another case it may help us to come to a better understanding. Twenty-year-old E.M. (Schilder, 1930), with a great number of neurasthenic symptoms, complained about itching on his penis, on his anus, and on his hands and feet. These are the very parts which are in the center of his sexual activities. The feet had a particular erogenic significance for him. The sight of naked feet excited him. Anal irritations played an important part in his earliest remembrances. It is of extreme importance to note that the patient had an itching disease in earliest childhood. When his mother gave birth to a younger sister he imagined that the doctor was torturing her and brushing her toenails with a hard brush. Later on he also had an opportunity to see his father rubbing his feet when he came home tired, and later he observed his father scratching his back because of an itching.

I do not want to go into psychological details of this rather completely analyzed case. But we find here the basis of the conversion symptom in the disease, the libidinal structure of the total personality. Such a structure is not merely an abstraction but is a part of the individual life situation, especially in connection with the Oedipus complex. In a very deep layer we find the organic disease in early childhood, the experience of the senses. It seems that the organic disease of another person, the itching and scratching of the father, has an important influence on the final formation of the symptom. I come, therefore, to the formulation that the basis of the conversion symptom is (1) the organic disease in the past of one's self as well as of others with whom one is in libidinal contact, and (2) the libidinal structure in connection with the life situations of the past and of the present. This formulation holds true, not only for itching and conversion symptoms of the skin, but also for conversion symptoms in general. I do not know, of course, whether the organic disease in the past is indispensable. We shall come back to this problem later.

I have made the assumption that even psychogenic itching is connected with organic changes in the skin. The cases quoted do not offer definite proof in this respect. But I have observed a 35-year-old man who complained, among other symptoms, about a distressing pruritus ani. He had in very early childhood thrombosed hemorrhoids. He also complained that there was always moisture around his anus. A series of dreams, dreamed in one night, may give a superficial insight into his psychosexual structure:

1. "I am shriveling up. Finally I was a small child with naked buttocks standing up. It was mostly anus. I think it was me.

Later on I felt washed and cleaned, and my genitalia were tweaked by the person who washed me."

2. "I am holding a girl by a cut in the back. The child seemed to be dead, but started to cry."

3. "My older brother had become a doctor. I found him operating on a sacral cyst." (All the dreams have been shortened.)

Castration fear and the wish to be castrated were outstanding features of the psychology of this patient. He wanted a masochistic, passive, and homosexual relation with his father and mother. I cannot here go into the details of his psychosexual structure, which are in close relation to his early history and to the attitudes of his parents. Anal elements seemingly also played an important part in the psychology of his father. I mention the case chiefly because there is not only itching around the anus but also moisture. The conversion in this case is therefore connected with so-called organic changes in the skin. I may add that the patient complained about sweating and vasomotor phenomena after intercourse. Such cases offer the proof that the centrifugal stream, going from the center of the personality to the periphery, is indeed an organic process affecting the peripheral organ.

It is my firm conviction that a deeper understanding of conversion phenomena and psychopathological phenomena in general can be reached when we study the processes of imagination in the normal subject. Out of this conviction I have studied (1933a) and with my co-workers Kanner (Kanner and Schilder, 1930), Bromberg (Bromberg and Schilder, 1932), and Parker (Parker and Schilder, 1935) willfully produced imaginations in the various senses. I refer here especially to the investigations of Bromberg and myself on tactile imaginations and the tactile aftereffects. The general tendencies of irradiation of the formation of the background, of the effacement of certain parts of the images, of the building up and the destruction of form [*Gestalten*] of movements, of curving of lines, and the tendency against the perception of angles, are identical in the aftereffects with the tendencies noted in imagination. Benussi (1914), by successive irritation of two points on the skin, produced an impression that an object had moved from one point to the other. It is, of course, necessary that the time between the two touches be short. The same phenomena can be observed, according to our investigations, in the successive imagination of two points and in the aftereffect of two touches. There is an inner link between the aftereffect of perceptions, perceptions of very short duration, and the imagination. We do not know in what way the imagination reaches the skin. Sack (1926, 1933) speaks about an antidrome irritation which may lead to production of histamin or acethylcholin. But one may ask whether or not vasomotor phenomena may be of importance in this respect. We have studied a case of extreme vasomotor irritability in a catatonic from this point of view, and we found in the vasomotor phenomena the tendency to irradiation, wandering of connecting two points, and of effacing sharp angles. The relation between the vasomotor phenomena and the tactile aftereffect is more of a similarity than an identity. The vasomotor phenomena may be parallel in part to the central tactual phenomena. It may be that the vasomotor changes increase the activity of the tactual imaginations, which are almost constantly connected with temperature sensations.

In the experiments quoted, the imagination provoked sensations on the skin which fulfill the conscious intention of the imagination. It is not a general excitation, but it is the production of a specific experience on the skin with a specific meaning. The conscious wish can therefore be effective. In experiments which I (1918) conducted I ordered my subjects to imagine that their hands were increased to a size twice as large as the normal, or that a second hand was growing out of their forearm. The tactile sensations which occurred corresponded exactly to the order. They conformed with a specific meaning of the order. This went so far that men ordered to imagine that they had female breasts felt specific sensations fitting to such a change in their bodies. Unconscious problems and strivings lead, of course, to still more obtrusive sensations of the skin. One of my patients felt pain in his penis, in his arms, in his anus, and in his palate (1931b). He felt the pain in those parts where, in his imagination, the penis of another man touched him. The literature contains many instances where willful or instinctive imaginations may produce hemorrhages and blisters on the skin. I am reminded here of the well-known experiments in hypnosis of Mabille (1885), Dumont-pallier (1885), Heller and Schultz (1909), and others. I mention especially the observation of Schindler (1927) concerning the psychogenic origin of spontaneous hemorrhages on the skin. In a case of Kreibich and Sobotka (1909), urticaria blisters appeared on the body when the patient was exposed to disagreeable excitement. The centrifugal process provoked not only sensations on the skin but actual changes on the skin.

In the instance of Kreibich and Sobotka, the question arises why the manifestation was spread all over the body. Does that not contradict our statement that a manifestation on the skin has a specific meaning? A 40-year-old married woman complained about itching all over her body, but especially in her vulva. "It is a burning sensation." This patient had never had sexual satisfaction in her marriage, remained excited after marital intercourse, and felt the itching especially after sex relations. The widespread itching had a specific meaning in spite of the fact that it was seemingly diffuse. Another patient, a paranoid schizophrenic, felt itching on his penis only after intercourse. We come, therefore, to the formulation that psychogenic sensations and manifestations on the skin always have a meaning even if they seem to be diffuse and widely spread. Not only does the localization have a specific meaning but also the character of the manifestation on the skin. Even if we deal with seemingly localized and isolated phenomena on the skin, they are never really isolated. Always, something is going on in the totality of the experiences. When we produce in our experiments a willful imagination, the willful imagination is never isolated; it has a distinct background. There is always a foreground and background in every psychological and biological phenomenon. I observed a patient with spontaneous heat sensations which came in attacks. Such attacks were observed and were connected with a temperature of 38.1° C. His face was extremely flushed, the left arm was cool and of a livid color. These attacks developed after he had witnessed the death of his nephew when he was run over by a truck. One leg was torn from the body, and the child died soon afterward. Following the accident, he dreamed that his own arm was cut off in a machine. In hypnosis, the accident was revived and led to the same phenomena and also to the rise in temperature. It was not possible to suggest directly a rise in temperature or the vasomotor phenomena. One sees that the phenomena in the face and on the arm have a very distinct meaning in a total situation; the rise in temperature is the background of the total experience.

A. Weinberg (1923, 1924) has studied the plethysmogram, the electrocardiogram, the galvanogram, pupillary reaction, and breathing at the same time under the influence of important experiences. The phenomena in all these spheres corresponded to an excitation of the sympathicus. A short excitation of the parasympathicus follows and, finally, a long-lasting excitation of the sympathicus. According to Weinberg, elevation of the level of consciousness is accompanied by increased sympathicus influence, depression by an increased parasympathicus influence. Before Weinberg, de Jong (1921) emphasized that every psychic experience leads to basically similar somatic changes in the plethysmogram and in the galvanogram. But the expression of this general psychosomatic change is dependent upon the psychic attitude toward the different parts of the body in general and of the skin especially.

This psychic attitude has a long history which only psychoanalysis can reveal. Furthermore, the body has a history and a constitution. In the case of psychogenic fever, the patient had gone through a long-lasting autumnoesteval malaria. The mother of the patient and the patient himself showed a constitutional vasomotor lability. The biological history and the life history of the individual determine, therefore, the final shape into which the general psychosomatic irritation is built. Heilig and Hoff (1928) could produce herpes labialis by suggestion in persons who spontaneously reacted with herpes to exciting experiences.

The herpes could be inoculated in the cornea of rabbits. The organism and its psychic manifestations are always in connection with the outer world (in this case infection), and the final manifestation of the psychosomatic change is therefore also dependent on the outer world. In the genesis of the diverse skin manifestations, therefore, not only psyche and body participate, but also their relations to the outer world. This may be true not only for allergic reactions of the skin but also for eczemas and the final result of mechanical irritations of the skin. One sees that the final borderline between the so-called psychogenic and organic case is unclear.

I have already mentioned that an early somatic disease offers the best basis for conversion symptoms in later life. We have spoken about the relation of the diverse skin diseases to the psychology of the individual. The variety of such skin diseases is very great. There is itching, blushing, sweating, impetigo, hemorrhages, urticaria, allopecia, psoriasis, eczema, herpes, acne, warts (Bunnemann, 1927). It is not very probable that the same conflicts find expression in so many different skin affections. A differential psychology must exist of the various affections of the skin. There must, finally, also be the possibility that specific conflicts manifest themselves in a specific way in the skin. We are far from a final solution of this problem.

The first case of psychogenic itching I mentioned was always particularly interested in health and was in narcissistic relation to his body. But this case was not psychoanalyzed. The neurasthenic case allows a deeper understanding. The sadomasochistic attitudes are in a very close relation with the itching. Anal components are of special importance.

Even in a rather completely analyzed case, some doubt remained whether the itching in early childhood was due to an organic disease as an indispensable factor. It must also be emphasized that the frequency of itching diseases of the skin in early childhood has to be considered from this point of view. These itching diseases provoke an enormous tendency to scratch, to break the skin, and in some way to disrupt the unity of the body. Children so afflicted also become restless, aggressive, and sadistic. The early skin disease of organic origin brings with it a definite set of psychic attitudes which certainly must have an important influence on later psychic attitudes. The relation between itching and pruritus to sadomasochistic and anal tendencies seems to be rather obvious. It has often been observed (cf., for instance, Fenichel, 1931) that neurotic blushing and perspiration are often connected with paranoid trends. These individuals feel continually that people are watching them. I have in my material a case in which the fear of blushing and perspiring and the actual blushing and perspiring are in the foreground of the picture. The blushing proved, as it is analytically well known, a substitute for erection. Not only masturbation but also erection is an extremely social phenomenon and concerns the body image of others as well as one's own. Our patient tried frantically to hide his erection and his penis. The blushing transferred them to his face. The face became the focus of the body image which attracts the attention of other people. It is the tool by which the patient brought the body image of others nearer to himself. All the other people looked at him and gave him attention. This is the attention he primarily wanted for his defecation and for his erection. Analysis revealed that anal tendencies were very strong in early childhood. At four years of age he was afraid to be observed by others when defecating. A genital castration threat by the father had, furthermore, increased the genital, anal, and passive homosexual trends. Blushing was the illicit satisfaction of a close anal and genital relation to other human beings. It was therefore not tolerated by the ego system. He avoided other people and was afraid of them, although primarily he wanted to be in relation with everyone. All human beings were in the same way threatening or admiring. I have seen very similar trends in another case in which psychogenic sweating was one of the minor symptoms. The patient felt that all people should admire him, and his neurosis chiefly consisted of a continual self-observation, of measuring himself against an unobtainable ideal. Narcissistic trends were in this case in the foreground, with tendencies to visual observation of libidinal type. The number of cases observed does not allow definite conclusions, but we surmise a specific psychosexual structure in the various psychogenic manifestations on the skin. The case with the paling of the arm, reddening of the face, and psychogenic temperature definitely belongs to the hysterical group with strong object relations. The cases of hemorrhages on the skin observed by Schindler (1927) belong in a similar group.

I do not think that we have the right to expect a general formula concerning the different psychogenic manifestations on the skin. Itching, for instance, may not always have the same meaning. The localization, the type of itching, has to be considered. The dermatological manifestation of a neurosis is, after all, only one of the manifestations of a total personality, which cannot be understood from one symptom alone even if this symptom should be the leading one.

If one considers the relation between psyche and skin, one should not forget that every affection of the skin must have a profound psychic influence. General experiences make it very probable that a set of psychic attitudes is connected with every organ. So the organic diseases can provoke attitudes similar to those which can be provoked psychogenically. As stated above, the organic disease goes from the periphery (the organ) to the center (the personality of the subject); the psychogenic disease goes from the center to the periphery. Skin diseases do indeed deeply affect our relations to other human beings, and every skin disease provokes attitudes very similar to those described in the case of psychogenic blushing. There is a leveling of relations to other human beings. A particular attention is given to one's own body. But the whole personality will again participate in the evaluation of the skin disease. There are not only the different aspects of the skin, there are also the different sensations connected with the change in the function of the skin. This self-perception of the skin and its changes is a very complicated process. In a hyperthyroid condition of a 31-year-old patient, the basal metabolism was at first increased to plus 42. After an operation, a slight dryness of the skin developed, with a rapid pulse. Her basal metabolism three years after the operation was still plus 19. Her pulse was rapid. Her skin was inclined to be dry and rough. This patient had, psychologically, the complete picture of myxoedema. For two months she had imagined that her head was changing, that her ankles had become larger, that her face had become thinner, that her hair had become dry, that her eyes had become smaller, that her scalp had become hard and wooden. She also stated that her heart did not palpitate any more, that her nails were broken. The patient showed otherwise the picture of a depression. She felt that other people observed and laughed at her. She was deeply worried about a leukorrhea and about the fact that she had no children. In this case, the patient perceived an actual change in her skin in an exaggerated way due to her total attitude, the problems of her life, and probably also due to the organic influence of the dysthyroidism on the central nervous system. The case reminds one of the well-known fact that, in dreams, organic changes may appear in an exaggerated way and show the presence of the disease before it is perceived otherwise. Every perception of an organ of the body, and, therefore, also of the skin and its changes, is not merely a mechanical act, but goes through the various symbolic stages by which it is brought in connection with the individual's total experience. The self-perception of the body—I speak about the body image—is therefore a highly symbolic act, not less symbolic than the expression of the problems of the personality in functional and organic changes of the skin. Psychogenic manifestations of the skin have always a meaning. This meaning may be conscious, it may lie in a symbolic and instinctive sphere. There is no fundamental difference between a change imagined on the skin, between a merely so-called psychogenic manifestation, and a so-called organ neurosis. They are all centrifugal, but reach the periphery, the organ, as such. No emotions and imaginations are merely psychic. The psyche is an organic agent. But there is no change in the body which is not reflected in the psychic attitudes. There exists only one organism, and this is a psychophysical one (Schilder, 1924, 1925b, 1931a).

CHAPTER SIXTEEN

On Homosexuality

This is a report on some cases of homosexuality which I have observed. It is not a comprehensive study, and I do not intend to "solve" the problem. But these are interesting cases that afford us a psychological approach to this important problem.

I shall begin with a case that I had the opportunity of analyzing for seven months. The patient came to me with the complaint that he felt attracted only to men and in no way to women and girls. Once, when he was fifteen years old, he had relations with a servant girl, but after that he had never succeeded with any social contact. Just before he came for treatment he was in a brothel, but could not get an erection and felt very dejected about it. In none of his relations with men had he ever had sexual intercourse. All his relations with men had been of the social type and were associated with many fantasies.

At the time he came for treatment he had a special friend who was very virile and masculine, as were his other men friends. He was not fond of homosexuals who made a more feminine impression. He preferred friends of the distinctly masculine type, and he wanted to feel superior to them. He achieved this by being very amiable, by being necessary to them, and by his intellectual superiority. In his relations with these friends he displayed a double attitude. On the one hand, he wanted to take the place of their girl friends. Sometimes he imagined that he had

---

Appeared originally in *The Psychoanalytic Review*, 16:377-389, 1929. Reprinted through the courtesy of the Editors and the Publisher, National Psychological Association for Psychoanalysis, New York, N.Y.

intercourse with one of his friends, thus taking the place of the friend's girl. He therefore never had friends who were real homosexuals. On the other hand, he wanted to make his friend inferior to himself by putting his friend in the feminine position.

It was interesting to observe that this double attitude toward his friends developed from his feelings toward his father. The patient's father was a man of a decidedly masculine type. The patient had hated him as a child and hated him still. He wanted to be superior to his father, but was fearful that he would not achieve this. He had always feared his father, always felt that his father was much stronger than he, and that he would never become as strong as his father.

It is important from a theoretical point of view that all his tendencies toward superiority and inferiority were based on sexual scenes that he had witnessed when he was a very little child. He slept in bed with his mother. He observed frequently that during the night his mother would go to his father's bed, after which he heard noises that made him surmise that something was going on. Once, when he was seven or eight years old, he went to his father's bed where his mother and father were cohabitating and was promptly sent back by his father. This event was very likely of the greatest importance in his life. In puberty he had many fantasies of men and women having intercourse, and in these fantasies he himself sometimes played the part of the woman, sometimes the man. He wanted to play the part of the father, but he always had the feeling that his father was stronger than he, that he would never equal him. He felt that if he could not "play the part of my father then I will play the part of my mother." He identified himself with his mother because he feared that he could not identify with his father.

His father had often beaten him and had ridiculed him because of his feminine attitude. He, in turn, grew to despise his father because of his many promiscuous relations. The father once had a gonorrheal infection with much pain during urination, which the patient had observed. In puberty, the patient built up the idea that he did not want to be like his father, that he did not want to have sex relations with women. He built up an ascetic ideal which, it should be noted, derived partly from the feeling that he was weak in comparison to his father. But he never gave up this struggle for superiority against his father. He tried to get this superiority by being very clever and more educated than his father. This carried over into his attitude toward his friends. He did not want to be like his father in relations with girls, fearing that he might not be dominant enough.

In almost every homosexual this is an important motive, namely, that the heterosexual partner seems somehow too distant, too difficult to reach, and therefore the individual decides to take what is apparently the line of least resistance. At the same time, however, my patient did not want to give up his masculinity, which, by being superior to very masculine men, he could still retain. Even though his masculinity was somehow threatened, he could retrieve it in this roundabout way. This "detour" is, I think, one of the most important rules in homosexuality.

As psychoanalysts we cannot believe that events in the seventh and eighth year of life can be of such importance for later development. We assume that something must have taken place in an earlier period of life which pointed in the same direction. The patient's first memories were revealed in connection with a dream which he reported in one of the first analytic hours I had with him. "I am in a grey suit and have a knife in my hand. I press the knife to my heart. This knife is not made of metal, however, but of paper mâché, and collapses slowly and falls together." The associations to this dream led quickly to the fact that the grey suit was one belonging to his current friend. The next association involved the following memory. When he was about four years old, his father once came home drunk and was violent toward his mother. His mother became very agitated and frightened. She made an attempt at suicide, taking the kitchen knife and trying to stab it into her chest. In this dream we see clearly the role of the father; the father violent and pressing the knife, the phallus, into the mother, and the mother suffering and falling down. The patient wanted to bring his friend into this same position, and he himself wanted to be in the superior position. In other words, it was very likely that at an early age (before five) he had an opportunity to observe the sex life of his parents, the activity of his father, the passivity of his mother. He grew up feeling that his father might be very dangerous, very violent, that perhaps it might not be possible to be the same as his father. We can also say that basically there is a tendency to double identification. He wants to take the place of his father, but, feeling himself too weak, he takes the second course of identification with the mother. That does not satisfy him, and so he tries to regain his superiority in a roundabout way, by being superior to the most masculine man, his father.

This patient also had a strong love for his mother and his sister. This is always found in homosexual cases. There is no case of homosexuality in which we do not find a phase where heterosexuality also plays a great part. In this case it appeared clearly: in the quarrels between his mother and father he had always fought against his father, taking the part of his mother. In an interesting dream, which he reported, he dreamed about a man in a parcel with strings around it which was being pulled from the water. It turned out that in some way that parcel was a symbol of the mother's uterus. He was always interested in his mother's uterus and in operations she had undergone, as well as in the womb of his sister who had also been operated on. The same hostile attitude that he had for his father he also had for his brother-in-law. As in every other patient of this type, we find a very strong heterosexual tendency which appeared clearly in many little psychic love affairs he had in early puberty. He had completely forgotten these affairs when he began the analysis, but he then gave the typical history of homosexuals. When he was a little boy he was interested only in the things that girls and women were interested in. "I played only with little girls, and I have always had only an interest in men." It is this sort of history that has caused some psychiatrists to believe that homosexuality is a fate one has from birth and can never change.

In this whole picture there was one point which was of great importance, and that was the particular attitude this patient had toward his penis, which he always felt was inferior. We find that these patients are in despair that they can never equal their fathers, and in the concrete way of childish thinking, never have as big a sex organ as the father. It is also very important to hear from our patient that he was very much concerned at the time of puberty because he felt that he did not have enough hair around his penis. He masturbated in front of a mirror and always observed that he did not have enough pubic hair. He took cotton and put it around the penis as a substitute. This is indeed an important feature, and we see here that the feeling of inferiority was not really a general feeling but related to a special organ, the penis. We find this almost invariably in cases of homosexuality.

Some other features did not appear quite so clearly in this analysis, although the practical result was satisfactory. Our experiences in other cases made it very likely that these factors were also present in this patient, especially the fact that he wanted a love object who possessed the beloved phallus. The "parcels" dream related above suggests that he wanted it in the mother, but did not find it there. When our patient was in his masculine attitude, he might find in his friend the mother with the phallus, while he himself played the part of the father.

I will pass directly to the second case, a boy of 22 whom I did not analyze for as long a time as I did the first patient. I can, however, prove that this patient, too, had a strong interest in heterosexuality. He had a great interest in his mother, a great interest during puberty in girls, but he was afraid that he might not be strong enough to maintain this relation to girls, and during puberty he built up the fantasy that it would be easier to have intercourse with a cow, the introitus of which is not so narrow. Again, we meet the idea that sexual intercourse is too difficult, that he might not be dominant enough to have such a sex relation. This patient already had very strong sex interests at a very early age. When he was about five years old he gave money to a little girl of four years to induce her to allow him to put his genital organ into hers.

Something very interesting happened in this case. When he was about six years old he went to a school and was seduced by a rabbi, who, after the lesson, took some of the boys into the classroom and ordered them to touch his erect penis.

It is interesting from the general point of view of the psychology of seduction to know how this one took place. Our patient had heard from some of the other boys that something of the kind was going on. He arranged it so that he could be alone with this teacher. When he saw this man's erect penis, he got a feeling of inferiority, comparing his small organ with his teacher's big one. His whole childhood was filled with interest in the penises of other people and with measuring his against those of others. He developed an enormous sex activity, and had relations with almost every boy in his class. At this time he did not have the feeling that these homosexual actions were really sexual. He felt that heterosexual actions were quite as important but something different. This is characteristic in the psychology of some homosexuals: when they are children, in puberty, and later, they do not regard their perverse actions as real sexuality. I have seen female patients who were rather prudish in heterosexual relations, but did not feel that homosexual relations had anything to do with sex. This is of very great significance in the psychology of homosexuality and perversions.

To continue with the second case, in his later life he continued his extensive homosexual activities, always in fear that he was too weak to have relations with girls. His attitude was sometimes active and sometimes passive. In the latter attitude he often had passive anal intercourse with others. His passive attitude was not primarily chosen, but was resorted to because he did not feel himself strong enough to be active. The passivity culminated in an interesting delusion which he developed at about eighteen years of age. He believed that by anal intercourse he would get a child and he would then get the Nobel prize because he, a boy, would give birth to a baby. He developed this idea at a time when he suffered very much from inflamed hemorrhoids. We see here again a great interest in the penis, a feeling of inferiority based on the idea that his penis was insufficient, and a consequent regression to passivity, which in this case was closely related to the anal attitude. In the course of the treatment he had heterosexual intercourse, but he experienced his sexual excitement chiefly through the fantasy that another man's phallus was in his partner's vagina also having intercourse. Feeling his own semen in the vagina, he immediately had a second emission without withdrawing.

I mentioned in connection with the first case that most homosexuals who come for treatment come with the homosexual legend that they have been homosexual since the beginning, that they have always had sexual interest only in boys and have never had interest in girls. In both these cases I have demonstrated that the homosexuals originally had strong heterosexual interests. There is another homosexual legend, that the homosexual is not really interested in the anus of his partner, but that he is merely interested in coitus inter femoro, and that only a few attempt anal intercourse. That might be true in the consciousness of the homosexual. Indeed, it is true that many homosexuals abhor anal intercourse, but not so many as stated in some of the literature. When one analyzes homosexuals, one finds that every one of them has a primary interest in anal intercourse. If we have someone with a tendency to passivity, there must be an organ for this passivity, an organ which takes in something. Passivity and anal sexuality must be very closely connected, and if we analyze any homosexual, we find that the feeling of not being strong enough to be active or, to put it more concretely, the feeling that "my phallus is not strong enough to be active" must be connected with the feeling that "I must be passive, and I have the organ for this passivity." I would say that male homosexuality and anal eroticism are always connected with each other, but in consciousness the process of repression often makes it appear as if the homosexual abhors anality.

Before discussing these problems from a purely theoretical

point of view, I want to report a third case. The man began treatment when he was about 37 years old. He liked to talk to boys about the age of twelve to fourteen. He was not at all interested in older boys. He did not do very much with the boys he liked. He merely talked with them, and during such conversation he asked them to tell him something about what happened at school. He was especially glad when the boys told him that the teachers had been dissatisfied with them, had punished them, had put them in the corner, etc. Sometimes the patient experienced the desire to beat these boys himself, or he felt a tendency to pull their ears. At such times he experienced sexual satisfaction. He never performed real sexual actions with these boys.

This patient was a rather wealthy man, and whenever he met such a boy and had spoken with him, he felt somehow obliged to care a little more for the boy. He approached the boy's parents, spoke with them, and very often arranged to pay for the boy's education, or, as he himself put it, he behaved toward the boy like a mother. This was his sex life.

He had never shown any interest in women, but it appeared in the course of his analysis that he was very much interested in his mother. This relation to his mother was of a special type. He came to this topic in the following way. In the course of the analysis it became clear that this patient had no idea what sex life was, which was the more astonishing for he was the owner of an estate where he had cows and bulls, etc. Once he asked whether the erection was not a sign of shame. He believed that one got an erection only if one were ashamed. In connection with that, it appeared that he had his first erection when he was about eight years old and had been beaten by his mother. Thus it was that he wanted to hear that the boys had been shamed. He felt that the boys would have an erection telling about it, and he himself at such a moment also got an erection. It appeared that in his fantasies as a boy he supposed that something similar took place in his mother when she was beating him. In other words, this scene which took place between him and his mother, i.e., being beaten, getting an erection, and supposing some sex excitement in his mother, had become the scene after which his later sex life had been patterned. When he wanted to beat the boys or pull their ears, he wanted to take the part of the mother. In other words, in his sex life he identified himself with his mother. Now we understand why this man had the intention of caring for these boys, paying for their education, etc.

We can say that in the first case the patient identified himself with his mother because he felt himself too weak to identify with his father. In the present case, the identification was different. The patient began to identify himself with his mother when he was about twelve years old. At that time his older brother became schizophrenic, and his mother and father (especially the mother) withdrew their affection from our patient. He had never been shown much tenderness by his mother, but even that little had been taken from him. He felt very lonely, felt that he would not have the love of his mother, and at that time resolved to take her place. We see this mechanism very frequently, that, in the moment of a great disappointment, the disappointed person terminates the love relation by identification. It was at such a moment that the patient took the place of the mother, feeling that he would be loved by the boys of this age in the same way that he had loved his mother. We identify ourselves with other persons in order to gain the love and esteem the other person possesses, or as Freud (1910) put it, we identify ourselves with other persons on the basis of the same wish. We identify ourselves with others when we want to get what the others have. We now understand why the patient played the part of the mother, why he began to play this part when he was twelve years old, and why throughout his life he was interested in boys of this age.

I want to stress one point. The patient had had a great many relations of the type described. In fact, two of the patients of whom I speak were very promiscuous. My general impression is that perverse persons are, for the most part, much more promiscuous than heterosexuals usually are, although I do not underestimate the promiscuity of heterosexuals. This might have something to do with the fact that it is only at the highest, the heterosexual level, that we find the development of tenderness which makes it possible to cling to the love object for a longer period of time.

To return to our third case, a special interest in his own penis was also present in this patient. He had phimosis and had resolved, on the advice of his family physician, to rid himself of the phimosis by operation. It was a long time before he could decide to have the operation. On the day before he was to have the operation, he caught a cold and could not be operated on. After that the patient never again considered having the operation. During the night before he was to be operated on, he dreamed that he broke his leg and was very much frightened about it, a rather clear symbolism. At a very early age, about four or five years, our patient felt that to break one's leg was the most terrible thing. Along with that, the idea came to him that he had heard something in old Greek myths of castration, breaking the penis. This special interest in his penis appeared in the way he cared for this organ. In the winter time he always had a sensation of cold in it. Therefore he wrapped it up to keep it warm and well cared for.

We have found similar attitudes toward the penis in other patients. No psychology of homosexuality can neglect the interest of the homosexual in his own penis. He does not want a partner in his love life who does not have the same valuable organ. Or we could say that every homosexual has some narcissism, some self-love which centers on the penis.

To formulate briefly, we may say that the male homosexual identifies himself with his mother, but the identification differs in different cases. There can be a disappointment in the love object, as in the third case. There can be a feeling that it is impossible to equal the father and therefore the mother's part is taken, as in the first case. There can be the feeling of insufficiency in regard to the phallus, as in the second case. In the third case, the incomplete psychoanalysis pointed to an identification with the mother, but the identification was not proven. Taking the mother's part did not necessarily lead to passivity. In the first case, the impossibility of equaling the father led to a roundabout effort to become superior to him and to place him in the position of the female. The hated father then took the place of the mother (with the phallus). It may also be possible that great tenderness on the part of the father forces the boy into an identification with the mother. Besides the identification with the mother, the love for and interest in the individual's own phallus and the phallus of the partner play an important part. With the passivity is connected a strong anality, the anus substituting for the phallus of the mother. In another one of my cases (not analyzed) the homosexuality was at least precipitated by the fact that a beloved boyish female teacher used to pull the patient's ears while standing behind him. The picture was marked by an anal tenderness.

In cases of female homosexuality, the idea of not being able to accomplish the female sex functions (narrowness of the vagina, ugliness) leads to identification with the father. In Freud's case of female homosexuality (1920b), this identification was reached in another way. In one of my cases, a 26-year-old girl, rough playing with the father instilled in her a desire to be superior to him. His phallus had made a great impression on her when, as a child of four, she had observed him urinating. Her distrust in her female sex ability led to an identification with the beloved father. She therefore chose masculine love objects and struggled with them for superiority. In another case of female homosexuality, the child feared the severe father, but found in the mother, with whom she slept, a suitable love object. In a case of schizophrenia, the patient complained that her vagina was being obliterated and that in this way she was being made homosexual. It is not yet clear what part anal eroticism plays in female homosexuality. We also do not know enough about the role of self-love and the narcissistic pride in the genitals in these cases. I would suppose that the female homosexual would show an exaggerated pride in the care of her body. It seems that the female as well as the male homosexual tries to take the masculine part when she wants to achieve superiority over her father.

When we consider homosexuality from this point of view, we cannot agree that it is based on hormones in the testicles (Steinnach, 1913). We cannot expect homosexuality to be cured if we replace the patient's testicles with the testicles of a heterosexual individual. We must say that every case of homosexuality is based on a psychic development, and only on such a basis can we understand the great variety in homosexual trends. In one of the cases I have reported, there is, for instance, an interest only in twelve- to fourteen-year-old boys. That cannot be due to a special type of cell in the testicles. We know, for example, that the first patient about whom I have reported was interested only in men of a very masculine type. Others are interested in men of a very feminine type, and still others only in men who have reached a certain age, the senile phase, etc. In short, we must also take the pathological development of the individual into consideration, and then we shall find that first there was a heterosexual tendency and that, because of the development of some infantile conflicts, heterosexuality had been replaced by homosexuality. We have found that perversions, too, are due to childhood conflicts. In other words, a perversion is the result of an infantile neurosis. What is true for perversions generally is especially true for homosexuality (cf. Rank, 1924; Freud, 1922).

Now, what is the role of the body in homosexuality? It may be that the constitution plays a definite part. We should never deny, from a psychoanalytical point of view, that there is a deviation in the sexual constitution as well, but the sexual constitution alone never produces homosexuality if it has not been shaped by what takes place in psychological development.

We may now go a step beyond these formulations on homosexuality and draw some conclusions about activity and passivity in sex life. We may ask what homosexuality teaches us about the essence of femininity and masculinity. In the instances I have given, it is clear that we cannot say generally that the male homosexual is passive or feminine. We find only that, in the course of his psychic development, passive or feminine trends can be increased. In addition, we find many active tendencies.

But we have to assume that what appears in the homosexual must be present in the heterosexual also. It is one of the principles of psychoanalysis that we never find mechanisms in neurosis which cannot be found in the normal person. The differences are merely quantitative. We must reckon with passive tendencies and the tendency to anality in every male individual. A definition of masculinity as activity and femininity as passivity is wrong to begin with. We must presuppose bisexuality in every person. We may say that bisexuality is somewhat characteristic of the basic constitution of every human being, and consequently we must suppose that female, passive, and anal characteristics must be present in every male, just as we must suppose that active tendencies are present in the female.

K. Schneider (1921) stated that the active attitude is one which somehow consists only of looking down from above, looking down toward the woman in a protecting way, being stronger than she is. I think such a definition is wrong. It is absolutely erroneous to believe that the masculine principle consists in activity. There are active as well as passive tendencies in every individual, but it may be that the manner in which the active or passive tendencies are combined in the male is different from the way they are combined in the female. It is thus perhaps of advantage to consider the psychology of sex action in intercourse from a more general point of view. We may reckon with the general principle that the sex organ and the body generally may lead us to a better understanding of what the psychology of these organs may be.

We may say that in the first phase of sex activity the shape and action of the male sex organ show that there is a sadistic active tendency of intrusion into the other person's body; but that is only the first phase of intercourse. In the culmination of intercourse, when the intrusion has taken place, the activity decreases, the organ of activity is, as it were, given away. In other words, male sexuality consists of an initial phase of great activity, the activity being followed by passivity, by the feeling of being given into the power of the female and the female genitals. Male sexuality can be recorded in a curve in which there is at first activity and then a succeeding passivity. The curve of female sexuality is perhaps the converse. First, passivity of receiving followed by the triumph of having the valuable organ of activity. There is a state of superiority, of holding the man and his organ like holding a child, of having him in her arms helpless, powerless like a child. The female curve is passivity in the beginning, activity toward the end. The shape of the sex organs in both sexes expresses this clearly, and we can say that sex psychology reflects itself in the sex organs, as psychology generally expresses itself in the organism. In the male body, there are organs of passivity, or receiving, i.e., the anus, and we could therefore say that in the male, too, there must be some passivity in the initial phase of sex activity. I believe that in really satisfactory sex life not only the activity but also the passivity of the male has to be gratified.

We may say that what we meet in homosexuality is not something completely new, but an exaggerated form of what can also be found in the sex life of the normal male and female. Activity and passivity are characteristic of every human being. Everyone's body is prepared to be only active to protrude with something into the other's body—the clitoris, the tongue, the penis; but everyone's body also has parts which are ready to receive—the mouth, the vagina, the anus. We may therefore say that we can understand the psychology of sex only if we consider it under the double aspect of the desire to intrude and the desire to be intruded. Intruding and being intruded, being strong and being weak, these are the two poles of every sexual activity (see also Schilder, 1920, 1923, 1942a).

CHAPTER SEVENTEEN

The Psychogenesis of Alcoholism

In order to understand the psychogenesis and psychodynamics of alcoholism, one has to understand the effects of alcoholic intoxication. What happens when an individual is intoxicated? The experimental literature has been reviewed by Jellinek and McFarland (1940), who came to the conclusion that alcohol had a depressing effect on all psychological functions measured and that such stimulation as has been reported for some psychological variables is a pseudostimulation. The psychological picture of the effect of alcohol is one of reduced efficiency. The simple psychological functions are less affected than the complex ones. The ability to judge relations and to grasp concepts suffers greatly under the influence of alcohol. The associations are impoverished, and there is a tendency toward egocentric concepts. The authors conclude that the main effect of alcohol is cortical with an added subcortical effect. The experimental results concerning the influence on volition, emotion, and personality are very meager.

People, however, do not drink in order to produce an impairment in cortical function or to reduce their critical faculty; they drink in order to feel different. We are accordingly chiefly

---

Appeared originally in *The Quarterly Journal of Studies on Alcohol*, 2:277-293, 1941.

interested in the emotional manifestations of alcoholic intoxication. Turning to clinical experience, Fleming (1935) has collected material on acute alcoholic intoxication. There is no question but that the higher degrees impair perception, judgment, and motor function. The fundamental change, however, is in mood. There is, at first, euphoria and increased confidence in one's mental and physical powers. If the intoxication progresses, lack of judgment combines with the increased feeling of one's own importance, and actions occur which show the weakening of inhibitions.

A description like this leads to the fundamental problem. In acute alcoholic intoxication one can love oneself. One has the feeling that one is good, both morally and intellectually. Accordingly, one is ready to receive the love of others and one feels more loved. The term "love" means not only sexual desirability but also admiration and appreciation. One becomes a valuable citizen. Hand in hand with this increased self-esteem is increased love for others to whom one is ready to grant love, appreciation, and admiration. The appreciation of one's own conversation and intelligence increases irrespective of the objective impairment of judgment. When one feels so valuable, there is no need to control one's activities. Free rein is given to impulses, especially the sexual ones. No doubt, the individual who is drunk has not completely lost the awareness that his claims for eminence and gratification are not justified in reality. An underlying anxiety leads to an increased emphasis on one's claims, and even to irritability and pugnaciousness. There is clinical evidence of a fundamental change in sexual attitudes. Sexual desire is increased. Sexual wishes, otherwise hidden, find more or less open expression. The forms of sexuality that appear are often of a more or less primitive character, and even infantile forms of sexuality may prevail.

It is vain to speculate whether the impairment of judgment and reality sense, with the lessening of one's critical faculty, liberates the sexual tendencies, or whether alcohol as such has a direct influence on the sexual function. Dynamically speaking, alcohol produces a change in the relation between the ego and the id. One may say that the function of the superego is impaired. Such formulations are unsatisfactory, however, since they neglect the finer psychological structures and especially because they lead away from the all-important concrete situations of life. With the progress of the intoxication and its aftereffects, the individual is more and more overcome by the insight that he really does not deserve love and appreciation. The euphoria changes into feelings of depression and worthlessness.

Intoxications vary not only in severity but also in form, according to individual differences and according to the changes of the total situation in a single individual. However, it seems that we always deal with the same basic picture and that what varies is merely the accent on the different facets of the intoxication. The same is true of the problem of tolerance. There is no doubt that both psychological and physiological factors contribute to the differences in the pictures of acute alcoholic intoxication.

The so-called pathological intoxication occurs in individuals with labile perceptive (cortical) mechanisms. Difficulties in perception and memory disturbances are in the foreground, with violent outbursts resulting from confusion. These types have a close clinical relation to epilepsy and head injury. The intoxication releases a dissociation in cortical function. The effects of alcoholism will differ according to the total situation. The effects are not merely the sum of two psychopathological disturbances, but an interaction.

So-called pathological intoxication is merely an exaggerated expression of the fact that alcoholic intoxication does not occur in the ideal average person, who obviously does not exist, but in a specific individual who lives in a specific way. One may expect that a tendency to self-depreciation and a feeling of not being loved and not deserving love will enhance the pleasure of feeling sure of one's own esteem and of the esteem of others in the acute intoxication. This surmise is amply substantiated by clinical experience. The return to soberness will be particularly bitter in such cases, resulting in the "blues."

One may expect that those with a reasonable amount of self-assurance will enjoy the intoxication without having a definite need for it.

One will expect that people of cyclothymic temperament as well as many depressives will show a comparatively strong reaction when intoxicated since their basic psychology is so closely related to the problem of love and self-esteem.

There is no special relation between the paranoid attitudes of individuals who live in tense relations with the outside world and the psychological effects of alcohol. Alcoholic intoxication in paranoids is therefore generally uneventful. The same is true regarding the fantastic dreamer and the schizophrenic.

Individuals who are accustomed to fight against their drives and urges and who have repressed strong sexual urges persistently will enjoy the release offered by intoxication and will express sexuality with gusto. One can make similar statements about those who have been persistently careful not to experience hate and have otherwise conformed to social proprieties such as tact, cleanliness, and orderliness. However, it seems that obsessional types with their deeply destructive hate, which is usually related to social ambitions and maintenance of prestige, do not find any particular gratification in alcoholic intoxication.

The general principle is that individual differences must be considered in the approach to the problem of alcoholic intoxication.

Acute alcoholic intoxication in one who drinks regularly and in one who generally does not drink is certainly not identical. We have very little evidence about what happens psychologically in someone who is intoxicated often and acutely. We may surmise that we deal then with one whose perceptive and thinking apparatus is dulled and whose emotions are more and more pressed into a pattern of striving for admiration and appreciation, which he can gain subjectively and objectively only by being intoxicated. The underlying awareness of this very deficiency will make him crude, irritable, and overbearing, and the characteristics of the bully will come more and more into the foreground.

It is not our problem to decide whether this progressive alcoholic deterioration is due to the cumulative effect on the brain of alcohol or whether the various vitamin deficiencies play an important role here (see Bender and Schilder, 1933). I may also mention that the physical signs of acute alcoholic intoxication are different in persons who are chronic alcoholics. There is, for instance, a type of coarse tremor which occurs only in the acute intoxications of the severe chronic alcoholic.

I cite here three cases of so-called alcoholic hallucinosis.

The first one was a 40-year-old man who had been repeatedly admitted to psychiatric institutions because of alcoholism. He had been drinking for twenty years. His childhood was sheltered and strictly supervised. His marriage was unsatisfactory. There was a passing episode of impotency. In the course of heavy drinking he saw himself in a bus surrounded by men and women trying to stab one another. He himself felt threatened and hit them over the head with a bottle, thus defending himself until the Naval Intelligence Service should arrive. This was a visual dreamlike experience which faded from reality as a dreamlike memory. It seems that the patient had some concern regarding his regained potency, which he wanted to utilize in a second marriage. The problem, which should be an individual one, became the problem of a general mix-up in which persons of the same sex participated, as well as persons of the opposite sex. The social situation was obviously filled with fear, and he maintained the role of eminent hero with some difficulty. One has the impression that there is always some correlation between problems of social prestige and physical attachments to persons of the same sex.

The second case was a 31-year-old man who heard that a girl in the apartment nearby had sex relations with a boy and was surprised by her mother, who felt that this patient was responsible for the incident. The patient, a chronic alcoholic for ten years, had been on a spree since his sister's marriage several weeks before. The hallucinatory episode expresses seemingly incestuous desires concerning his sister, otherwise hidden from himself. The patient was very proud that he had so many friends. His sex activity, however, was limited. The psychotic episode, causing a distorted breaking through of incestuous impulses, could just as well be termed a pathological intoxication as an alcoholic hallucinosis.

The third case was a 39-year-old alcoholic of long standing who had attempted to jump into the East River. He had heard voices threatening to shoot him in the chest and in the legs; the President and the Mayor were talking about him, discussing a plan for his execution. He was also supposed to meet President Roosevelt on a boat where he was to get his final citizenship papers. This was a more or less typical case of alcoholic hallucinosis. He was in the center of a social situation and was undergoing something comparable to a distorted and terrifying initiation rite. The community insisted upon shooting him or, in the terminology of Bromberg and myself (1933b) he was about to be dismembered. Interestingly, the shots were aimed all around his genitals, but not at the genitals themselves. This is somewhat contrary to the usual picture, in which castration is often the main motive. Nevertheless, it is the same problem, which can be characterized as the idea that the community will demand the sacrifice of the integrity of the body, and especially of the sex parts which have sinned.

Indeed, the alcoholic has not reached the durable heterosexual attachment which is socially demanded. Caught in problems of prestige, inferiority and superiority, self-esteem and social esteem, he has often found himself in close relation to persons of the same sex with whom he may even have had sexual contact in early childhood and later. Or at least he may have wished so. His early education may have inhibited him from sexuality in general. This led him to an insufficient heterosexual adjustment. This was followed by impulses of a primitive sexual order—urethral, anal, oral, sadistic, and homosexual—which obviously could not be tolerated by an individual conscious of his social obligations. The newly gained awareness that heterosexual adaptation was demanded was not strong enough to overcome the severe feelings of guilt which in childhood were connected with every sexual activity, due to faulty education. The description of these processes is fairly uniform in the recent literature on alcoholism, which has been collected by Crowley (1939). The studies by Wall (1936, 1937) and Curran (1937) are of particular importance from our point of view. Curran formulates as follows (pp. 666-667):

> . . . a strong attachment to a parent of the same sex, strong narcissism and strong inner-tensions making social contact difficult are the outstanding features in the alcoholic women. The alcoholic women are always striving for social recognition and fear that this will not be given. In their acute psychosis they often experience an attack of criticism from others, which is a projection of the self-criticism which is at the base of their social shyness. The alcoholism also influences the aggressive and sadistic tendencies, so that in the acute hallucinosis they believe relatives or others have been killed off. The alcoholics experience feelings of sexual inferiority and project it in hallucinations to the outside world.

The results of Wall are basically similar. The correlation between these findings concerning the character structure of alcoholics and the experiences in acute intoxication is a close one if we put into the foreground the potential alcoholic's increased wish for admiration and love. Alcoholic intoxication gives to the socially insecure individual the fulfillment he desires.

With these statements we have already approached the central problem in the psychodynamics of the chronic alcoholic. In my opinion, the central social problem of an alcoholic transgresses the boundaries of homosexuality. The struggle for prestige and the close attachment to the person of the same sex, especially the parent of the same sex, also evokes sexual repercussions. Sexual attachments of this type will lead, in turn, to prestige problems even if the homosexual attachment comes from other sources. However, as mentioned earlier, the possibility that alcoholism, as such, disturbs the libidinal balance must be seriously considered.

It is an interesting thought, which cannot be substantiated at the present time, that human beings choose addiction drugs which physiologically will increase tendencies already present. Homosexuality can be almost experimentally produced by cocaine intoxication, which in turn is mostly resorted to by those with latent homosexual cravings. Hartmann (1925) presents clinical evidence which makes it seem plausible that a similar relation exists between the organic influence of alcohol in sexuality and the so-called psychological processes. The formulations given so far make it clear that placing the emphasis in alcoholism on oral and anal libidinal trends cannot exhaust the problem. It seems more or less accidental that the alcoholic ingests the alcohol by mouth, and the satisfaction received from drinking has no deeper relation to the oral gratification of eating. Rado (1926) has spoken of alimentary orgasm. This concept overrates not only the oral-libidinal gratification of alcoholics, but also the libidinal gratification connected with the process of eating. However, in a later paper (1933) Rado stresses the complicated dynamics of the tense depression which results from frustration and drives the ego to a desire to return to a stage of magical omnipotence. This formulation considers the problem too much from the point of view of the isolated individual and neglects the social aspects. There are two dimensions to the social aspects in the psychology of alcoholism: the alcoholic primarily has deep relations to the society around him and is at least psychologically in continual contact with it. (I think this is even true concerning the lonely drinker, although I have never had the opportunity of analyzing one.) He furthermore commits a social act in drinking and is fully aware that he needs an agent which acts in reality, namely, the drug, for the fulfillment of his desires. To stress the self-destructive tendencies of alcoholism, as Menninger (1938) does, overlooks the deep striving of the alcoholic to be loved and appreciated by society, which would grant to him the integrity of his body and his sex parts. He feels that without alcohol he will be exposed to criticism and destruction. It is true, however, that in the deeper layers the alcoholic experiences the striving for prestige as a struggle for life and death. He may feel that by incapacitating himself with alcohol he may gain a greater claim for mercy.

The problem remains: what are the forces which give to the individual the feeling of such a deep-seated social insecurity? The answer has always been sought in the patient's individual history. Knight (1937a, 1937b) and Chassell (1938) discuss, similarly to Wall and Curran, the family situation of the alcoholic. They stress the inner need to be loved by the parent of the other sex if the parent of the same sex is overaggressive and severe. The alcoholic strives to restore his sex value and his strength in connection with the restoration of his prestige. We have less evidence in this respect concerning women. According to the material of Curran (1937), it seems that women maintain great pride in their body, not only concerning its strength, but also concerning its function and beauty.

These general remarks may help us in the understanding of cases which have been studied from the point of view of psychogenesis.

F.R. was a man of 41, of Irish descent, and a Catholic. He was married, had a boy of five and a girl of ten. He was particularly attached to the boy. Sex relations with his wife were satisfactory, although he was not enthusiastic about them. He was a lawyer of great capacities who worked at first in a firm where the somewhat older employees used to drink. He finally decided that he would not drink continually, but would merely have an alcoholic bout at spaced intervals. These bouts, however, became more and more frequent until they finally endangered his position, which resulted in his stopping for a while. But after laborious work, failure or success, more often after failure in court, he would decide to refresh himself by only one drink. Having once started, he drank continually, did not go home, drove wildly, picked up women without caring very much about what they were like, was rather reckless in having sex relations with them, and finally was being picked up in hotels, completely drunk, psychotic, or stuporous. He was otherwise a very meticulous and clean person and an overcareful dresser. He was extremely polite and overcareful in everything. When he had sex relations with his wife he was very careful not to be disturbed by the least suggestion of uncleanliness on either his or her part. The preparations for this took almost an hour, and very often he was too tired to go through the somewhat complicated procedure. There was no question that his sexual and social behavior during the alcoholic intoxication were the complete reversal of his usual attitudes. In the psychotic episodes he dreamed of machinery falling on one of his children and of big horses jumping on him. In one of the dreams he had after such a spree he saw colored laughing faces which looked like little artists' models in red and yellow. "They were grotesque and in different shapes. They came close to my bed. There were scattered colors and movements. A theatrical village appeared. There were phony Chinese and Italians with hatchets and beams battling each other. People were cut up; horses and a big bull ran away. I ran up a flight of stairs, afraid to be crushed." The patient had been afraid throughout his whole childhood. He was afraid of being attacked by others who were fighting. He was afraid of horses. He was afraid of fights in general. This was partially due to the fact that he had always been very tall and felt that he would not gain any social prestige if he were to win but would lose prestige if he did not win. In addition to this, he was continuously cautioned by his father to be careful, and he was beaten by his father whenever he had an accident. He practiced the same method with his own children. The motive of prestige was one of the leading motives in his entire life. He came from a very large family in which he was the second oldest. His father was strict, and his mother also enforced discipline. He was beaten, for instance, by his mother when he was five when he left a smaller child alone. He saw his father drunk rather often. He had to start working very early; responsibilities were soon thrust upon him. However, due to his intelligence, he assumed leadership inside and outside of the family very early and even threatened to hit a younger brother with a hammer when he resisted him. He often induced other children in school to do what he organized. At the time of treatment he was also active in all kinds of organizations. However, he was always a failure in dramatic plays and in debating societies. In spite of being an excellent talker at the present time he always had to take careful notes when he talked and felt insecure. He wanted to be a good baseball and football player, but he was afraid of getting hurt. It is interesting that in spite of his fear of accidents from earliest childhood on, he was decidedly accident-prone and had had a great number of minor as well as major accidents. He was always afraid of criticism, and when a teacher proved to be unsympathetic to him, he played truant for long periods of time. It may be worthwhile mentioning that during his sober periods he was also particular concerning food. Since he was not allowed to eat candies as a child, he had an enormous urge for them, and overate them whenever he had the opportunity. He had some disgust concerning food that was shiny, such as butter.

The details of this case history could be easily multiplied. However, the basic pattern is obvious. A child rather harshly treated and restricted in sex developed a particular interest in prestige, showed outbursts in fighting against everything he was supposed to do, but felt threatened continually, taking over some of the fears of his father whom he later on also imitated in drinking. Prestige and fighting, particularly with persons of the same sex, and the change between the utmost consideration for social order and a complete neglect of it, were the outstanding features. His interest in women was restricted to a rather primitive type of sexual gratification. The psychogenesis of his alcoholism in the family constellation and the social constellation is obvious. In the single bout he rebelled against the restriction imposed upon him. There was fighting in some of the psychotic episodes; there was no breaking through of homosexuality in the libidinal sense and there was very little indication of an increase of homosexual tendencies in early childhood. Alcohol was here a release. He felt that he would not be condemned even if he did let out his reckless and sexual tendencies. The family factors and the social factors were of equal importance. It is significant that his father and his superiors were alcoholics. The alcoholic is socially sensitive, and for this reason the social customs change the type of drinking. It is also in connection with this fact that there are fewer women alcoholics and fewer Jewish alcoholics.

I have observed a similar type of drinking in a 30-year-old lawyer of good intelligence in whom social shyness was in the foreground. He had a very severe conscience, which was due to a very rigid education, especially in relation to sex problems. His feelings of inferiority extended particularly to his body. Drinking relieved him from an ever-present social tension and allowed casual sex contact of which he would otherwise have been afraid. In his early sex history, urination and defecation played an important part. He urinated with other children repeatedly and was discovered and punished. (As an adult, he wet the bed when drunk.) He was punished by spanking his bare buttocks. His parents said it hurt them more than it did him. He yelled loudly when spanked. Everything was forgiven after the punishment. He always felt that he was socially not popular enough. He always wanted to be praised for his looks, wanted to be considered well built, and wanted to stand out in sports. He wanted to be intellectually brilliant and to be praised for this. He felt that he was disliked in high school as a sissy. His parents warned him particularly against drinking. He was always afraid to look into the eyes of people, particularly his mother's, after masturbation or intercourse, He preferred to blame himself for his drinking and for his sex activities, and blamed the alcohol for his sexuality. He was very much concerned about his body. He always worried that his parents lacked social graces. In this patient, the alcoholism was less important than his social fears. However, the social neurosis unquestionably had a close relation to alcoholism, since alcohol is, as mentioned, specific in relieving social tensions.

It seems doubtful whether drinking may not serve different purposes. B., a man of 31 years, drank rather heavily; he always had a very high opinion of himself. However, he felt continually mistreated by his father, who also mistreated his mother. Both father and mother showed, from his earliest childhood on, an enormous interest in the boy's alleged masturbation. Since he was born after a mentally deficient sister, his mother gave him an extraordinary amount of attention. However, he was beaten by his mother as well as by his father, especially by the latter. Around puberty his sexuality developed with a decidedly masochistic trend, which persisted. He was intellectually vain. He worked only very irregularly and drank excessively without being strictly an alcoholic. One may expect that his drinking allowed him to maintain his feeling of intellectual superiority and gave him the feeling that he could hold his own in relation to his father and mother. The sexual conflict was more manifest in this case. However, even in such a case, which seemed to differ so much in structure from the other cases, the prestige problem in relation to his family played the leading part in his drinking. This prestige-seeking was the counterpart of a deeply masochistic attitude acquired from the family situation.

We deal with variations of the same basic motive, and it does not seem necessary, from our point of view, to assume as varied a genesis of alcoholism as Seliger (1938) has stated. One may, of course, list many apparent reasons for drinking. From a general point of view, I would not think that such a well-characterized picture as chronic alcoholism should not have a psychogenesis in which basic features are common in spite of all kinds of variations. I have observed the following case.

L.R. was a white man of 35, married twice (divorced from his first and separated from his second wife), and an artist by occupation. On admission he was acutely alcoholic and had a three-inch laceration at the base of the penis with two healed scars distal to it. His history revealed that he had been drinking and, on awakening, had found his penis cut. This had happened on two previous occasions, and he believed they were self-inflicted because he had been alone. He persistently denied ever having had a delirious or hallucinatory episode. No signs of such a state were ever found, despite several subsequent hospital admissions for alcoholism. No explanation was ever offered by him for his actions.

When sober, he was shy and ill at ease and had a tremendous sense of guilt. This sense of guilt had been with him since early childhood and arose out of his father's harsh and punishing attitude toward him. When alcoholic, he was witty and friendly and lost all his self-consciousness. However, he would seduce the wives of his friends, for which he suffered with a great intensification of his guilty feelings. He related many memories concerning feelings of inferiority, both physically and mentally. Following intercourse with his wife, he invariably felt ashamed and guilty, though he claimed to have satisfactory potency. There had never been any special preoccupation with sex, death, or suicide.

The patient wrote a detailed report of his early memories. They consisted mostly of being slapped or scolded or derided by his father. The following is typical. (Age five or six): "I had a whistle and I allowed a colored boy to blow it. My father whipped me for this. I was always punished bodily; never sent to bed or deprived of meals. My father would slap my face with his open hand. I did not resent it, but accepted it as a matter of course." When asked about his feelings of guilt, he wrote: "This is difficult for me to write about or explain. Neither can I determine if the feeling is of guilt, or shame, or embarrassment, or a sense of inferiority, or of a combination of these. As far back as I can remember, I was never free of this feeling. Punishment does not seem to have had as much to do with this feeling as being ridiculed or laughed at, which my parents and others often did. When very young, I was ridiculed for physical weakness, cowardice, misfit clothing, and many other things. I made good marks in school, so my schoolmates called me 'teacher's pet.' This made me feel guilty."

It would appear that his attempt at self-castration was a gesture to regain the passive state into which his father had forced him. At the same time it satisfied his guilt feelings toward his father in regard to his homosexual love for him. It also served as a punishment for his incestuous desires, as indicated in his repeated seductions of his friends' wives.

In contrast to the other patients, this man gave in to his desire for passivity in his alcoholic state. However, the family problems of prestige and social shyness are again outstanding. He owed his success with his friends' wives to his increased self-confidence in the first stages of his alcoholism.

In men and women, the fear of loss of sexual prestige may become of paramount importance. In E., a 33-year-old very good-looking woman alcoholic, this motive came out in voices which called her hermaphrodite, "which would be the same thing as homosexual, which certainly would be one form of split-personality unless it was natural." This patient reported that she remembered that at four or five she hid under a woodpile and masturbated. However, she said that her mother had always told her that she had masturbated since her birth. She had a very extensive and promiscuous sex life, and "I have not fulfilled my duties as a citizen. I feel sometimes not worthy to talk to others. It is exactly like when my mother told me at the age of five that I would be like a defective woman who could not walk and floundered along with the help of one or more nuns." Her mother accused her father very often. She had separated from him when the patient was around seven. It is not necessary to add further details, since sufficient material can be found in the case histories reported by Curran (1937).

There is a tendency to believe that the drinking of psychotics has mechanisms fundamentally different from the mechanisms discussed here. However, the drinking of psychotics, including schizophrenics, is comparatively rare and can be understood on the basis of mechanisms discussed here, which are in connection with the particular personality structure of the psychotic individual. This, at least, is the impression I have received from the clinical observation of schizophrenic alcoholics. However, I have never analyzed cases of this type deeply.

I cannot believe that alcoholism consists, in some cases, of an attempt to get over the effects of previous drinking by new imbibing. I am much more inclined to believe that those who suffer from occasionally drinking too much are persons who have a very low opinion of themselves and suffer from social tensions (cf. Moore, 1939).

Summary and Conclusions

An acute alcoholic intoxication gives to the individual the desire to be loved and appreciated. He feels accepted by others because of his capacities, appearance, and sexual qualities. At the same time he feels ready and willing to give the same appreciation to others. The perceptive and intellectual spheres are impaired.

Hand in hand with this impairment and increased self-confidence goes a lack of inhibition which leads to a breaking through of sexual striving otherwise repressed.

This basic pattern varies with the total situation. There may be a lability of the perceptive and intellectual inhibitory (cortical) mechanism. This may lead to more or less dissociated breaking through of sexual and aggressive impulses. The social situation may demand particular drinking habits. Early experiences in childhood may have enforced one or the other variation in sexuality, which then appears during the intoxication. For similar reasons violence may break through. The total situation will determine the psychological picture of the acute alcoholic intoxication, the basic pattern of which, however, is a heightened feeling of one's being connected in love and admiration with other human beings so that one can even allow oneself the breaking through of one's sexual impulses. An underlying anxiety that one's social perfection may merely be assumed is never completely absent and may lead to self-assertion, irritability, aggressiveness, and the attempt to bully others. The psychological gain by intoxication points to the personality structure of those who badly need this psychological gain. These are people with feelings of great social insecurity and social tension.

Acute alcoholic intoxication in persons who are chronic alcoholics differs from those who are intoxicated for the first time. It seems that in the chronic alcoholic the acute intoxication brings forward more primitive material with a corresponding increase in anxiety. Such an acute intoxication in the chronic alcoholic leads him imperceptibly to delirious and hallucinatory episodes in which he experiences primitive sexuality in a distorted form and feels particularly threatened in his social function. The threat does not remain in the sphere of social insecurity, but extends from there to sexual threats and even to the threat of dismemberment and castration. Society has become completely hostile and destructive, and the patient may not even blame his environment for the attempt to destroy him.

The chronic alcoholic person is one who, from his earliest childhood on, has lived in a state of insecurity. This insecurity in childhood is necessarily insecurity in relation to parents and siblings. The child has felt ridiculed and pushed into a passive position, sometimes by threat, sometimes by corporal punishment, and sometimes by deprivation. This threat may come from both parents or from one parent only. In men the threat by the father seems to be more effective. It seems that help and consideration from the other parent cannot counteract the tendency to submission and the development of a severe superego which takes over the part of the punishing and repressing parent. The punishing parent is particularly intolerant toward sex in any form. The community is experienced as an agent similar to the restrictive parents. Individuals are generally ready to submit to these influences in a passive and masochistic way. Men generally blame themselves for their "femininity" and have to seek redress in ideals of heightened masculinity and strength. In women, this process may be similar, or the women feel that they are not capable of fulfilling their feminine functions. The characteristic of the alcoholic is social tension, with the tendency to give in passively to the assumed pressure or to react by overcompensation.

Alcoholism reverses this process. It gives social security and acceptance as long as the intoxication lasts. With the wearing off of the intoxication the underlying tensions and terrors reappear in increased form and demand renewed drinking.

The alcoholic is dependent upon his society, since he has a striving for social acceptance beyond the norm. The sociological and economic factors in alcoholism should therefore not be underrated. To be sure, no problem is merely an individual problem. Human beings live in communities. However, alcoholism is, even beyond this, a problem of society. Not only is there the problem of social competition, in which the alcoholic does badly, but society continually exposes the socially insecure individual to the temptation of a seemingly easy escape by encouraging drunkenness. Alcoholism is not only a problem of individual treatment but of social attitudes, and it seems, therefore, that individual treatment has to be complemented by offering to the alcoholic a social group in which competition is diminished and in which the use of alcoholic beverages is not foisted upon him. It seems, indeed, that all modern treatments of alcoholism stress the community factor. However, beyond that, the alcoholic needs a deeper understanding of his problem, which very often is only possible by continued and intensive psychoanalytic work. The basic psychology of the alcoholic is preordained by the psychological effect of the acute intoxication, and all forms of alcoholic intoxication and patterns of chronic alcoholism center around the psychological effect of the drug. In some types of chronic alcoholism, the personality difficulty is chiefly in the sphere of sexual adaptation. In others, the family situation or community situation seems to offer the chief difficulty. However, these variations are merely facets of the same basic problem. The best prevention of alcoholism will lie in an attitude of the parents which does not increase the insecurity and passivity of the child and guarantees a reasonably free development of sexual adaptation. If the family, and later on the community, does not stress superiority, perfection and blamelessness, and offers, beyond that, friendly help and understanding, individuals will not need alcohol as an escape for insecurities, but may be able to enjoy it as a method of heightening one's appreciation of oneself and of others on rare occasions of festivity.

CHAPTER EIGHTEEN

The Sociological Implications of Neuroses

There cannot be any doubt that cultural factors influence the occurrence and the type of neurosis. The great dancing epidemics of the Middle Ages, for instance, have not been repeated in modern times. It is the common opinion of all observers that the manifestations of hysteria have changed considerably in the last 50 years. During World War I particular types of neurosis occurred. A neurosis has been described by Ochimara of the Psychiatric Clinic of the Imperial University of Tokyo (Tokyo Psycho-Analytic Soc., 1935) which was observed only in the Ainu people of Northern Japan. In this "Imu" syndrome the individuals felt possessed by a fox. Severe confusion, echo symptoms, and catalepsy occurred following a fright usually due to a snake. In a population of 17,500 people, 111 cases were reported, all women but one. The condition was more frequent in the older generations and was rarely to be found in areas which bordered upon civilization. Imitation played a great part. Similar reactions have been observed in other primitive communities.

Wechsler (1929) writes: "The neurologic department of the Vanderbilt Clinic with its yearly admission of over two thousand new patients showed in one statistical study an incidence of 27.5 percent of neurosis among Negroes and 55.5 per cent among

Appeared originally in the *Journal of Social Psychology*, 15:3-21, 1942.

whites. But what is equally pertinent is that among British West Indian Negroes, who are generally better educated, more intelligent, and socially superior to their American brothers, the incidence of neuroses was 37.5 per cent, that is, 10 (actually 30) per cent higher.... I do not know what the incidence of neurosis is among the Chinese who are an even older and also civilized people" (pp. 150-151).

J. Schottky (1937) has collected, without much insight, material concerning the incidence of neurosis in different races. J. H. Otto (1930) and R. Schaltenbrand (1931) reported on neuroses among the Chinese. These seem to be common and seem to be similar to the types of neuroses seen among Europeans and Americans. Otto reported that the outward expression of their neuroses may be different, since they exercise their ideal of self-restraint. Obsessional pictures center on food. A particular type of hysteria was concerned with the retraction of the penis. This also occurred in Java.

It is of course difficult to evaluate material of this type. One might point to racial factors. However, these preliminary remarks have shown that an older culture often has a different type of neurosis from a younger one. The population of the same race nearer to more civilized centers shows a type of neurosis different from the types of neurosis which appear farther from the centers of civilization.

Of particular interest are the studies of Cohen et al. (1939). They studied a comparatively small health district in Maryland of 56,000 persons and came to the following conclusion concerning personality deviates:

"Of the principal race and sex groups, white and Negro male and female, this difference is reflected in all except Negro females. Male rates are consistently higher than female rates. Negro rates exceed the white rates.... The two major geographical sections of the district ... differ appreciably in their rates.... Within each ward the white rates for smaller subdivisions are highest in those subdivisions with largest proportions of Negroes.... The difference in white rates between the two wards is found in both Jews and non-Jews. The association of the higher rates with Negro neighborhoods within wards is seen in both non-Jews and Jews.... The rate of personality deviation increases with increasing size of household. The rate increases as the economic status of the household decreases" (p. 128).

It cannot be denied that these investigations point strongly to the importance of social factors in the incidence of personality disorders. The personality deviates include, in addition to psychotics, psychoneurotic and psychopathic personalities, some postpsychotics and epileptics, and 47 percent of so-called maladjusted persons. However, W. L. Neustatter (1938) found that only 20 percent of children of poorer districts in London showed neuroses, whereas 38 percent of the children of wealthier families showed neurotic trends. Neustatter wrote: "Case histories showing even very bad social conditions left children unaffected psychologically, provided the psychological home situation was good. Therefore there was no *direct psychological* effect . . . . There is a statistically significant relationship between the presence of a worrying disposition in the parents and the presence of anxiety and a tendency to worry in the children, irrespective of class" (p. 1441).

The difference between the results of Neustatter and Cohen et al. may be due to the difference in the material. Neustatter spoke of neuroses, whereas the other authors spoke of personality deviates in general. Neustatter, furthermore, deals only with children. The following discussion is restricted to the problem of neurosis.

Whatever the influence of the sociological process on the neurosis may be, the neurosis changes the situation of the individual in society fundamentally. Every neurosis impairs social contact in general and, specifically, the capacity to work and to love. Almost every neurosis starts with difficulties concerning one's work. This incapacity is due partially to direct inhibitions concerning work and partially to the difficulty of adapting to companions in the work situation. A neurosis has very different sociological effects depending on the individual's economic position. I may point to the studies of W. Eliasberg (1928). In times of crises even the milder degrees of neurotic difficulties in work and adaptation will be of decisive influence, and the neurotic will be the first to be pushed into a helpless economic situation. He will then add to the general disorganization of society, as I have shown (1938b). Horney (1937) has given particular attention to these problems. Sullivan's studies (1937) should be mentioned, and it is also pertinent to call attention to the contributions of Franz Alexander on "Psychoanalysis and Social Disorganization" (1936-1937) and especially to the American Orthopsychiatric Association's symposium on Culture and Personality of which Alexander was chairman and in which the findings of Saul (1938) and Hall (1938) were of particular significance for this discussion. These investigations were concerned with the way the neurosis influences the sociological process and also the manner in which the sociological and cultural process determines the appearance and type of neurosis. There appears, furthermore, the fundamental problem, which concerned K. Birnbaum (1924), of how the neurotic individual may be the originator and carrier of far-reaching cultural movements.

A final answer to these fundamental questions, of course, cannot be expected, since this whole field has not been adequately investigated. As a preliminary approach it seems to be more advantageous not to work with large statistics of cases incompletely studied, but to use material which has been well studied from a psychological and particularly from a psychoanalytic point of view. As a basis for discussion I therefore use 85 cases which have had extensive psychotherapy in the mental hygiene clinic of Bellevue Hospital. Some of these cases were in individual psychoanalysis, some of them in group psychoanalysis, and in all of them attempts were made to come to a deeper understanding of the underlying psychological and sociological factors. These were not consecutive cases, but were selected on the basis of need for treatment and of the possibility for deeper psychotherapy. I have compared the results with material from my private practice, consisting of 35 cases in which either psychoanalysis or short psychotherapy with a basic analytic approach was used. The difference in the economic status in these two groups was rather marked. However, it must be stated that there was no fundamental difference in these two groups in any trend in the symptomatology. The cases could even be matched with each other in corresponding intimate details.

The first case, Hugh S.,[1] came from a very wealthy family, and his economic insecurity was merely a question of how much luxury he could afford. The second case, Dave B.[2] never had any economic security, and, although the family had not been on public relief, the patient never had more than the bare necessities of life. Both patients were Jewish. The parents of both were immigrants, in the one case from Germany and in the other from Russia. Both neuroses were dominated by suffering in social contacts. Each had been pushed by earlier experiences into passive and dependent positions by one parent. The passivity was not merely sexual. There was a considerable cultural difference between the two families.

It might be of interest to note that among my private cases two females showed this picture, whereas only one female of my hospital patients suffered from a social neurosis. Both female patients in my private practice demanded of themselves a particularly high degree of achievement.

Similarly, there was no difference in the type of anxiety neurosis, hysteria, obsessional neurosis, or character difficulties in the two groups. It was merely due to my specific interest in the depersonalization problem that my private practice contained a comparatively large number of depersonalization cases in the previous few years; these are not included among the 35 cases of this discussion. I could not see any difference in the course of the neurosis in these two groups. In the economically dependent group, the improvement in the neurosis led mainly to a better social adaptation and to an improvement in the economic status

[1] [See pp. 163-167].
[2] [See pp. 167-171].

of the patients. The hospital cases included in this study comprised one case of traumatic neurosis following head injury, whereas cases of this type were not seen in my private practice. In a study concerning neurosis following head and brain injuries (1940, see Ch. 10) I have shown the importance of social and economic factors for these particular types of neurotic disturbances. This seems to be the only form in which the resentment concerning social injustice finds a clear expression in the neurosis.

There is no question of the severe consequences of a neurosis for persons in bad economic circumstances. The social difficulties encountered by the poor are used as secondary elaboration by the neurotic in bad economic circumstances, and the neurosis can be used more effectively as an economic weapon against his family. However, the basic structure of the neurosis in the wealthy as well as in the poor is based upon the family situation in early childhood. This fundamental contribution of Freud's becomes particularly clear if one compares groups in different economic circumstances. It is an established fact that the final symptomatology of the neurosis, and especially the use of the fundamental neurotic symptoms from a social point of view, is modified by the economic situation. I want to point to the report of René Spitz (1937) at the ninth Congress of French Analysts, in which the problem of the family was discussed from an analytic point of view. The work of Laforgue (1938) and Leuba (1925) show that every family forms a cultural and neurotic unit. From the wealth of material offered, it is noteworthy that Leuba has described the specific problems of economically secure families who do not show obvious neurotic symptoms but nevertheless are still badly adapted in the deeper human aspects. The problem of the pathology of successful social adaptation in different economic levels, however, goes beyond the frame of this paper.

Recently, in a paper on "Cultural Patterns and Constructive Psychology" (1940), I arrived at the conclusion that our present methods are not sufficient to determine fundamental emotional differences in different races. S. D. Porteus and Marjorie E. Babcock (1926), for instance, found that at the age of thirteen the highest test averages in maze-test investigations were shown by Anglo-Saxon boys, while decreasing scores were shown by Japanese boys, Chinese boys and Japanese girls, Portuguese boys, Filipino boys and Chinese girls, in that order. However, American boys were inferior to the Japanese at all ages up to twelve years. According to these authors, the test does not merely measure intelligence but also emotional characteristics, especially planning capacities. If one studies the book by Porteus (1931) on the Australian aborigines one becomes still more doubtful concerning the question about the fundamental emotional differences between primitives and cultured people. Róheim's (1932) description of Australian children corresponds very closely to observations of European and American children. The chief difference is that the latency period, by no means absolute in our culture, was reported absent among primitives (compare also B. Malinowski, 1929).

Among the 85 neurotic patients from the mental hygiene clinic of Bellevue Hospital, 70 were Jewish. Among the wealthier patients, 21 of 35 were Jewish. The prevalence of neurosis in Jews has been found by other observers (M. Sichel, 1909; R. Becker, 1918; J. Schottky, 1937). It is difficult to evaluate this pronounced statistical difference. In order to understand it one would have to take into consideration the fact that the percentage of Jews presenting criminality and alcoholism is comparatively low. A study like this, of course, cannot exhaust problems of this kind. One has to keep in mind that the difference in race is also connected with difference in social and cultural background. Only one of the 120 cases treated in this study was a Negro. In the mental hygiene clinic, no type of neurosis was seen among Negroes whose condition required or who were willing to accept extended treatment. However, neurosis among Negroes was observed on the hospital wards, and one of these was a case of depersonalization treated with metrazol and subsequently followed in the mental hygiene clinic. (See Ch. 13.)

It is worth while reviewing the different types of neuroses

from a racial point of view. I have given special attention to the picture of depersonalization for many years. The clinical picture is identical all over the world. It has been observed among Jews, Negroes, Italians, French, Germans, English, Irish, and Japanese (1935a). The pictures correspond in every detail.

Anxiety neuroses did not show any specific differences whether observed in Irish, Jewish, or English patients. Among the cases of social neuroses I found Jews, Irish, Italians, and Finns. Furthermore, they have been observed all over the earth in identical forms.

I could not find any differences in cases of obsessional neuroses in different members of the white race. Even the difference between those who have been brought up as Catholics and those who have been brought up with a different creed are negligible and pertain merely to unimportant details of contents.

The prevalence of symptoms concerning food and the gastrointestinal tract in Jews has been repeatedly stressed, most effectively by Dorothy E. Hall (1938). My own material, without being conclusive, points in the same direction.

Everything considered, the basic structure of neuroses in persons belonging to the modern cultures does not seem to be very dissimilar in the different races. There is no question that the numerous races in the United States have a different cultural background. However, the frequency of neuroses among Jews has to be stressed.

In this formulation, Negroes are not included. It goes without saying that the social conditions under which they live and their racial and cultural background are fundamentally different from the background of whites. Lauretta Bender (1939) has shown that specific reaction patterns occur in the Negro child in the form of narcolepsy, blocking, mutism, catalepsy, negativism, and stubbornness. Dramatic motility pictures with spontaneous dancing may be a part of the socially acceptable, or in extreme cases nonsocially acceptable, behavior of the child. "Racial conflicts due to recognition ... [of being a member] of the unpopular, underprivileged race whose physical beauty is not accepted as standard at present, find ready expression among the children.... Sexual delinquencies and problems arise from the unsuitable social and economic situations, associated with overcrowding, poor recreational facilities, early maturity, inadequate protection and perhaps from a certain casual attitude of a special group ideology" (Bender, 1939, p. 228). Similar observations can be made concerning the neuroses in adult Negroes. Dramatic pictures with a plastic or primitive motility are more often seen in Negroes than in whites (Parker et al., 1939).

The number of total admissions in the Psychiatric Division of Bellevue Hospital in the year 1938 was 25,909. Of these, 20,099 were whites, 3,722 were Negroes, and the remainder were Orientals and others. This corresponds to the general experience of the greater percentage of Negroes in mental institutions compared with the population as a whole. Of these admissions, 1,647 were classified as neuroses. One hundred eighty-five of these were Negroes. The percentage of neuroses among Negroes is therefore 11.2, compared with 14.4 percent of Negroes among the total admissions. This difference would probably be still more striking if one took into consideration the fact that 127 of these cases among Negroes were reactive depressions. However, even then, the percentage of admissions of neurotic Negroes admitted to the wards is high in relation to the percentage of Negroes in the total population. Wechsler (1929) reported different results. If one looks over statistics, it is particularly striking that obsessions and compulsions are completely absent in Negroes (Tables 3-5). There was, in 1938, only one case which could be classified as neurasthenia. This checked exactly with my nine years of clinical experience in New York in which I did not see any cases of true obsessional neurosis among Negro patients. One would be inclined to believe that individuals belonging to an economically and educationally different class might suffer more from symptoms of the hysterical type when they get a neurosis. Although it is difficult to decide to what extent racial factors are involved, it is at least worth mentioning that the Imu reaction of the primitive Ainus (*Amer. J. Psychiat.*, 1938) could be classified

TABLE 3
ADMISSIONS TO BELLEVUE HOSPITAL IN 1937 (25,260)

Total of Neurosis	Total	White	Black	Not Stated
Anxiety Hysteria	49	43	6	—
Conversion Hysteria	76	64	7	5
Anesthetic Type	4	4	—	—
Paralytic Type	3	3	—	—
Hyperkinetic Type	23	20	2	1
Paresthetic Type	1	1	—	—
Autonomic Type	1	1	—	—
Amnesia Type	81	75	4	2
Mixed Hysterical Psychoneurosis	18	15	3	—
Obsession	32	30	0	—
Compulsive Tics and Spasms	7	6	0	—
Phobia	2	2	—	—
Mixed Compulsive States	10	9	—	1
Neurasthenia	16	16	—	—
Hypochondriasis	101	97	4	—
Reactive Depression	943	831	80	30
Mixed Psychoneurosis	102	95	7	—
Anxiety State	121	105	16	—

as hysteria. Van Brero (1895) reported about Latah among the Malays, which consists of a transient automatic imitation. This neurosis was also hysterical.

We may therefore conclude that there are statistical differences concerning neurosis in different races. There cannot be any question that neurosis among Jews is more frequently observed than in the non-Jewish whites. But there is no fundamental difference in the dynamics of the neuroses when they are studied sufficiently.

TABLE 4
ADMISSIONS TO BELLEVUE HOSPITAL IN 1938 (25,909)

	Male	Female	Total
Catholic	9,229	3,419	12,648
Hebrew	1,507	1,078	2,585
Protestant	4,603	2,282	6,885
Others	33	6	39
Undetermined	2,776	976	3,752
	Color		
White	15,712	6,387	22,099
Black	2,360	1,372	3,732
Yellow	57	—	57
Others	19	2	21

The types of neuroses, however, in races which live under very different social conditions show characteristic differences. It is at the present time impossible to say whether these differences are due to social and economic factors only or whether racial factors are involved. The evidence in the case of Negroes certainly speaks very much for a participation of racial factors. The question is still undecided whether neuroses are comparatively infrequent in groups which we may call more primitive, since we lack better designation.

There have been a great number of attempts to understand the neuroses in terms of a constitutional deviation of the nervous system, of the endocrine glands, and of the constitution in general. However, the results, although suggestive, are inconclusive. If cases are studied from a psychoanalytic point of view, there is indeed the impression that a specific family constellation in early childhood does not have the same effect in every case. A constitutional factor would explain why experiences of similar type are traumatic, producing a point of fixation, in one case and not in another. In psychoanalysis this problem appears repeat-

TABLE 5
(YEAR 1938)

Type of neurosis	Male	Female	Black	White	Nativity	Status
Hysteria						
Anxiety	8	32	4	32	25 U.S.; 2 Puerto Rico; 1 Russia; 1 Italy	13 M 8 S
Conversion	36	29	9	56	28 U.S.; 1 Poland; 2 Italy; 2 Puerto Rico; 1 Russia; 1 Germany; 1 Cuba; 2 Austria; 1 Spain	13 M 27 S
Anesthetic Type	—	3	—	—		
Paralytic Type	1	2	—	3		
Hyperkinetic Type	10	8	5	13	11 U.S.; 1 Greece; 2 Puerto Rico; 1 Italy	3 M-7 S
Paresthetic Type	2	1	1	2	3 U.S.	2 M
Amnesic Type	40	24	2	17	4 U.S.; 1 Poland; 2 England	3 S
Mixed Psychoneurotic	12	9	3	24	16 U.S.; 1 Canada	5 M-10 S
Psychasthenia or Compulsive States						
Obsession	8	9	1*	21	14 U.S.; 1 Poland; 1 Russia; 1 Ireland; 1 Hungary	5 M 12 S
Compulsive Tics and Spasms	3	—	—	3	2 U.S.; 1 Germany;	2 M-1 S
Phobia	2	—	—	2	1 U.S.; 1 Greece	1 M-1 S

Mixed Compulsive States	10	3	—	13	4 U.S.	4 S
Neurasthenia	9	3	1	16	11 U.S.; 2 Puerto Rico; 1 Austria	11 M-5 S
Hypochondriasis	46	37	9	80	28 U.S.; 2 Ireland; 3 Russia;	
					3 Italy; 2 Greece; 1 Belgium;	34 M
					1 Brazil; 3 Poland; 1 Austria;	14 S
					1 Germany; 3 Puerto Rico; 1 Canada	
Reactive Depressive	471	545	127	905	417 U.S.; 4 Hungary; 30 Puerto Rico;	348 M
					22 Italy; 6 Ireland; 13 Poland;	236 S
					21 Russia; 18 Germany; 15 England; 14 Austria	
Anxiety State	72	42	13	104	90 U.S.; 4 Puerto Rico; 3 Italy	33 M
					1 Russia; 1 Poland; 1 Hungary;	50 S
					1 Germany; 1 Greece	
Mixed Psychoneurosis	78	92	10	150	75 U.S.; 5 Russia; 2 England;	
					1 Poland; 2 Germany; 3 Austria;	50 M
					2 Puerto Rico; 1 Italy; 1 Scotland;	59 S
					1 Ireland	

* This turned out to be a case of schizophrenia.
(The discrepancies in the sum totals are due to the fact that in many cases not all the data were stated.)

edly under the heading of the quantitative factors in the libido situation. But psychoanalysis assumes this constitutional factor only after the psychological investigation has been more or less exhaustive. Even then, doubts often remain as to how important the constitutional factor is if one considers merely neuroses and not psychoses. Doubtless, there are functional changes in neuroses which can be understood from the point of view of brain pathology and endocrinology. However, these may still be due to the influence of psychological factors on the sensorimotor and vegetative systems. We have the right to assume that early childhood experiences, especially when they use the pattern of a preceding organic disease, can have very outspoken somatic influence, as I reported in my paper "The Somatic Basis of the Neurosis" (1929c) (See Ch. 2.).

L. Szondi (1936) summarized the results of his studies and the studies of others, especially German investigators, concerning the heredity of neurotics. He concluded that neurotics do not belong to a single hereditary group. They belong either to the hereditary circle of schizophrenia or manic-depressive psychoses or epilepsy. Thus, apathetic asthenic neurasthenia may have a hereditary relation to schizophrenia; irritative pyknic neurasthenia to the circular psychoses; hysteria, social maladaptation, and stammering to the hereditary group of epilepsy. He believed, therefore, that the choice of the neurosis was partially determined by genes. However, investigations of this type tend to neglect the problem of the family situation in early childhood. Szondi concluded that psychoanalysis as well as neuroendocrinology and the science of heredity point to the formulation that the neurotic is an extreme variant who has remained on a primitive, archaic, and infantile level of instinctual organization. Such a formulation, though, neglects the social factors and the interhuman relations, especially in the family. Lauretta Bender (1936) has shown how profoundly the occurrence of a psychosis influences the family structure. She concluded:

> Mental illness in one member of a family is a suggestion of a constitutional weakness and indicates that another member of the

> family is more liable to a breakdown than the average person, although the second psychosis need not be of the same category as the first. These are conclusions that we arrive at from hereditary studies. In addition there is a tendency for a second member of a family to respond to a mental illness in the family with an emotionality because of processes of identification, feelings of guilt and self-accusation, and feelings of aggressivity directed either at the sick individual or at other factors in the environment other than the family situation [p. 310].

She supplemented this study by one on behavior problems in children of psychotic and criminal parents (1937). Besides the hereditary factor, she pointed to the effects of the loss of the psychotic or criminal parent, the broken home, the unsuitable treatment of the child by the parents, and the disturbance of the parent-child relationship.

Leuba (quoted by Spitz, 1937) has shown how closely knit families can be and that frigidity might be inoculated from mother to daughter. Members of such families choose particular types for their mates. Attitudes of a family might be transmitted by identification through four generations. However, it is not only the mechanism of identification which is of importance in these families; there is a continuous interaction between the members of the family, and, especially, the choice of a mate is dictated by the inner structure of the family. Furthermore, every family develops ideologies of its own. Jewish families, for instance, develop specific food habits and are preoccupied with the importance of defecation. This may lead to neurotic symptoms but much more often to specific habits and convictions. In one of my female patients, the mother was considered sloppy by her in-laws, which led the patient to an exaggerated system of orderliness, but without manifest neurotic character. In another of my patients, the father as well as the mother admired strength and chose their friends accordingly. The boy, however, felt that he was too weak to comply with such demands and felt physically inferior. He admired the moral strength of the mother, who was intellectually superior, but finally found her substitute in men of the working class with strong muscles. By social and sexual contact with these men he achieved a strength similar to his mother's and one which might also satisfy her demands for a strong man. Homosexual adaptation difficulties followed.

Servants, as well as members of the family, contribute to the construction of family ideologies. A cook played an important part in the fate of one of my patients who admired his superior mother very deeply. Between the ages of four and five he asked the cook, who was very large, to roll over him. She answered that he was too weak, that only his father would be capable of withstanding her weight. The wish to be smothered by a heavy body, representing also the moral superiority of the beloved mother, remained paramount and led to impotency and homosexual experiences in which the "rolling over" repeatedly played an important part. Furthermore, the mother's anality was prominent. The patient in early childhood had repeatedly seen his mother and a heavily built nurse sitting on the toilet undressed. It may be that such events finally became significant because of constitutional factors.

There is nevertheless always a psychological and sociological cause for a neurosis in the family unit. Family ideologies are transmitted from one generation to another, and determine in large measure the libidinal and social development of human beings. There is no field of human endeavor for which family ideologies do not exist. They are prominent in every phase of sex life. They determine the relation to one's own body and the relation to others. The amount of aggressiveness which is allowed an individual is also dependent upon them. The ideology of father and mother may show different features and may place before the child particularly difficult tasks.

Freud has repeatedly pointed to the fact that children for a long time remain dependent upon their parents and that their relation to society is determined by the attitudes of their parents. According to the libidinal situation, ideologies of the parents may be accepted or they may be rejected and an opposite ideology might be chosen. Playmates bring in ideologies of different groups. Parents live in different cultural, educational, and economic conditions. Every one of these influences is decisive in the neurosis that may develop even before the child has an opportunity of getting in touch with the community on its own. The basis of a neurosis is set long before the child has had an intimate relation with the culture and the economic situation. However, it is influenced by cultural and economic factors through the parents.

Furthermore, there is no question but that the growing individual also has contact with social realities which are not dependent upon the parents. Many of the factors which have built up the structure of the personality in early childhood will modify the approach to and the effect of the immediate social surroundings. The unit in which the neurosis is constructed resides primarily in the family and only secondarily in the social structure. The social structure as such has already exerted its influence in building up the family. It seems that even in different cultures the basic human relations of affection and need for affection, the fear of aggression, and the wish to maintain one's integrity are fundamentally the same. It is true that different social structures emphasize more or less different sides of the interhuman relations. However, I do not believe that there are societies in which competition is completely absent or in which the relation of aggressiveness and submission is entirely different from that observed in our culture. I do not share the opinion of Ruth Benedict (1934), who believed in a far-going cultural relativism. Patterns of culture may look very different, but upon closer examination one may find many or all of the human trends which seemed at first to be absent. The structure of community culture is very similar to family ideology. Deeper roots are often very different from the superficial picture.

I therefore conclude that hereditary constitutional factors and organic factors in general may play a part in the genesis of neuroses, although the real value of these factors is unknown. As far as one can make out at the present time, they merely give dynamic value to the psychological conflicts determining the neurosis. This psychological conflict is basically dependent on the smaller sociological unit, in which the child gets love and protection—the family in its widest sense. The libidinal structure of the family is of fundamental importance. Nevertheless, the ideologies which the parents have built up in their social and cultural contacts are of fundamental importance in the process of conscious and unconscious education. Society acts on the child at first through the family units. In later development, the individual's more independent contacts with the community give the final elaboration to the ideological pattern. The relation of the adult to society and to the inanimate world has an immediate effect on the growing individual. The final pattern and the life style of the individual is doubly influenced by his cultural surroundings. Cultural patterns as such have a structure similar to the individual life style and cannot be understood merely by a superficial description.

A deep conflict exists among psychoanalysts over the question of the part which culture plays in behavior. Some are inclined to explain cultural phenomena, such as war, merely from the point of view of the psychology of those who participate in this process, as, for instance, Glover (1933). Róheim (1934) is inclined to consider the whole cultural process from a similar point of view. Others like Fenichel (1935) and Alexander (1938) insist on the independent importance of the cultural process. This latter point of view corresponds more closely to the Marxist point of view, which stresses the importance of economic factors. The discussion of this fundamental problem is beyond the scope of this paper and has been discussed elsewhere (1940). I merely want to emphasize here that a cultural pattern and an economic process, once created, although fundamentally related to the psychology of the participant, follow their own laws. They become in some way a part of nature, which can be modified by human endeavor but not in the same way as psychological processes. However, it would seem that this part of nature does not directly influence the psychological processes we call neuroses. We may conclude that what is specific for the neurosis is not specific for the cultural process. I have already stressed that the fundamental difficulty of the neurosis lies in the human contact with other human beings and the impairment of work. However, the neurotic shows a serious difficulty in his adaptation to the family. A reorientation of the family will sooner or later become necessary, in response to the demands of society. Furthermore, through his neurosis, the neurotic may get a deeper insight, which he may use in the social process and which may give him access to his fellow human beings and liberate him from his neurosis. It does not seem to me that the neurosis in the proper sense has a decisive influence on the cultural and economic process. It might be, however, the beginning of a reorientation to the community, either in the neurotic himself or in others. It is very doubtful whether one can call mass movements and social and cultural movements, as such, neurotic, and the connotation of a neurotic culture seems to be self-contradictory. The flagellantism of the Middle Ages and the child crusades are borderline phenomena between hysteria and mass movement. The neurotic will only have a deeper influence upon the structure of the society when his regression helps him to a new insight which he can use for better adaptation. He may be capable of seeing that rigid forms have only a relative value, and this may help the work of the community. However, in the long run, the neurotic does not help us, but needs help. His different style of living may give us a new insight into the relativity of cultural forms and may reinforce in us the insight that we have to help other human beings.

It seems to me that the neurotic, by his neurosis, is hindered from a deeper social contact. Part of his energies are bound by his symptoms. Neurosis means suffering. There is a fundamental difference in this respect between neurosis and so-called psychopathy. The psychopath has overcome some of his conflicts and acts in the community. He utilizes the insight he may have gained in his regression to rebuild the community. Something similar seems to be true for the psychotic in whom the regression did not involve all the forces of the personality. A superficial survey seems indeed to show that there is a rather close relation between psychopathy, psychosis, and genius (W. Lange-Eichbaum, 1928). However, there seems to be no close connection between genius and neurosis. I know only about three important personalities in which a neurosis was rather outspoken: Darwin (neurasthenia), Fechner (hypochondriac neurasthenic picture) and Elizabeth Barret Browning (hysterical picture on the basis of an organic disease). But we are only in the beginning of such studies. The borderline between neuroses and psychoses may be difficult to draw, and the borderline between neuroses and psychopathies is still more indistinct.

The psychiatrist is in danger of overlooking the existence of forces in the outer world and economic processes which follow their own laws. Culture is not merely dependent upon living human beings as carriers. The forces of economy and culture are inherent in the outer world. However, there still remain three realms to consider: the external physical world, the body or organism, and the ego or the psychic life in its widest sense. Some psychoanalysts seem to have forgotten that the organism has its own laws, and they show a lack of understanding of the nature of organic disease. Others neglect the aspects of the outer world which are cultural or economic. World, organism, and psyche are interrelated and will have to be so studied. One should respect the world and the organism no less than the psyche.

In a given culture the influence of economic factors upon the manifestations and the symptomatology of neuroses is not fundamental. However, the economic setting has importance in some forms of neuroses, especially the compensation neurosis, and has an influence upon the secondary manifestations of the neurotic psychological process.

The basic structure of neuroses among white people today is not different in different races, although their cultural backgrounds may be different. However, neuroses are more frequent among Jews. In Negroes and Orientals and generally in other economic, racial and cultural situations, hysterical pictures of particular types prevail. It is at present impossible to say whether these differences are due to social, economic or cultural factors alone or to racial factors or, what is most probable, to a combination.

Hereditary and constitutional factors in general may play a part in neuroses. The real value of these factors is unknown. Most probably they give the dynamic value to the psychological conflicts underlying the neurosis. This psychological conflict is basically dependent on small sociological units in which the child gets the love and protection of the family in its widest sense. The libidinal structure of the family is of fundamental importance. Society acts on the child at first through the family unit and its ideologies. The ideological pattern gets its final elaboration by the independent contact of the individual with the community.

Cultural and economic processes, once created, are a part of the outer world and follow their own laws. They are no longer dependent on the psychology of the single individual. They can only be changed by work. The neurotic individual, isolated and incapable of work, can receive from his regression merely a deeper insight, which he may use for a better adaptation, and only then can he influence the sociological process. His different styles of living may give us new insight into the relativity of cultural form and may reinforce the wish to help other human beings.

REFERENCES

Abeles, M. & Schilder, P. (1935), Psychogenic loss of personal identity: Amnesia. *This Volume,* Chapter 14.

Abraham, K. (1924), A short study of the development of the libido, viewed in the light of mental disorders. In: *Selected Papers of Karl Abraham.* New York: Basic Books, 1953, pp. 418-501.

Adler, A. (1907), *Study of Organ Inferiority and Its Psychical Compensations.* New York & Washington, D.C.: Nervous & Mental Disease Publ. Co., 1917.

Adler, Alexandra, Brezina, E., & Wastl, J. (1931), Über die Bedingtheit der Häufung gewerblicher Unfälle. *Arch. Gewerbepath. u. Gewerbehyg.,* 2:359-384.

Alexander, F. (1927), *Psychoanalysis of the Total Personality. The Application of Freud's Theory of the Ego to the Neuroses.* New York & Washington, D.C.: Nervous & Mental Disease Publ. Co., 1930.

______ (1936-1937), Psychoanalysis and social disorganization. *Amer. J. Sociol.,* 42:781-813.

______ (1938), Culture and personality. *Amer. J. Orthopsychiat.,* 8:587-626.

Amer. J. Psychiat. (1938), Editorial comment. The syndrome of *Imu* in the Aino Race. 94:1467-1469.

Astruk, P. (1923), Über psychische Beeinflussung des vegetativen Nervensystems in der Hypnose, I: Hypnotische Beeinflussung der Herztätigkeit und der Atmung. *Arch. f. d. ges. Psychol.,* 45:266-281.

Azam, C. M. E. (1887), Hypnotisme, Double Conscience et Altérations de la personalité. Paris: Ballière et fils.

Babinski, J. (1934), Hystérie-pithiatisme. In: *Oeuvre Scientifique.* Paris: Mason et Cie., pp. 457-546.

Beard, G. M. (1869), *Neurasthenia [nerve exhaustion].* New York: Appleton, 1879.

Bechterew, W. von (1911), Über die Anwendung der assoziativ-motorischen Reflexe als objectives Untersuchungsverfahren in der klinischen Neuropathologie und Psychiatrie. *Ztschr. ges. Neur. u. Psychiat.,* 5:299-318.

Becker, R. (1918), *Die jüdische Nervosität, ihre Art, Entstehung, und Bekämpfung.* Zurich: Füssli, 1919.

Bender, L. (1935), Anatomopathological data on personality function. *Amer. J. Psychiat.,* 92:325-351.

______ (1936), Reactive psychosis in response to mental disease in the family. *J. Nerv. & Ment. Dis.,* 83:143-165; 289-312.

______ (1937), Behavior problems in the children of psychotics and criminal parents. *Genet. Psychol. Monogr.,* 19:231-339.

______ (1939), Behavior problems in Negro children. *Psychiat.,* 2:213-228.

______ & Schilder, P. (1933), Alcoholic encephalopathy. In: Schilder, P., *On Psychoses.* New York: International Universities Press, 1976, pp. 193-258.

______ ______ (1940), Impulsions: A specific behavior disorder. In: Schilder, P., *Contributions to Developmental Neuropsychiatry.* New York: International Universities Press, 1964, pp. 218-241.

Benedict, R. (1934), *Patterns of Culture.* Boston & New York: Houghton Mifflin.

Bennett, A. E. (1938), Convulsive shock therapy in depressive psychoses. *Bull. Menninger Clin.,* 2:97-100.

Benussi, V. (1914), Kinematohaptische Scheinbewegungen und Auffassungsformung. *VI. Kongress für Experimentelle Psychologie.* Leipzig: Barth, pp. 31-35.
Bergler, E. (1935), Psychoanalysis of a case of agoraphobia. *Psychoanal. Rev.*, 22:392-408.
_____ (1936), Bemerkungen über eine Zwangsneurose in Ultimis. Vier Mechanismen des narzisstischen Lustgewinns im Zwang. *Internat. Ztschr. Psychoanal.*, 22:238-248.
_____ & Eidelberg, L. (1935), Der Mechanismus der Depersonalization. *Internat. Ztschr. Psychoanal.*, 21:258-285.
Bergmann, G. von (1930), Klinische funktionelle Pathologie des vegetativen Nervensystems. In: *Handb. d. norm. u. pathol. Physiol.*, ed. O. Bumpke. 16:1019-1070. Berlin: Springer.
Bergson, H. (1910), *Time and Free Will: An Essay on the Immediate Data of Consciousness.* Atlantic Highlands, New Jersey: Humanities, 1971.
Beritoff, J. (1926), Über die Individuellerworbenetätigkeit des Zentralnervensystems. *Arch. ges. Physiol.*, 213:370-406.
Bernheim, H. (1889), *Suggestive Therapeutics.* 2nd ed. New York: Putnam, 1903.
Bing, R. (1926), Die unfallneurologische Bedeutung des prätraumatischen Gesundheitszustandes. *Schweiz. med. Wochenschr.*, 56:1233-1237.
Birnbaum, K. (1924), *Grenzfragen des Nerven und Seelenlebens.* Munich: Bergmann.
Blau, A. (1936), Mental changes following head trauma in children. *Arch. Neur. & Psychiat.*, 35:723-769.
Bogaert, L. van (1935), L'hystérie et les fonctions diencéphaliques, étude neurologique. *Congrès des médecins aliénistes de France.* XXXIX Session. Paris: Masson et Cie., pp. 169-229.
Braun, E. (1928), Psychogene Reaktionen. In: *Handbuch der Geisteskrankheiten,* ed. Bumke. Berlin: Springer, 5:112-226.
Brero, P. C. van (1895), Über das sogenannte Latah. *Allg. Ztschr. Psychiat.*, 51:939-948.
Breuer, J. & Freud, S. (1893-1895), Studies on hysteria. *Standard Edition,* 2:1-105. London: Hogarth Press, 1953.
Bromberg, W. (1930), Mental states in chronic encephalitis. *Psychiat. Quart.*, 4:537-566.
_____ & Schilder, P. (1932), On tactile imagination and tactile aftereffects. *J. Nerv. & Ment. Dis.*, 76:1-24.
_____ _____ (1933a), Death and dying. *Psychoanal. Rev.*, 20:133-185.
_____ _____ (1933b), Psychologic considerations in alcoholic hallucinations—castration and dismembering motives. *Internat. J. Psycho-Anal.*, 14:206-224.
_____ _____ (1936), The attitude of psychoneurotics toward death. *Psychoanal. Rev.*, 23:1-25.
Brown, W. (1934), *Psychology and Psychotherapy.* Baltimore: Williams & Wilkins, 1944.
Bunnemann, O. (1927), Tatsachen dermatologischer Psychogenese. *Bericht. allg. ärztl. Kong. Psychother.*, 2:133-144.*
Bürger, H. (1928), Über Encephalitis und Zwang. *Ztschr. ges. Neur. u. Psychiat.*, 113:239-245.
Buzzard, E. F. (1924), Traumatic neurasthenia. *Ment. Hyg.*, 8:425-437.

* The Editor was unable to verify or complete those references marked with an asterisk.

Cannon, W. B. (1932), *The Wisdom of the Body.* New York: W. W. Norton, 1963.
Charcot, J. M. (1873), *Clinical Lectures on Certain Diseases of the Nervous System.* Detroit, Mich.: G. S. Davis, 1888.
Chassell, J. (1938), Family constellation in the etiology of essential alcoholism. *Psychiat.*, 1:473-503.
Cohen, B. M., Fairbank, R. E., & Greene, E. (1939), Statistical contributions from the mental hygiene study of the Eastern Health District of Baltimore; III, Personality disorder in the Eastern Health District in 1933. *Human Biology,* 11: 112-129.
Crowley, R. M. (1939), Psychoanalytic literature on drug addiction and alcoholism. *Psychoanal. Rev.*, 9:39-54.
Curran, F. J. (1937), Personality studies in alcoholic women. *J. Nerv. & Ment. Dis.*, 86:645-667.
______ (1938), A study of fifty cases of bromide psychosis. *J. Nerv. & Ment. Dis.*, 88:163-192.
Dana, C. L. (1920), Wounds of the head and compensation laws. *Arch. Neur. & Psychiat.*, 4:479-483.
Dattner, B. (1929), Analysen zur Somatogenese der Neurosen. *Klin. Wochenschr.*, 8:554-559.
Deutsch, F. (1922), Psychoanalyse und Organkrankheiten. *Internat. Ztschr. Psychoanal.*, 8:290-306.
______ (1933), Studies in pathogenesis: biological and psychological aspects. *Psychoanal. Quart.*, 2:225-243.
Deutsch, H. (1928), Agoraphobia. In: *Neuroses and Character Types.* New York: International Universities Press, 1965, pp. 97-116.
Dumontpallier, V. A. (1885), De l'action vaso-motrice de la suggestion chez les hystériques hypnotisables. *Compt. Rend. Soc. de Biol.*, 2:458-597.*
Eliasberg, W. (1927), Ist die Unfallneurose ein rein medizinisches Problem? *Klin. Wochenschr.*, 6:1388-1392.
______ (1928), Der Arzt und das Wirtschaftsleben. *Psychol. u. Med.*, 3:198-220.
Eppinger, H. & Hess, L. (1911), *Die Vagotonie.* Berlin: Hirschwald.
Erickson, M. H. (1937), Development of apparent unconsciousness during hypnotic reliving of a traumatic experience. *Arch. Neur. & Psychiat.*, 38:1282-1288.
Federn, P. (1926), Some variations in ego feeling. In: *Ego Psychology and the Psychoses.* New York: Basic Books, 1952, pp. 25-37.
______ (1928), Narcissism in the structure of the ego. In: *Ego Psychology and the Psychoses.* New York: Basic Books, 1952, pp. 38-59.
______ (1933), Die vier Frongesetze der Zwangsneurose. *Ztschr. f. Psychoanal.*, 19:616-620.
Feigenbaum, D. (1926), A case of hysterical depression. Mechanisms of identification and castration. *Psychoanal. Rev.*, 13:404-423.
Fenichel, O. (1931), *Hysterien und Zwangsneurosen.* Vienna: Internationaler Psychoanalytische Verlag.
______ (1934), *Outline of Clinical Psychoanalysis.* New York: Norton.
______ (1935), Review of G. Róheim's *The Evolution of Culture. Internat. Ztschr. Psychoanal.*, 21:300-305.
______ (1945), *The Psychoanalytic Theory of the Neuroses.* New York: Norton, pp. 117-147.
Ferenczi, S. (1925), Psycho-analysis of sexual habits. In: *Further Contributions to the Theory and Technique of Psychoanalysis.* New York: Basic Books, 1955, pp. 259-296.

______ (1926), Organ neuroses and their treatment. In: *Final Contributions to the Problems and Methods of Psychoanalysis.* New York: Basic Books, 1955, pp. 22-28.

Fetterman, J. E. (1928), Traumatic neurosis. *JAMA*, 91:315-319.

Fischer, S. (1925), Die Intelligenz und ihre Prüfung bei leichten Schwachsinnformen. *Ztschr. Neur. Psychiat.*, 97:53-105.

Fleming, R. (1935), A psychiatric concept of acute alcoholic intoxication. *Amer. J. Psychiat.*, 92:89-108.

Freud, A. (1927), Four lectures on child analysis. *The Writings of Anna Freud.* 1:3-69. New York: International Universities Press, 1975.

Freud, S. (1894), The neuro-psychoses of defence. *Standard Edition*, 3:43-61. London: Hogarth Press, 1962.

______ (1905a), Fragment of an analysis of a case of hysteria. *Standard Edition*, 7:3-122. London: Hogarth Press, 1953.

______ (1905b), Three essays on the theory of sexuality. *Standard Edition*, 7:125-243. London: Hogarth Press, 1953.

______ (1910), Five lectures on psycho-analysis. *Standard Edition*, 11:3-56. London: Hogarth Press, 1957.

______ (1911), The handling of dream-interpretation in psycho-analysis. *Standard Edition*, 12:89-96. London: Hogarth Press, 1958.

______ (1914), On narcissism: An introduction. *Standard Edition*, 14:69-102. London: Hogarth Press, 1957.

______ (1915), Repression. *Standard Edition*, 14:143-158. London: Hogarth Press, 1957.

______ (1917), Introductory lectures on psycho-analysis. Part III, General theory of the neuroses. *Standard Edition*, 16:243-463. London: Hogarth Press, 1963.

______ (1918), From the history of an infantile neurosis, Part VII, Anal eroticism and the castration complex. *Standard Edition*, 17:72-89. London: Hogarth Press, 1955.

______ (1919), Lines of advance in psycho-analytic therapy. *Standard Edition*, 17:158-168. London: Hogarth Press, 1955.

______ (1920a), Beyond the pleasure principle. *Standard Edition*, 18:3-64. London: Hogarth Press, 1955.

______ (1920b), The psychogenesis of a case of homosexuality in a woman. *Standard Edition*, 18:147-172. London: Hogarth Press, 1955.

______ (1922), Some neurotic mechanisms in jealousy, paranoia and homosexuality. *Standard Edition*, 18:221-232. London: Hogarth Press, 1955.

______ (1923), The ego and the id. Part III, The ego and the super-ego (ego ideal). *Standard Edition*, 19:28-40. London: Hogarth Press, 1961.

______ (1926), Inhibitions, symptoms and anxiety. *Standard Edition*, 20:77-174. London: Hogarth Press, 1959.

Friedjung, J. K. (1925), Akute Psychoneurosen in der Kinder. *Ztschr. Kinderheilk.*, 40:126-132.

Friedmann, M. (1892), Über eine besondere schwere Form von Folgezuständen nach Gehirnerschütterung und über den vasomotorischen Symptomenkomplex bei derselben im Allgemeinen. *Arch. Psychiat. u. Nervenkrankheiten*, 23:230.

Froebe, J. (1923), *Lehrbuch der experimentellen Psychologie.* Freiberg: Herder.

Gabrio, M. R. (1920), A case of traumatic hysteria. *Arch. Neur. & Psychiat.*, 3:569.

Gigon, A., Aigner, E., & Brauch, W. (1926), Über den Einfluss der Psyche auf körperliche Vorgänge. Hypnose und Blutzucker. *Schweiz. med. Wochenschr.*, 56:749-750.

Glaser, F. (1924), Psychische Beeinflussung des Blutserumkalkspiegels. *Klin. Wochenschr.*, 3:1492-1493.

Glover, E. (1933), *War, Sadism, and Pacifism.* New York: Macmillan, 1948.
Glueck, B. (1936), Induced hypoglycemic state in the treatment of the psychoses. *N.Y. State J. Med.*, 36:1473-1489.
Goldman, G. S. (1938), An act of compulsive handwashing. *Psychoanal. Quart.*, 7:96-121.
Goldstein, K. (1924), Über die gleichartige funktionelle Bedingtheit der Symptome bei organischen und psychischen Krankheiten; im besonderen über den funktionellen Mechanismus der Zwangsvorgänge. *Monatsschr. Psychiat. u. Neur.*, 57:191-209.
_____ (1927), Das Kleinhirn. *Handb. Norm. u. Path. Physiol.*, 10:227-317.
_____ & Riese, W. (1923), Über induzierte Veränderungen des Tonus bei normalen Menschen. *Klin. Wochenschr.*, 2:1201-1206.
Gordon, A. (1926), Dual personality apropos an unusual case of amnesia. *Med. J. & Record*, 124:12-14.
Groddeck, G. (1923), *The Book of the It.* New York: International Universities Press, 1976.
Guttmann, E. & Maclay, W. S. (1936), Mescalin and depersonalization. *J. Neur. & Psychopath.*, 16:193-212.
Hall, D. E. (1938), Culture and personality. *Amer. J. Orthopsychiat.*, 8:618-622.
Hall, G. W. & Mackay, R. P. (1934), The posttraumatic neuroses. *JAMA*, 102: 510-513.
Hamill, R. C. (1925), Amnesia and pathological stealing. *Internat. Clin.*, Phil., 1:114-126.
Hansen, K. (1927), Zur therapie der Symptombildung in der Neurose. *Bericht. allg. ärztl. Kong. Psychother.*, 1:86-93.*
Hartmann, F. (1902), *Die Orientierung.* Leipzig: Vogel.
Hartmann, H. (1925), Kokainismus und Homosexualität. *Ztschr. ges. Neur. u. Psychiat.*, 95:79-94.
_____ & Schilder, P. (1927), Körperinneres und Körperschema. *Ztschr. ges. Neur. u. Psychiat.*, 109:666-675.
Hartshorne, C. (1934), *The Philosophy and Psychology of Sensation.* Washington, D.C.: Catholic University of America Press, 1941.
Haug, K. (1936), *Die Störungen des Persönlichkeitsbewusstseins.* Stuttgart: Enke.
Hauptmann, A. (1926), Krieg der Unfalls-Hysterie! *Dtsch. Ztschr. Nervenh.*, 88:186-193.
Heilig, R. & Hoff, H. (1925), Beiträge zur hypnotischen Beeinflussung der Magenfunktion. *Med. Klin.*, 21:162-163.
_____ _____ (1928), Psychische Beeinflussung von Organfunktionen. *Allg. gerstl. Ztschr. Psychother.*, 1:268-280.*
Heller, F. & Schultz, J. H. (1909), Über einen Fall hypnotisch erzeugter Blasenbildung. *Münch. med. Wochenschr.*, 56:2112.
Henderson, D. K. (1918), War psychoses: Amnesia as a defence reaction for desertion. *Rev. Neur. & Psychiat.*, 16:151-178.
Herrmann, G. (1922), Zwangsmässiges Denken und andere Zwangserscheinungen bei Erkrankungen des striären Systems. *Monatschr. Psychiat. u. Neur.*, 52: 324-330.
Hess, W. R. (1925), On the interrelationship between psychic and vegetative functions. *J. Nerv. & Ment. Dis.*, 74:300-320, 511-528, 645-655, 726-735.
Hitschmann, E. (1920), Urethralerotik und Zwangsneurose. *Internat. Ztschr. Psychoanal.*, 6:263-264.
_____ (1937), Bemerkungen über Platzangst und andere neurotische Angstzustände. *Internat. Ztschr. Psychoanal.*, 23:393-401.
Hoff, H. & Schilder, P. (1927), *Die Lagereflexe des Menschen.* Vienna: Springer.

_____ _____ (1928), Zur Kenntnis der Symptomatologie vestibulärer Erkrankungen. *Dtsch. Ztschr. Nervenh.*, 103:145-175.

Hoffman, J. (1931), Entwicklungsgeschichte eines Falles von sozialer Angst. *Internat. Ztschr. Psychoanal.*, 17:99-124.

Hollós, S. & Ferenczi, S. (1925), *Psychoanalysis and the Psychic Disorder of General Paresis.* New York & Washington, D.C.: Nervous & Mental Disease Publ. Co.

Hopmann, R. (1926), Die Beziehungen der galvanischen Muskelerregbarkeit zu Elektrolytstörungen und zur allgemeinen vegetativen Überregbarkeit. *Klin. Wochenschr.*, 5:1552-1555.

Hopwood, J. S. & Snell, H. K. (1933), Amnesia in relation to crime. *J. Ment. Science*, 79:27-41.

Horney, K. (1937), *The Neurotic Personality of Our Time.* New York: Norton.

Huddleson, J. H. (1932), *Accidents, Neuroses and Compensation.* Baltimore: Williams & Wilkins Co.

Jaensch, E. (1930), *Eidetic Imagery.* New York: Harcourt & Brace.

Jaensch, W. (1930), Persönlichkeitstypen, psychische. In: *Handwörterbuch der med. Psychol.*, ed. K. Birnbaum. Leipzig: Thieme, pp. 391-396.

Janet, P. (1889), *L'automatisme Psychologique.* 10th ed. Paris: Felix Alcan, 1930.

_____ (1894), *Major Symptoms of Hysteria.* New York: Hafner, 1965.

_____ (1898), *Neuroses et Idées Fixes,* 2nd ed. Paris: Felix Alcan, 1904.

Jelliffe, S. E. (1932), *Psychopathology of Forced Movements and the Oculogyric Crises of Lethargic Encephalitis.* New York & Washington, D.C.: Nervous & Mental Disease Publ. Co.

_____ (1933), Psychoanalysis and internal medicine. In: *Psychoanalysis Today,* ed. S. Lorand. New York: International Universities Press, 1944, pp. 12-22.

Jellinek, E. M. & McFarland, R. A. (1940), Analysis of psychological experiments on the effects of alcohol on the individual. *Quart. J. Stud. Alcohol.*, 1:272-371.

Jones, E. (1920), Recent advances in psycho-analysis. *Internat. J. Psycho-Anal.*, 1:161-185.

_____ (1929), The psychopathology of anxiety. In: *Papers on Psychoanalysis.* Baltimore: Williams & Wilkins, 5th ed., 1950, pp. 294-303.

Jong, H. de (1921), Die Hauptgesetze eineger wichtigen körperlichen Erscheinungen beim psychosen Geschehen von Normalen und Geisteskranken. *Ztschr. ges. Neur. u. Psychiat.*, 69:61-141.

Kanner, L. & Schilder, P. (1930), Movements in optic images and the optic imagination of movements. *J. Nerv. & Ment. Dis.*, 72:489-517.

Kardiner, A. (1932), The bio-analysis of the epileptic reaction. *Psychoanal. Quart.*, 1:375-483.

Karger, P. (1925), Die eidetische Anlage der Jugendlichen, ihre Bedeutung für die Klinik und die Schulleistungen. *Klin. Wochenschr.*, 4:2247-2249.

Kasanin, J. (1929), Personality changes in children following cerebral trauma. *J. Nerv. & Ment. Dis.*, 69:385-406.

Kauders, O. (1931), *Zur Klinik und Analyse der psychomotorischen Störung.* Berlin: S. Karger.

_____ & Schilder, P. (1923), A textbook of hypnosis. In: P. Schilder, *The Nature of Hypnosis.* New York: International Universities Press, 1956, pp. 45-184.

Kehrer, F. (1924), Spezielle Symptomatologie der Hysterie und Neurasthenie. *Handb. Neur.*, 3:72.*

_____ (1938), Die Verbindung von chorea und ticförmigen Bewegungen mit Zwangsvorstellungen und ihre Beziehungen zu den Zwangsvorgängen bei Zwangsneurose und Encephalitis epidemica. *Abhandl. Neur. u. Psychiat.*, 85. Basel: Karger.

Klauder, J. V. (1924), Psychoneurotic manifestations in dermatology with particular reference to treatment with suggestive and educative measures. *Arch. Neur. & Psychiat.*, 12:99-100.

______ (1925), The cutaneous neuroses. *JAMA*, 85:1683-1689.

Klein, E. & Schilder, P. (1929), The Japanese illusion and the postural model of the body. *J. Nerv. & Ment. Dis.*, 70:241-263.

Klein, M. (1932), *The Psycho-Analysis of Children.* New York: Delacorte, 1975.

Kleist, K. (1927), Zur Entschädigungsfrage bei der sogenannten Unfallneurose. *Klin. Wochenschr.*, 6:1317-1319.

Knauer, A. (1915), Über den Einfluss normaler Seelenvorgänge auf den arteriellen Blutdruck. *Ztschr. ges. Neur. u. Psychiat.*, 30:319-353.

Knight, R. P. (1937a), Dynamics and treatment of chronic alcohol addiction. *Bull. Menninger Clinic*, 1:233-250.

______ (1937b), The psychodynamics of chronic alcoholism. *J. Nerv. & Ment. Dis.*, 86:538-548.

Kraulis, W. (1931), Zur Vererbung der hysterischen Reaktionsweise. *Ztschr. ges. Neur. u. Psychiat.*, 136:174-259.

Kraus, F. (1927), Über das Neuroseproblem. *Klin. Wochenschr.*, 6:537-541.

Kreibich, C. & Sobotka, P. (1909), Experimenteller Beitrag zur psychischen Urticaria. *Arch. Dermat. u. Syph.*, 97:187-192.

Kretschmer, E. (1923), *Hysteria.* New York & Washington, D.C.: Nervous & Mental Disease Publ. Co., 1926.

Kretschmer, M. & Krueger, R. (1927), Über die Beeinflussung des Serumkalkgehaltes in der Hypnose. *Klin. Wochenschr.*, 6:695-697.

Laforgue, R. (1938), *Clinical Aspects of Psycho-Analysis.* London: Hogarth Press.

Landauer, K. (1927), Automatismen, Zwangsneurosen und Paranoia. *Internat. Ztschr. Psychoanal.*, 13:10-19.

Lange-Eichbaum, W. (1928), *Genie—Irrsinn und Ruhm.* Munich: Ernst Reinhardt.

Leavitt, F. H. (1935), The etiology of temporary amnesia. *Amer. J. Psychiat.*, 91:1079-1088.

Lemos, M. (1906), Parte de la vision mentale des objets dans la melancholie auxierse. *Ann. médicopsych.*, 4:9-64.*

Leuba, J. H. (1925), *The Psychology of Religious Mysticism.* New York: Harcourt Brace.

Loewi, O. (1921), Über humorale Übertragbarkeit d. Herznervenwirkung. *Arch. ges. Physiol.*, 189:239-242.

Mabille, H. (1885), Note sur les hémorrhagies cutanées par auto-suggestion dans le somnambulisme provoqué. *Progres. med.*, 2:155-156.

Magnus, R. (1924), *Körperstellung.* Berlin: Springer.

Malamud, W. (1934), Psychogenic motor disturbances. *Arch. Neur. & Psychiat.*, 32:1173-1188.

Malinowski, B. (1929), *The Sexual Life of Savages in Northwestern Melanesia.* New York: Liveright.

Marburg, O. (1936), Die traumatischen Erkrankungen des Gehirns und Rückenmarks. In: *Handb. Neur.*, ed. O. Bumke & O. Foerster. Berlin: Springer, 11:1-177.

Marie, P. (1916), La conduit à tenir vis-à-vis des blessures du crâne. *Rev. Neur.*, 23:453-476.

Martland, H. S. (1928), Punch drunk. *JAMA*, 91:1103-1107.

Mayer-Gross, W. (1935), On depersonalization. *Brit. J. Med. Psychol.*, 15:104-126.

______ & Steiner, G. (1921), Encephalitis lethargica in der Selbstbeobachtung. *Ztschr. ges. Neur. u. Psychiat.*, 73:283-309.

Meduna, L. J. (1937), *Die Konvulsionstherapie der Schizophrenie.* Halle: Marhold.
Menninger, K. A. (1938), *Man Against Himself.* New York: Harcourt Brace, pp. 160-184.
Minkowsky, E. (1923), Etude psychologique et analyse phénoménologique d'un cas de mélancholie schizophrénique. *J. de Psychol. Norm. et Path.*, 20:543-558.
Missreigler, A. (1932), Vierzig Lebensjahre in einem Traum. *Psychoanal. Praxis,* 2:114-122.
Moore, M. (1939), Treatment of alcoholism. *New Eng. J. Med.*, 221:489-493.
Moorhead, J. (1931), *Traumatotherapy.* Philadelphia: Saunders.
Neustatter, W. L. (1938), The effect of poor social conditions in the production of neuroses. *Lancet,* 234:1436-1441.
Nunberg, H. (1924), States of depersonalization in the light of the libido theory. In: *Practice and Theory of Psychoanalysis.* New York: Nervous & Mental Disease Publ. Co., 1948, pp. 60-74.
_____ (1932), *Principles of Psychoanalysis.* New York: International Universities Press, 1955.
Oberholzer, E. (1931), Zur Differentialdiagnose psychischer Folgezustände nach Schädeltraumen mittels des Rohrschachschen Formdeutversuchs. *Ztschr. ges. Neur. u. Psychiat.*, 136:596-630.
Oberndorf, C. P. (1934), Depersonalization in relation to erotization of thought. *Internat. J. Psycho-Anal.*, 15:271-295.
Oppenheim, H. (1889), *Die Traumatischen Neurosen.* Berlin: Hirschwald.
_____ (1923), *Lehrbuch der Nervenkrankheiten,* 7th ed. Berlin: Karger.
Orenstein, L. L. & Schilder, P. (1938), Psychological considerations of insulin treatment in schizophrenia. In: P. Schilder, *On Psychoses.* New York: International Universities Press, 1976, pp. 398-432.
_____ Rosenbaum, I. J., & Schilder, P. (1938), Application of convulsive therapy in schizophrenia. *N.Y. State J. Med.*, 8:1506-1508.
Osnato, M. & Giliberti, F. (1927), Postconcussion neurosis; traumatic encephalitis; conception of postconcussion phenomena. *Arch. Neur. & Psychiat.*, 18:181-214.
Otto, J. H. (1930), Über Neurosen bei Chinesen. *Ztschr. Psychother.*, 3:5-12.
Parker, S. & Schilder, P. (1935), Acoustic imagination and acoustic hallucination. *Arch. Neur. & Psychiat.*, 34:744-757.
_____ _____ Wortis, H. (1939), A specific motility psychosis in Negro alcoholics. In: P. Schilder, *On Psychoses.* New York: International Universities Press, 1976, pp. 263-284.
Pavlov, I. P. (1927), *Conditioned Reflexes.* London: Oxford University Press, 1941.
Pfeifer, B. (1924), Die psychischen Störungen nach Kriegsverletzungen des Gehirns. In: *Handb. Neur.*, ed. O. Bumke. Berlin: Springer, p. 493.*
Pfister, O. (1930), Schockdenken und Schockphantasien bei höchster Todesgefahr. *Internat. Ztschr. Psychoanal.*, 16:430-455.
Pick, A. (1908), Zur Pathologie des Selbstbewusstseins. *Ztschr. Psychol. u. Physiol.*, 1:275-288.
Pick, E. P. (1919), Über Änderung der Adrenalinwirkung nach Erregung d. vagalen Endapparate. *Arch. ges. Physiol.*, 184.*
Pisk, G. (1936), Über die Änderung der hysterischen Symptome in den letzten Jahren. *Wien. klin. Wochenschr.*, 2:938-939.*
Pötzl, O. (1917), Über einige Wechselwirkungen hysterieformer und organischzerebraler Störungsmechanismen. *Jahrbüch. f. Psychiat. u. Neurol.*, 37:269-373.
Poppelreuter, W. (1917), *Die Psychischen Schädigungen durch Kopfscruss im Krieg.* Leipzig: Voss.

Porteus, S. D. (1931), *The Psychology of a Primitive People*. New York: Longmans, Green.
_____ & Babcock, M. E. (1926), *Temperament and Race*. Boston: Badger.
Price, G. E. & Terhune, W. B. (1919), Feigned amnesia as a defense reaction. *JAMA*, 72:565-567.
Prince, W. F. (1916), The Doris case of quintuple personality. *J. Abnorm. Psychol.*, 11:73-122.
Rado, S. (1926; 1928), The psychic effects of intoxication: Attempt at a psychoanalytic theory of drug addiction. *Internat. J. Psycho-Anal.*, 7:396-413; 9:301-317.
_____ (1933), The psychoanalysis of pharmacothymia. *Psychoanal. Quart.*, 2:1-23.
Rank, O. (1924), *The Trauma of Birth*. New York: Harcourt Brace, 1929.
Reich, W. (1927), *The Function of the Orgasm*. New York: Farrar, Strauss & Giroux, 1974.
_____ (1933), *Character Analysis*. New York: Touchstone Press, 1974.
Reichardt, M. (1928), Der heutige Stand der Beuteilung der sogenannten Unfallneurosen. *Deutsch. med. Wochenschr.*, 54:213-215, 261-264.
Reik, T. (1925), *Geständniszwang und Strafbedürfnis*. Leipzig: Internationaler Psychoanalytische Verlag.
_____ (1927), *Wie man Psychologe wird*. Leipzig: Internationaler Psychoanalytische Verlag.
Ribot, T. (1881), *The Diseases of the Personality*. Philadelphia: Boericke & Tafel, 1909.
_____ (1882), *The Diseases of Memory*. New York: Humboldt Library of Popular Science.
Riese, W. (1928), Grundsätzliche Bemerkungen zu einer "Nachuntersuchung von Unfallkranken mit traumatische Neurose." *Acta Psychiat. et Neur.*, 3:153-164.
_____ ed. (1929), *Unfall-Neurose als Problem der Gegenwartsmedizin*. Stuttgart: Hippokrates Verlag.
Roheim, G. (1932), Psycho-analysis of primitive cultural types. *Internat. J. Psycho-Anal.*, 13:2-224.
_____ (1934), *The Riddle of the Sphinx*. New York: Harper & Row, 1974.
Sachs, H. (1909), *Die Unfallneurose*. Breslau: Preuss & Jünger.
Sack, W. (1926), Psychotherapie und Hautkrankheiten. *Ber. allg. ärztl. Kong. Psychother.* Halle: Marbold, pp. 133-144.*
_____ (1933), Psyche und Haut. *Handb. der Haut—u. Geschlechtskrankh.*, 4: 1302-1382.
Sadger, J. (1920), Neue Studien zum Kastrationskomplex. *Fortsch. Med.*, 37:1-32.
_____ (1928), Über Depersonalisation. *Internat. Ztschr. Psychoanal.*, 14:315-351.
Sands, I. J. (1936), Anatomic consideration in clinical interpretation of brain injuries. *Amer. J. Psychiat.*, 92:771-789.
Saul, L. (1938), A Chinese man. *Amer. J. Orthopsychiat.*, 8:609-610.
Schaltenbrand, G. (1931), Psychiatrie in Peking. *Ztschr. Neur.*, 137:168-232.*
Schilder, P. (1914), *Selbstbewusstsein und Persönlichkeitsbewusstsein*. Berlin: Springer.
_____ (1918), *Wahn und Erkenntnis*. Berlin: Springer.
_____ (1920), Über Identifizierung auf Grund der Analyse eines Falles von Homosexualität. *Ztschr. ges. Neur. u. Psychiat.*, 59:217-249.
_____ (1923), *Das Körperschema*. Berlin: Springer.
_____ (1924), *Medical Psychology*. New York: International Universities Press, 1953.

______ (1925a), *Introduction to Psychoanalytic Psychiatry.* New York: International Universities Press, 1951.
______ (1925b), Die organischen Grundlagen der Neurose. *Dtsch. Ztschr. Nervenh.*, 88:237-247.
______ (1929a), Conditioned reflexes. In: P. Schilder, 1942b, 10:153-172.
______ (1929b), Zur Kenntnis der Psychosen bei chronischer Encephalitis epidemica. Nebst Bemerkungen über die Beziehung organischer Strukturen zu den psychischen Vorgängen. *Ztschr. ges. Neur. u. Psychiat.*, 118:327-345.
______ (1929c), The somatic basis of the neuroses. *This Volume,* Chapter 2.
______ (1930), Neurasthenic hypochondriac character. *This Volume,* Chapter 4.
______ (1931a), *Brain and Personality.* New York: International Universities Press, 1951.
______ (1931b), Notes on the psychopathology of pain in neurosis and psychosis. *Psychoanal. Rev.*, 18:1-22.
______ (1933a), Experiments on imagination, after-images and hallucinations. *Amer. J. Psychiat.*, 13:597-611.
______ (1933b), The vestibular apparatus in neurosis and psychosis. In: P. Schilder, 1942b, 8:83-134.
______ (1934a), Psychic disturbances after head injuries. In: P. Schilder, 1976, pp. 152-192.
______ (1934b), Self-consciousness and optic imagination in a case of depression. *Psychoanal. Rev.*, 21:316-328.
______ (1935a), *The Image and Appearance of the Human Body.* New York: International Universities Press, 1950.
______ (1935b), Psychoanalysis of space. In: P. Schilder, 1942b, 12:75-82.
______ (1936a), The analysis of ideologies as a psychotherapeutic method, especially in group treatment. *Amer. J. Psychiat.*, 93:601-617.
______ (1936b), The psychology of geometry and physics. In: P. Schilder, 1942b, 22:350-360.
______ (1937), The relationship between social and personal disorganization. In: P. Schilder, 1951a, pp. 52-60.
______ (1938a), *Psychotherapy.* New York: Norton, 1951.
______ (1938b), The social neurosis. *This Volume,* Chapter 9.
______ (1940), Cultural patterns and constructive psychology. In: P. Schilder, 1951a, pp. 332-351.
______ (1942a), *Goals and Desires of Man.* New York: Columbia University Press.
______ (1942b), *Mind: Perception and Thought in Their Constructive Aspects.* New York: Columbia University Press.
______ (1951a), *Psychoanalysis, Man and Society.* New York: Norton.
______ (1951b), *Psychotherapy.* New York: Norton.
______ (1964), *Contributions to Developmental Neuropsychiatry.* New York: International Universities Press.
______ (1976), *On Psychoses.* New York: International Universities Press.
______ & Eisinger, K. (1929), Träume bei Labyrinthläsionen. *Monatschr. Psychiat. u. Neur.*, 73:314-330.
______ & Wechsler, D. (1934), Children's attitudes toward death. In: P. Schilder, 1964, pp. 293-295.
______ ______ (1935), The child's concept of the inside of his body. In: P. Schilder, *Contributions to Developmental Neuropsychiatry.* New York: International Universities Press, 1964, pp. 54-60.
Schindler, W. (1927), *Nervensystem und Spontanblutungen.* Berlin: Springer.

Schneider, K. (1921), Bemerkungen zu einer phänomenologischen Psychologie der invertierten Sexualität und erotischen Liebe. *Ztschr. ges. Neur. u. Psychiat.*, 71:346-351.
Schnyder, P. (1936), Commotio cerebri, posttraumatische Neurosen und Störungen der Sexualfunktionen. *Schweiz. med. Wochenschr.*, 66:242-244.
Schottky, J. (1937), *Rasse und Krankheit.* Munich: Lehmanns Verlag.
Seliger, R. V. (1938), The problem of the alcoholic in the community. *Amer. J. Psychiat.*, 95:701-716.
Sichel, M. (1909), *Die Geistesstörungen bei den Juden.* Leipzig: M. W. Kaufman.
Sidis, B. & Goodhart, S. P. (1905), *Multiple Personality.* New York: Appleton & Co.
Simmel, E. (1919), *Psychoanalysis and the War Neuroses.* London: International Psychoanalytic Press, 1921, pp. 30-40.
Sperling, O. (1929), Die Unfallneurose. In: *Handbuch des Unfallneurose,* ed. W. Riese. Stuttgart: Hippokrates Verlag, pp. 87-98.
Spitz, R. (1937), Familienneurose und neurotische Familie. *Internat. Ztschr. Psychoanal.*, 23:548-559.
Steinnach, E. (1913), Feminierung von Männchen und Maskulierung von Weibern. *Zentralbl. Physiol.*, 27:717-723.*
Stekel, W. (1923), *Conditions of Nervous Anxiety and Their Treatment.* New York: Liveright, 1952.
______ (1943), *The Interpretation of Dreams: New Developments and Technique.* New York: Liveright.
Stengel, E. (1928), Zur Klinik und Pathophysiologie des postenzephalitischen Blickkrampfes. *Monatschr. Psychiat. u. Neur.*, 70:305-338.
______ (1930), Weitere Beiträge zur Kenntnis des postenzephalitischen Blickkrampfes. *Ztschr. ges. Neur. u. Psychiat.*, 127:441-453.
______ (1935a), Über psychische Zwangsphänomene bei Hirnkranken. *Jahrb. Psychiat. u. Neur.*, 52:236-248.*
______ (1935b), Zur kenntnis der Triebstörungen und der Abwehrreaktionen des Ichs bei Hirnkranken. *Internat. Ztschr. Psychoanal.*, 21:544-560.
Stern, E. (1919), Beiträge zur Psychologie und Psychopathologie des Selbstwerterlebens. *Ztschr. Pathopsychol.*, 3:500-553.
Stern, F. (1928), *Die Epidemische Encephalitis.* Berlin: Springer.
Stier, E. (1926), *Über die sogenannten Unfallneurosen.* Leipzig: Thieme.
Stockert, F. G. von (1929), Klinik und Ätiologie der Kontaktneurosen. *Klin. Wochenschr.*, 8:76-79.
Straus, E. (1928), Des Zeiterlebnis in der endogenen Depression. *Monatschr. Psychiat. u. Neur.*, 68:640-656.
______ (1930), Die Formen des Räumlichen. *Nervenärzt.*, 3:633-656.
Strauss, I. & Savitsky, N. (1934a), Head injury: Neurologic and psychiatric aspects. *Arch. Neur. & Psychiat.*, 31:893-955.
______ ______ (1934b), The sequelae of head injury. *Amer. J. Psychiat.*, 91:189-202.
______ ______ (1937), The sequelae of head injury. *N.Y. State J. Med.*, 37:1181-1188.
Sullivan, H. S. (1937), A note on the implications of psychiatry. *Amer. J. Sociol.*, 42:848-861.
Szondi, L. (1936), Der Neurotiker im Lichte der psychoanalytischen, neuro-endokrinen und erbpathologischen Forschungen. *Schweiz. Arch. Neur. u. Psychiat.*, 37:313-334.
Taine, H. (1870), *De l'intelligence,* 2nd ed. Paris: Hachette, 1906.

Tokyo Psycho-Analytic Society (1935), Report. *Internat. Ztschr. Psychoanal.*, 21:161-162.
Vogt, C. & Vogt, O. (1920), Zur Lehre der Erkrankungen des striären Systems. *J. Psychol. Neur.*, 25:627-846.
Wagner, M. (1932), Die Erbanlage bei Rentenneurotikern. *Dtsch. Ztschr. Nervenh.*, 123:230-273.
Wall, J. H. (1936), A study of alcoholism in men. *Amer. J. Psychiat.*, 92:1389-1402.
______ (1937), A study of alcoholism in women. *Amer. J. Psychiat.*, 93:943-956.
Watson, J. B. (1924), *Behaviorism*. New York: Norton.
Wechsler, I. S. (1929), *The Neuroses*. Philadelphia: Saunders.
______ (1935), Trauma and the nervous system. *JAMA*, 104:519-525.
Weinberg, A. A. (1923, 1924), Psyche und unwillkürliches Nervensystem. *Ztschr. ges. Neur. u. Psychiat.*, 85:543-565; 86:375-390; 93:421-445.
Wernicke, C. (1906), *Grundriss der Psychiatrie*. Leipzig: F. Barth.
Wexberg, E. (1929), Die Grundstörung der Zwangsneurose. *Ztschr. ges. Neur. u. Psychiat.*, 121:236-255.
______ (1937), Remarks on the psychopathology of oculogyric crises in epidemic encephalitis. *J. Nerv. & Ment. Dis.*, 85:56-69.
Weygandt, W. (1936), Hysterie als Erbkrankheit. *Ztschr. ges. Neur. u. Psychiat.*, 155:758-782.
Wilder, J. (1935), Änderung in den Manifestationen der Hysterie in Deutschland und Oesterreich in den letzten Jahren. *Giornale di Clin. Med.*, pp. 239-248.*
Wilson, G. W. (1934), Report of a case of acute laryngitis occurring as a conversion symptom during analysis. *Psychoanal. Rev.*, 21:408-414.
______ (1935), The analysis of a transitory conversion symptom simulating pertussis. *Internat. J. Psychiat.*, 16:474-480.
Winterstein, E. E. (1937), Head injuries attributable to boxing. *Lancet*, 2:719-720.
Wulff, M. (1933), Über den hysterischen Anfall. *Internat. Ztschr. Psychiat.*, 19:584-612.
Yaskin, J. C. (1936), The psychoneuroses and neuroses. *Amer. J. Psychiat.*, 93:107-125.
Zondek, S. G. (1923), Die Bedeutung des Antagonismus von Kalium und Calcium für die Physiologie und Pathologie. *Klin. Wochenschr.*, 2:382-385.

NAME INDEX

SUBJECT INDEX